Thin Calcium Phosphate Coatings for Medical Implants

Betty León · John A. Jansen
Editors

Thin Calcium Phosphate Coatings for Medical Implants

Springer

Editors
Betty León
Depto. de Física Aplicada, E.T.S.I.
Industriales
Universidad de Vigo
Vigo, Spain
Bleon@uvigo.es

John A. Jansen
Radboud University Medical Center
Nijmegen, The Netherlands
j.jansen@dent.umcn.nl

ISBN: 978-0-387-77718-4 e-ISBN: 978-0-387-77719-1
DOI 10.1007/978-0-387-77718-4

Library of Congress Control Number: 2008936512

Printed on acid-free paper

springer.com

Preface

Calcium phosphate coatings ($\sim$50 μm thick), especially those made with hydroxyapatite (HA), produced by the plasma-spraying process have been successfully used on orthopedic and dental implants to improve fixation of these implants in bone. Thin calcium phosphate coatings ($\leq$ 10 μm thick) formed by various techniques other than plasma spraying may be the successor of the current thick plasma-sprayed coatings because of their improved properties. Like plasma-sprayed HA coatings, these alternative calcium phosphate thin coatings are capable of enabling bone formation on their surfaces and forming a bond with the newly formed bone. In addition, the thin calcium phosphate coatings have shown better adhesion to substrates and are more stable in the biological environment because they have more uniform structure and composition than plasma-sprayed HA coatings. Moreover, some of these thin calcium phosphate coatings can be formed on all kinds of substrates including polymers and on the entire surfaces of complex geometries such as porous surfaces.

This book presents, for the first time, the once scattered novel results that have been achieved in recent years in studies on various thin calcium phosphate coatings produced by diverse techniques. Comparisons of thin calcium phosphate coatings with the thick plasma-sprayed ones are included. Readers will find a comprehensive collection of work that reviews the state of the art of the field, with critical assessments of the achievements of the various preparation techniques. Emphasis is placed on the benefits of special characterization techniques for this type of thin coating, which may be particularly useful to graduate students. The information is also considered extremely valuable for industrial applications.

This comprehensive effort summarizes the state of the art in bioactive calcium phosphate coatings and reviews the physicochemical properties and *in vitro* and *in vivo* performance of thin calcium phosphate coatings prepared by various techniques. It can be valuable not only to students involved in studying biomaterials but also to engineers in the design, development, and manufacture of medical implants.

Contents

Contributors

C. Mauli Agrawal
Department of Biomedical Engineering, University of Texas at San Antonio, One UTSA Circle, San Antonio, TX 78249, USA, mauli.agrawal@utsa.edu

Mark Appleford
Department of Biomedical Engineering, University of Texas at San Antonio, One UTSA Circle, San Antonio, TX 78249, USA, mark.appleford@utsa.edu

Serena M. Best
Department of Materials Science and Metallurgy, University of Cambridge, Pembroke Street, Cambridge, CB2 3QZ, United Kingdom, smb51@cam.ac.uk

Susanne Bierbaum
Institute of Materials Science, Max-Bergmann-Center of Biomaterials, Technische Universität Dresden, 01062 Dresden; now Biomet GmbH, Gustav-Krone-Str. 2, 14167 Berlin, Germany

Jeol Bumgardner
Department of Biomedical Engineering, University of Memphis, 328D Engr Tech Bldg, Memphis, TN 38152, USA, jbmgrdnr@memphis.edu

David L. Carnes
Department of Periodontics, University of Texas Health Science Center at San Antonio, San Antonio, TX 78229, USA, carnes@uthscsa.edu

Weihui Chen
Department of Biomedical Engineering, University of Texas at San Antonio, One UTSA Circle, San Antonio, TX 78249, USA; Department of Oral Surgery, Union Hospital, Fujian Medical University, 350001 Fujian, China, dr.whchen@yahoo.com

Stefano Chiussi
Departamento de Física Aplicada – E.T.S.I.I., University of Vigo, Lagoas-Marcosende s/n, E-36200 Vigo, Spain, schiussi@uvigo.es

Guy Daculsi
INSERM, U791, Laboratory for Osteo-articular and Dental Tissue Engineering, Faculty of Dental Surgery, University of Nantes, 1 Place Alexis Ricordeau, 44042 Nantes, France, gdaculsi@sante.univ-nantes.fr

Bas Feddes
Philips Research, High Tech Campus 34, 5656 AE, Eindhoven, The Netherlands, bas.feddes@tiscali.nl

Pío González
Departamento de Física Aplicada – E.T.S.I.I., University of Vigo, Lagoas-Marcosende s/n, E-36200 Vigo, Spain, pglez@uvigo.es

Ulrich M. Gross
Institute of Pathology, Free University of Berlin, Campus Benjamin Franklin, Hindenburgdamm 30, D 12200 Berlin, Germany, and Institute of Cardiac Diagnostics and Therapy (IKDT), Moltkestrasse 31, D 12203 Berlin, Germany, ugross@zedat.fu-berlin.de

Warren Haggard
Department of Biomedical Engineering, University of Memphis, 328D Engr Tech Bldg, Memphis, TN 38152, USA, whaggrd1@memphis.edu

Ernst B. Hunziker
Center of Regenerative Medicine for Skeletal Tissues, Department of Clinical Research, University of Bern, P. O. Box 54, Murtenstrasse 35, CH – 3010 Bern, Switzerland, ernst.hunziker@dkf.unibe.ch

Christian Jäger
Federal Institute of Materials Research and Testing, Division I.3, Richard Willstaetter Strasse 11, D-12489 Berlin, Germany, christian.jaeger@bam.de

John A. Jansen
Department of Periodontology and Biomaterials, Radboud University Nijmegen Medical Center, Philips van Leijdenlaan 25, 6525 EX Nijmegen, The Netherlands, j.jansen@dent.umcn.nl

Kyo-Han Kim
Department of Dental Biomaterials, College of Dentistry, Kyungpook National University, 2-188-1 Samduk-dong, Jung-gu, Daegu, South Korea, kyohan@mail.knu.ac.kr

Dirk Lassner
Institute of Pathology, Free University of Berlin, Campus Benjamin Franklin, Hindenburgdamm 30, D 12200 Berlin, Germany, and Institute of Cardiac Diagnostics and Therapy (IKDT), Moltkestrasse 31, D 12203 Berlin, Germany

Pierre Layrolle
INSERM, U791, Laboratory for Osteo-articular and Dental Tissue Engineering, Faculty of Dental Surgery, University of Nantes, 1 Place Alexis Ricordeau, 44042 Nantes, France, Pierre.layrolle@nantes.inserm.fr

Sander C.G. Leeuwenburgh
Department of Periodontology and Biomaterials, Radboud University Nijmegen Medical Center, Philips van Leijdenlaan 25, 6525 EX Nijmegen, s.leeuwenburgh@dent.uncn.nl

Betty León
Departmento de Física Aplicada, E.T.S.I. Industriales, University of Vigo, Lagoas-Marcosende s/n, 36200 Vigo, Spain, bleon@uvigo.es

Yongxing Liu
Center for Biomaterials, MC-1615, University of Connecticut Health Center, 263 Farmington Ave, Farmington, CT 06030-1615, yoliu@uchc.edu

Yuelian Liu
Section of Oral Implantology, Department of Oral Function, Academic Centre of Dentistry Amsterdam (ACTA), Louwesweg 1, 1067 EA, Amsterdam, The Netherlands; ITI Research Institute for Dental and Skeletal Biology, University of Bern, Switzerland, y.liu@acta.nl

Namsik Oh
Inha University Hospital, Department of dentistry, College of Medicine, 7-206, 3rd Street, Shinheung-dong, Choong-gu, Incheon 400-711, South Korea, onsdo@inha.ac.kr

Sunho Oh
Department of Biomedical Engineering, University of Texas at San Antonio, One UTSA Circle, San Antonio, TX 78249, USA, daniel.oh@utsa.edu

Joo L. Ong
Department of Biomedical Engineering, University of Texas at San Antonio, One UTSA Circle, San Antonio, TX 78249, USA, anson.ong@utsa.edu

Sangwon Park
College of Dentistry, Chonnam National University, Hak-Dong 8, Dong-Ku, Gwang-ju 504-190, South Korea, psw320@chonnam.ac.kr

Juan Pou
Departamento de Física Aplicada – E.T.S.I.I., University of Vigo, Lagoas-Marcosende s/n, E-36200 Vigo, Spain, jpou@uvigo.es

Dieter Scharnweber
Institute of Materials Science, Max Bergmann Center of Biomaterials, Technische Universität Dresden, Budapester Str. 27, 01069 Dresden, Germany, Dieter.Scharnweber@tu-dresden.de

Joop Schoonman
Laboratory for Inorganic Chemistry, Delft University of Technology, Julianalaan 136, 2628 BL Delft, The Netherlands, j.schoonman@tudelft.nl

Julia Serra
Departamento de Física Aplicada – E.T.S.I.I., University of Vigo, Lagoas-Marcosende s/n, E-36200 Vigo, Spain, jserra@uvigo.es

Marijke C. Siebers
Department of Periodontology and Biomaterials, Radboud University Nijmegen Medical Center, Philips van Leijdenlan 25, 6525 EX Nijmegen, The Netherlands, m.siebers@dent.umcn.nl

Eng San Thian
Department of Materials Science and Metallurgy, University of Cambridge, Pembroke Street, Cambridge CB2 3QZ, United Kingdom, est23@cam.ac.uk

Joop G.C. Wolke
Department of Periodontology and Biomaterials, Radboud University Nijmegen Medical Center, Philips van Leijdenlan 25, 6525 EX Nijmegen, The Netherlands, m.siebers@dent.umcn.nl

Yunzhi Yang
Department of Biomedical Engineering, Imaging University of Tennessee Health Science Center, 920 Madison Avenue, Suite 1005, 38163, Memphis, TN 38163, USA, yyang19@utmem.edu

Masao Yoshinari
Oral Health Science Center and Department of Dental Materials Science, Tokyo Dental College, Chiba 261-8502, Japan, yosinari@tdc.ac.jp

List of Abbreviations

A	apatite
α-TCP	α-Tricalcium phosphate
ACP	Amorphous calcium phosphate
AES	Auger Electron Spectroscopy
AFM	Atomic force microscopy
Ag	Silver
ALP	Alkaline phosphatase
Ar	Argon
ArF	Argon fluor excimer
ASTM	American Society for Testing and Materials
β-TCP	β-Tricalcium phosphate
BCP	Biphasic calcium phosphate
BD	biomimetic deposition
BMPs	Bone Morphogenetic Proteins
BR	brushite
BSA	Bovine Serum Albumine
Ca	Calcium
CA	Carbonate Apatite
CaP	Calcium Phosphate
Cbfa1	Core binding factor a 1
CDA	Calcium-deficient apatite
cDNA	complementary DNA
CFU	Colony forming units
CHA	Carbonated HydroxyApatite
CICP	C-terminal type I procollagen
CLST	Constant Load Scratch Test
C-O/CO_3	Carbonate
CPC	Calcium phosphate ceramics
CPP	Calcium phosphate phases
CPS	Calcium Phosphate Supersaturated Solution
CRT	Cathode Ray Tube
CSF-M	Colony stimulating factor-macrophage
c-Src	a transcriptional activator

CV	cell voltage
DBM	Demineralized Bone Matrix
dc	direct current
DCP	Dicalciumphosphate, monetite
DCPA	Dicalcium phosphate anhydrous (monetite)
DCPD	Dicalcium phosphate dihydrate (brushite)
DMEM	Dulbecco's minimal essential medium
DNA	Desoxyribonucleic acid
EBSS	Earl's balanced salt solution
ECAD	Electrochemically assisted deposition
ECM	Extracellular matrix
EDS	Energy Dispersive X-ray Spectrometry
EDTA	Ethylenediaminetetra acid
EDX	Energy dispersive X-ray spectroscopy
EP	Electrophoretic
EPMA	Electron probe microanalysis
ERD	Elastic Recoil Detection
ERDA	Elastic Recoil Detection Analysis
ERK	Extracellular signal-related kinase
ESCA	Electron Spectroscopy for Chemical Analysis
ESD	Electrostatic Spray Deposition
FA	Fluoroapatite
FcR	Fc-receptor
5xSBF	Five Times Concentrated SBF
FHG	Fourth harmonic generation
FOS	a transcriptional activator
FRS	Forward Recoil Spectrometry
FTIR	Fourier Transform Infrared Spectroscopy
GAPDH	Glyceraldehyde-3-phosphate dehydrogenase
GDFs	Growth and Differentiation Factors
GS	Galvanostatic
HA	Hydroxylapatite, Hydroxyapatite
HaCat	human keratinocyte cell line
Hap	Hydroxyapatite
HBDC	Human bone derived cells
HBP	Human Blood Plasma
hFOB	Human fetal osteoblast-like cell line
HOB	Human osteoblast
IBDM	Ion beam dynamic mixing
ICP-OES	Inductively coupled plasma optical emission spectroscopy
IHH	Indian hedge hog
IL-1b	Interleukin 1 beta
Il-1ra	Interleukin 1 receptor antagonist
Il-6	Interleukin 6
IL-8	Interleukin 8

IMDM	Iscove's modified Dulbecco's medium
IP	Ion plating
IR	Infrared
IS	Ion sputtering
JUN	a transcriptional activator
KrF	Krypton fluor excimer
LEIS	Low Energy Ion Scattering
LEP	Lung embryonic fibroblasts
MAPK	Mitogen activated protein kinase
MCPA	Monocalcium phosphate anhydrous
MCPM	Monocalcium phosphate monohydrate
MEM	Minimal essential medium
Mg	Magnesium
MMA	MethylMethAcrylate
MPST	Multi Pass Scratch Test
mRNA	messenger RNA
MTT	3-(4,5-dimethylthiazole-2-yl)-2,5-diphenyl tetrazolium bromide
Na	Sodium
Nd:YAG	Neodymium:Ytrium Aluminium Garnet
NFATs	Nuclear factor of activated T-cells
NF-kB	Nuclear factor kappa B
NMR	Nuclear Magnetic Resonance
OCP	Octacalcium Phosphate
O-H	hydroxyl
OPG	Osteoprotogerin
P	Phosphorus
PCL	Poly-ε-caprolactone
PCR	Polymerase chain reaction
PDA	Phase Doppler Anemometry
PDGF	Platelet derived growth factor
PDMS	PolyDiMethylSiloxane
PE	Polyethylene
PET	Poly(Ethylene Terephthalate)
PI	Polyimide ISion sputtering
PIXE	Proton Induced X-ray Emission
PLA	Poly-L-lactide
PLD	Pulsed Laser Deposition
PLST	Progressive Load Scratch Test
P-O	Phosphate
PS	Polystyrene
PS	Potentiostatic (chapter 5e: Electrochemical ...)
PTFE	Polytetrafluoroethylene (Teflon®)
PTH	Parathyroid hormone
RANK	Receptor activator of nuclear factor kappa B
RANKL	RANK ligand

RAS	Reflection-absorption spectroscopy
RBM	Rat bone marrow cells
RBS	Rutherford Backscattering Spectrometry
rf	radio frequency
RNA	Ribonucleic acid
RT PCR	Real-time Polymerase chain reaction
RT	Reverse transcriptase
SAGE	Serial analysis of gene expression
SBF	Simulated Body Fluid
SEM	Scanning Electron Microscopy
SHG	Second harmonic generation
SiHA	Silicon-substituted Hydroxyapatite
SIMS	Secondary Ion Mass Spectrometry
SiO_4	Silicate
SNP	single nucleotide polymorphism
SR	Silicon rubber
TCP	Tricalcium Phosphate
TCPS	Tissue culture polystyrene
TEA	Transversely excited atmospheric
TEM	Transmission Electron Microscopy
TGF-β	Transforming Growth Factor beta
TGF-β1	Transforming growth factor beta 1
THG	Third harmonic generation
Ti	Titanium
TNF	Tumor necrosis factor
TRAF6	TNF receptor associated factor 6
TRAP	signal transduction protein (chapter 4: *in-vitro* & *in-vivo*)
TRAP	Tartrate resistant acid phosphatase
TRITC	Tetramethyl rhodamine iso-thiocyanate
tRNA	transfer RNA
TTCP	Tetra calcium phosphate
UST	Universal Surface Tester
XPS	X-ray Photoelectron Spectroscopy
XRD	X-Ray Diffraction

Chapter 1
Introduction

John A. Jansen and Betty León

The 2004 global dental implant market was estimated to be € 1.2×10^9 and is expected to grow 15% to 18% annually, resulting in market duplication within 4 to 5 years. The main factors contributing to this expected growth include the simplification of implantation methods and the aging of the population. The estimated numbers of implant pillars placed in Europe, the United States, and Japan for 2005–2010 are shown in Table 1.1.

Orthopedic implants also constitute a main element in the (bio)medical implant market. Among the orthopedic implants, those used for joint replacement constitute the largest segment, estimated at € 7.6×10^9 globally in 2004. In Europe alone, this market is estimated at € 1.2×10^9. The expected annual growth of this market during the next 5 years is 7% to 9%. The number of primary hip implants is around 2 million worldwide, and the number of knee implants is about 1 million. Approximately 10% of these implants (depending on the type) will ultimately fail yearly. The number of revisions is thus about 300,000 each year, which attracts attention owing to the continuous aging of our population and the consequent steep increase in health care costs in relation to the gross domestic product.

The final success and lifetime of dental and orthopedic implants is determined by the quality of the bone–implant reaction, which is characterized by a tight bond of the bone with the implant surface without the occurrence of an intervening fibrous tissue layer. In addition to patient- and surgery-related factors, the interfacial bone reaction to medical and dental implants depends on the surface topography and chemistry and the mechanical properties of the implant material used.

The best available materials for bone-replacing devices are titanium and calcium phosphate ceramics. Titanium and its alloys are mainly used for their strength, although the thin oxide layer that naturally forms on their surface also acts as a passivating protective barrier, conferring on this metal its known

J.A. Jansen (✉)
Department of Periodontology and Biomaterials, Radboud University Nijmegen Medical Center, Philips van Leijdenlaa 25, 6525 EX Nijmegen, The Netherlands
e-mail: j.jansen@dent.umcn.nl

B. León, J.A. Jansen (eds.), *Thin Calcium Phosphate Coatings for Medical Implants*,
DOI 10.1007/978-0-387-77718-4_1, © Springer Science+Business Media, LLC 2009

Table 1.1 Estimated development of implant pillar placement

Year	No. of implant pillars (×1000) Europe	USA	Japan	*Sum*
2005	1730	938	316	*2984*
2006	1883	1030	355	*3268*
2007	2037	1137	397	*3571*
2008	2200	1239	441	*3880*
2009	2376	1351	489	*4216*
2010	2566	1459	543	*4568*

corrosion resistance under physiological conditions. Moreover, titanium oxide is thought to improve the response of bone. Calcium phosphates, however, are chosen for their unrivaled compatibility with human bone: they initiate a rapid biological response, improving adhesion between the bone and the implant and providing a scaffold for bone growth.

Apart from living cells and collagenous extracellular matrix (ECM), the main constituent of bones and teeth is a calcium phosphate called hydroxyapatite (HA), or $Ca_5(PO_4)_3OH$; the ideal surgical implant would thus be made from the same material. However, bulk calcium phosphates are weak and brittle, making them unsuitable for replacing parts of the body, such as teeth, that experience large stress. To eliminate this problem, it was suggested that implants could be improved by coating them with *titanium*, with calcium phosphate *ceramic*. This approach would combine the mechanical strength of titanium with the biological properties of calcium phosphate.

1.1 Plasma-Sprayed Calcium Phosphate Coatings

Currently, the most popular biomedical application of the plasma-spray technique is the production of calcium phosphate (CaP) ceramic coating on dental root implants and hip and knee orthopedic prostheses [1, 2]. Hermann provided a detailed description of the plasma-spray technique [3]. Briefly, the plasma-spray process requires roughening the metallic implant surface (e.g., by grit blasting) to obtain retention of the coating through mechanical interlocking. Plasma spraying is a technique in which a so-called plasma gun creates an electric arc current of high energy between a cathode and an anode. An inert gas is directed through the space between these electrodes, and subsequently the arc current ionizes the gas, and a plasma is formed. The electrons and ions in this plasma are separated from each other and are accelerated toward the cathode and anode, respectively. These rapidly moving particles then collide with other atoms or molecules in the gas, which results in expansion owing to the temperature increase. Then, a plasma flame is formed that emerges from the gun toward the substrate at velocities approaching or exceeding the speed of sound. Next, HA ceramic powder particles are fed into the plasma flame. The particles melt and are deposited on the substrate at which the gun is aimed.

The quality of plasma spray-deposited coatings can be influenced by several parameters, such as the temperature of the plasma, the nature of the plasma gas, the particle size of the powder, and the chemical nature of the ceramic powder [4]. In this context, it must be recognized that the CaP coating deposited by the plasma process is quite different from bone mineral apatite. During plasma spraying, overheating and melting can change the synthetic HA powder. As a result, the deposited coating consists of HA as well as amorphous and other crystalline CaP components [5–7]. Therefore, it has been suggested that all manufacturers of HA-coated implants perform relevant chemical and analytical tests to ensure the quality of their coatings [1, 2, 8]. This analysis should include information about chemical composition, the Ca/P ratio, crystallinity, density, tensile strength, thickness, and uniformity. There should also be a trace element analysis.

Irrespective of the apparent importance of such an accompanying report, these control tests are no guarantee of the final biological performance of the coated implants. For example, although high crystallinity decreases the extent of coating dissolution, faster bone bonding can probably be expected with coatings that have a high level of more soluble amorphous phases [9–11]. Therefore, biological evaluations are required for such certified coatings.

Currently, not all of the above-mentioned information is available, making comparisons between plasma-sprayed CaP coatings produced by different manufacturers difficult. Still, various short- and long-term animal studies performed up to now have demonstrated faster and greater bone adaptation to plasma-sprayed CaP-coated implants [1, 9, 11, 12–25]. Histological results have shown (1) higher percentages of bone contact along CaP-coated implants compared to noncoated implants; and (2) greater stability as measured by higher fixation strengths after short and prolonged implantation periods. On the other hand, it must be noted that occasionally less favorable results have been reported. For example, during a 6-month study in rabbits, Gottlander et al. [26] observed significant numbers of giant cells and macrophages around HA-coated implants. The presence of these cells was associated with partial disappearance of the HA coating. In addition, there was significantly less bone around HA-coated implants than was seen with noncoated commercially pure titanium implants.

1.2 Clinical Perspective of CaP-Coated Implants

The promising results from the earlier mentioned animal studies formed the base for the use of plasma-sprayed CaP-coated implants in human patients. However, two decades after the introduction of HA-coated implants, most oral implantology studies still report only about the first 5 to 8 years of clinical performance [27–29]. In addition, the number of studies published in peer-reviewed international journals is limited, although there are more published studies on the clinical performance of HA-coated hip and knee implants, with follow-up periods of up to 20 years [30–37].

For general acceptance and clinical use of plasma-sprayed CaP-coated implants, it is important to note that reported data must be confirmed by analysis of HA-coated implants that have been retrieved from human patients. A few histological studies of HA-coated dental implants under loaded conditions are already available [38–41]. Examination of the bone–implant interface of these retrieved implants showed intimate contact of the bone–HA coating. Furthermore, it was found that bonding of the HA coating to the metal was strong enough to resist loading forces. Retrieval of a bipolar coated hip prosthesis [42] from a patient whose hip had undergone revision because of severe mid-thigh pain 4 years after implantation showed scarce remnants of a coating-like material on the surface of the prosthesis. Histology of these remnants and of the bony side of the bone–HA interface failed to reveal any remnants of the HA coating. A large-scale study of retrieved failed HA-coated acetabular cups identified and quantified the residual HA area on the surface of the retrieved cup to understand the relevance between HA resorption and failure modes [35]. It showed that the HA coating resorbed significantly more slowly on the mechanically stable cups than on the unstable ones, substantiating the fact that acetabular cups need to be mechanically interlocked [33] to ensure strong and enduring fixation [34].

1.3 Clinical Concerns About Plasma-Spray CaP Coatings

In addition to the above-mentioned benefits, concerns have been raised regarding the viable use and clinical efficacy of plasma Spray-Coated implants [21, 43–57]. These concerns deal with: (1) thickness; (2) crystallinity; (3) biodegradation; (4) adhesion strength; (5) fatigue properties; and (6) third-body wear of the coating.

The thickness of a CaP coating is always, theoretically, a compromise between the dissolution and mechanical properties of the coating. The thickness of plasma-sprayed coatings, as applied by various manufacturers, varies between 50 and 200 μm. In view of this, it must be noted that a coating thickness > 100 μm can introduce fatigue under tensile loading. Moreover, the higher thermal expansivity of HA with regard to titanium alloy yields tensile stress that produces through-thickness cracking [48]. Moreover, residual stress increases with thickness, and its energy release may promote interfacial debonding. Therefore, de Groot et al. [49] proposed a 50 to 70 μm thick coating, whereas Osborn [50] recommended that it be 200 μm. Excessive thickness, however, can favor coating delamination and fragmentation, which in time can result in implant mobility. For example, Søballe [19] reported that a thin coating of 50 μm gave stronger fixation than a thick coating of 200 μm.

The degree of crystallinity influences the dissolution and biological behavior of plasma-sprayed CaP coatings. Several studies have shown that the more crystalline a CaP coating is, the lower its dissolution rate [20]. Furthermore, it was found that the combination of stress and dissolution had a dramatic influence on the integrity of the amorphous or glassy phase of the HA coating. The amorphous phase of a CaP coating demonstrates different fatigue behavior, whereas crystalline coatings did not show any changes.

The biodegradation of plasma-sprayed CaP coatings is controlled by numerous factors, including crystal structure, microporosity, crystallinity, chemical composition, Ca/P ratio, lattice defects, particle size, and the purity of the starting powder [49, 51]. During plasma spraying, the crystallinity of the starting material changes owing to the high temperature of the plasma, resulting in the formation of an amorphous or glassy phase in the finally obtained coating [4, 52–54]. This state of CaP ceramic is unstable and more susceptible to biodegradation [14]. In addition to physicochemical dissolution, degradation can result from cell-mediated processes [10, 55].

The adhesion strength between HA coating and substrate varies from 5 to 65 MPa depending on the plasma-spraying technique used. Filliaggi et al. [56] reported that the strength of HA coating is dependent on the coating thickness. Coatings of 50 μm gave higher adhesion strength than coatings of 240 μm. In addition, cyclic loading of the implants (dental and orthopedic) may affect the chemical and crystallographic characteristics of the thick plasma-sprayed coatings [57] as well as the corrosion resistance of the underlying substrate. Several studies have already demonstrated that cyclic loading might lead to fatigue failure. Coatings of $>$ 100 μm thickness reduce the fatigue resistance of the titanium alloy substrates, whereas 25 to 50 μm thick coatings did not delaminate during fatigue or final fracture [57]. Furthermore, it has been shown that a combination of aqueous environment and stress can result in delamination or accelerated dissolution of the HA coating, which can influence the long-term stability of the implant [58, 59].

The degradation of plasma-sprayed CaP coatings occurs by rapid dissolution of the relatively soluble amorphous phase followed by loosening of crystalline particles. Some studies demonstrated the appearance of loose crystalline CaP particles around the implant, which can cause a foreign body response [54]. Furthermore, it is suggested that an inflammatory response can contribute to HA particles' separation, which can cause third-body wear and associated osteolysis [60, 61]. Whether this phenomenon occurs frequently is difficult to determine. For example, Frayssinet et al. [55] found CaP particles inside bone tissue but noted no sign of localized osteolysis. Piatelli et al. [40] did not observe any relation between coating degradation and implant failure mechanisms.

1.4 Future Perspectives of CaP-Coated Implants

Controversies and concerns hamper the widespread use of plasma-sprayed CaP-coated implants. In view of this, new coating techniques are being developed. These new techniques focus mainly on the deposition of well characterized thin CaP layers. It is claimed that the current problems, as observed with the plasma-spray technique, can be overcome and can profit from the favorable bone biological properties of CaP ceramics. It is expected that thickness reduction will be advantageous in the sense that less material will be necessary, and there will be reduced residual stress, thus delivering better adhesion of the coating. Moreover, improved control of the overall physicochemical properties of the coatings (thin films) will allow a nano-technological approach of the coating design. The fact that no grit-blasting procedure is needed to ensure good mechanical adhesion allows conservation of a previously engineered surface topography.

Several of these new thin film technologies for the deposition of CaP coatings on medical and dental implants are discussed in the next chapters. This comprehensive work attempts to describe the state of the art in the study of bioactive CaP coatings, and it reviews the physicochemical properties and *in vitro* and *in vivo* performance of thin CaP coatings prepared by various techniques.

This book is meant to be valuable not only to students involved in the study of biomaterials but also to engineers active in the design, development, and manufacture of medical implants. Therefore, we included three introductory chapters that deal with the general physicochemical properties of calcium apatite and its related compounds, noting the benefits of special characterization techniques for this type of coating and the complexity of *in vitro* and *in vivo* testing of such material.

References

1. P. Serekian. in "Hydroxylapatite Coatings in Orthopaedic Surgery" (Raven Press, Ltd., New York: 1993).
2. J. E. Dalton and S. D. Cook. Journal Biomedical Materials Research 29 (1995) 239.
3. H. Hermann. Scientific American 9 (1988) 112.
4. J. G. C. Wolke, J. M. A. Blieck-Hogervorst, W. J. A. Dhert, C. P. A. T. Klein, and K. De Groot. Journal of Thermal Spray Technology 1 (1992) 75.
5. Z. Zyman, J. Weng, X. Liu, X. Zhang, and Z. Ma. Biomaterials 3 (1993) 225.
6. Z. Zyman, J. Weng, X. Liu, X. Li, and X. Zhang. Biomaterials 2 (1994) 151.
7. W. Tong, J. Chen, X. Li, Y. Cao, Z. Yang, J. Feng, and X. Zhang. Biomaterials 17 (1996) 1507.
8. K. A. Gross, C. H. C. Berndt, and V. J. Jacono. International Journal of Oral & Maxillofacial Implants 13 (1988) 601.
9. J. A. Jansen, J. P. C. M. Van Der Waerden, and J. G. C. Wolke. Journal of Biomedical Materials Research 279 (1993) 603.
10. C. A. Van Blitterswijk, Y. P. Bovell, J. S. Flach, H. Leenders, I. Brink, and J. De Bruijn, in: "Hydroxylapatite Coatings in Orthopaedic Surgery" (Raven Press, Ltd., New York, 1993).

11. M. T. Manley. in "Hydroxylapatite Coatings in Orthopaedic Surgery" (Raven Press, Ltd., New York: 1993).
12. R. G. T. Geesink, K. De Groot, and C. P. A. T. Klein. Clinical Orthopedics 225 (1987)147.
13. S. D. Cook, K. A. Thomas, J. F. Kay, and M. Jarcho. Clinical Orthopedics 232 (1988) 225.
14. D. Buser, R. K. Schenk, S. Steinemann, J. P. Fiorellini, C. H. Fox, and H. Stich. Journal of Biomedical Materials Research 25 (1991) 889.
15. C. P. A. T. Klein, P. Patka, H. B. M. Van Der Lubbe, J. G. C. Wolke, and K. De Groot. Journal of Biomedical Materials Research 25 (1991) 53.
16. M. Gottlander, T. Albrektsson, and L. V. Carlsson. International Journal of Oral & Maxillofacial Implants 7 (1992) 485.
17. M. Weinlaender, E. B. Kenny, V. Lekovic, J. Beumer, P. K. Moy, and S. Lewis. International Journal of Oral & Maxillofacial Implants 7 (1992) 491.
18. W. J. A. Dhert, C. P. A. T. Klein, J. A. Jansen, E. A. Van Der Velde, R. C. Vriesde, P. M. Rozing, and K. De Groot. Journal Biomedical Material Research 27 (1993) 127.
19. K. Søballe. Acta Orthopedica Scandinavia Suppl. 255 (1993) 1.
20. C. P. A. T. Klein, P. Patka, J. G. C. Wolke, J. M. A. Blieck-Hogervorst, and K. De Groot. Biomaterials 15 (1994)146.
21. T. Kitsugi, T. Nakamura, M. Oka, Y. Senaha, T. Goto, and T. Shibuya. Journal Biomedical Materials Research 30 (1996) 261.
22. G. H. Evans, A. J. Mendez, and R. F. Caudill. International Journal of Oral Maxillofacial Implants 11 (1996) 360.
23. B. Carr, D. A. Gerard, and P. E. Larsen. International Journal of Oral Maxillofacial Implants 12 (1997) 777.
24. H. Caulier, J. P. C. M. Van Der Waerden, Y. C. G. J. Paquay, J. G. C. Wolke, W. Kalk, I. Naert, and J. A. Jansen. Journal Biomedical Materials Research 29 (1995) 1061.
25. S. Vercaigne, J. G. C. Wolke, I. Naert, and J. A. Jansen. Clinical Oral Implants Research 9 (1998) 261.
26. M. Gottlander, C. B. Johansson, and A. Albrektsson. Clinical Oral Implants Research 8 (1997) 345.
27. J. Mau, M. Yong, C. U. Fritzemeier, A. Behneke, B. D'hoedt, N. Behneke, G. Gomez-Roman, H. Spiekermann, and V. Strunz, *Clinical Oral Implants Research* 13 (2002) 477.
28. M. Esposito, P. Coulthard, H. V. Worthington, P. Thomsen, and M. G. Grusovin, *International Journal of Oral and Maxillofacial Implants* 20 (2005) 557.
29. J. J. Lee, L. Rouhfar, and O. R. Beirne, *Journal of Oral and Maxillofacial Surgery* 58 (2000) 1372.
30. H. Effenberger, R. Graf, M. May, M. Lojpur, M. Imhof, and F. Lintner, *Biomedizinische Technik* 49 (2004) 290.
31. L. Palm, S. A. Jacobsson, and I. Ivarsson, *Journal of Arthroplasty* 17 (2002) 172.
32. P. R. Aldinger, S. J. Breusch, M. Lukoschek, H. Mau, V. Ewerbeck, and M. Thomsen, *Journal of Bone and Joint Surgery – Series B*85 (2003) 209.
33. W. N. Capello, J. R. Feinberg, J. A. D'antonio, and M. T. Manley, *Journal of Bone and Joint Surgery – Series A* 79 (1997) 1023.
34. K. G. Nilsson, J. Kärrholm, L. Carlsson, and T. Dalén, *Journal of Arthroplasty* 14 (1999) 9.
35. W. P. Hu, K. A. Lai, C. H. Lin, C. Y. Yang, and G. L. Chang, in Bioengineering, Proceedings of the Northeast Conference, edited by (2002).
36. J. A. Bojescul, J. S. Xenos, J. J. Callaghan, and C. G. Savory, *Journal of Bone and Joint Surgery – Series A* 85 (2003) 1079.
37. Y.-H. Kim, *Journal of Bone and Joint Surgery – Series B* 87 (2005) 623–627.
38. A. Piatelli and P. Trisi. Journal of Periodontology 64, (1993) 906.
39. A. Piatelli, P. Trisi, and M. Emanualli. International Journal of Oral & Maxillofacial Implants 8 (1993) 69.

40. A. Piatelli, A. Sarano, and M. Piatelli. Journal of Periodontology 89 (1998) 178.
41. H. Oguchi. Journal of Dental Research 73 (1994) 293.
42. P. Buma, *International Journal of Risk and Safety in Medicine* 8 (1996) 111.
43. I. M. O. Kangasniemi, C. C. P. M. Verheyden, E. A. Van Der Velde, and K. De Groot. Journal of Biomedical Materials Research 28 (1994) 563.
44. E. G. Hulshoff, K. Van Dijk, J. P. C. M. Van Der Waerden, J. G. C. Wolke, W. Kalk, and J. A. Jansen. Journal Biomedical Materials Research 31 (1996) 329.
45. H. Caulier, J. P. C. M. Van Der Waerden, Y. C. G. J. Paquay, J. G. C. Wolke, W. Kalk, I. Naert, and J. A. Jansen. Journal Biomedical Materials Research 35 (1997)19.
46. T. Albrektsson. Journal of Oral and Maxillofacial Surgery 56 (1988) 1312.
47. H. F. Morris and S. Ochi. Journal of Oral & Maxillofacial Surgery, 56 (1998) 1303.
48. Y. C. Tsui, C. Doyle, and T. W. Clyne, *Biomaterials* 19 (1998) 2015.
49. K. DE Groot, R. G. T. Geesink, C. P. A. T. Klein, and P. Serekian. Journal of Biomedical Material Research 21 (1997) 1375.
50. J. F. Osborn Biomedical Technics 32 (1987) 177.
51. C. P. A. T. Klein, A. A. Driessen, K. DE Groot, and A. Van Den Hooff. Journal of Biomedical Materials Research 17 (1983) 769.
52. B. Koch, J. G. C. Wolke, and K. De Groot. Journal of Biomedical Materials Research 24 (1990) 655.
53. S. R. Radin and P. Ducheyne. Journal of Material Sciences: Materials in Medicine 3 (1992) 33.
54. R. Y. Whitehead, W. R. Lacefield, and L. C. Lucas. Journal of Biomedical Materials Research 27 (1993) 1501.
55. P. Frayssinet, D. Hardy, J. S. Hanker, and B. L. Giamarra. Cells and Materials 5 (1995) 125.
56. M. J. Filliaggi, N. A. Coombs, and R. M. Pilliar. Journal of Biomedical Materials Research 25 (1991) 1211.
57. A. K. Lynn and D. L. Duquesnay, *Biomaterials* 23 (2002) 1937.
58. F. J. Kummer and W. L. Jaffe. Journal of Applied Biomaterials 3 (1992) 211.
59. R. L. Reis, F. J. Monteiro, and G. W. Hastings. Journal of Material Sciences: Materials in Medicine 5 (1994) 457.
60. R. D. Bloebaum and J. A. Dupont. Journal of Arthroplast 8 (1993) 195.
61. R. D. Bloebaum, D. Beeks, L. D. Dorr, C. G. Savory, J. A. Dupont, and A.A. Hofman. Clinical Orthopedics 298 (1994) 19.

Chapter 2
Physicochemistry of Apatite and Its Related Calcium Phosphates

Pierre Layrolle and Guy Daculsi

Abstract Hydroxyapatite and related calcium phosphates (CaPs) are similar in composition to the mineral part of bones and teeth. Synthetic CaPs are successfully used for filling bone defects in various clinical indications as they are considered bioactive and osteoconductive, guiding the bone healing process. Nevertheless, most of the synthetic bone substitutes lack the osteoinductive property for regenerating bone tissue over large defects. This chapter reviews the biological properties of CaP materials in relation to their chemistry, crystallographic structure, and solubility. Recent studies have shown that some macro and micro porous CaP ceramics have led to ectopic bone formation when implanted in muscles of animals. Although the interactions of these CaP materials with body fluids, cells, and tissues have been investigated at both the microscopic and ultrastructural levels, there is still a lack of understanding of the possible mechanisms leading to osteoinduction. Both the study of cell–material interactions *in vitro* and immunochemistry techniques after implantation may provide valuable information. These osteoinductive bone substitutes may be satisfactorily used in future as an alternative to autologous or allogenous bone grafts.

2.1 Biomaterials for Bone and Teeth Replacement

Biomaterials are synthetic materials used to replace parts of a living system or to function in intimate contact with living tissue [1]. They are intended to restore, replace, or treat any tissue, organ, or function of the body. Various biomaterials are used in bone and teeth replacement. Depending on their properties and functions in the human body, the materials range from ceramics to metals and polymers. Among ceramics, alumina (Al_2O_3) and zirconia (ZrO_2)

P. Layrolle (✉)
INSERM, U791, Laboratory for Osteo-Articular and Dental Tissue Engineering, Faculty of Dental Surgery, University of Nantes, 1 Place Alexis Ricordeau, 44042 Nantes, France
e-mail: Pierre.layrolle@nantes.inserm.fr

B. León, J.A. Jansen (eds.), *Thin Calcium Phosphate Coatings for Medical Implants*, DOI 10.1007/978-0-387-77718-4_2, © Springer Science+Business Media, LLC 2009

are employed as artificial dental crowns and the heads and inserts of hip joint prostheses because of their relatively high degree of toughness and resistance to abrasion. Metals such as stainless steel, cobalt-chrome alloys, and titanium and its alloys are used to manufacture dental implants (artificial roots) and hip and knee joint prostheses. Titanium and alloys are preferred over other metals owing to their corrosion resistance in the body and relative high strength and fatigue properties. Polymers such as ultra-high-molecular-weight polyethylene (UHMW PE) and polymethylmethacrylate (PMMA) found application in acetabular cups, patellar prostheses, and as cements for fixing hip and joint prostheses and fillers in dentistry or vertebroplasty. Upon implantation in bone, most of these biomaterials are tolerated by human tissues, leading to neither necrosis nor adverse inflammatory reactions. These artificial implants are simply encapsulated by fibrous tissue, not being in direct contact with bone tissue. The materials are classified as *bioinert* (e.g., zirconia, alumina) and *biotolerant* (e.g., PMMA, titanium, Co-Cr).

Hydroxyapatite (HA) and related calcium phosphates (CaPs) are of special significance in the field of biomaterials because they compose the mineral part of bones and teeth [2–6]. Calcium orthophosphates comprise a family of compounds having various chemical compositions, crystallographic structures, and solubility in water (Tables 2.1, 2.2). Synthetic CaPs are used as bone substitutes owing to their favorable biological properties [2–9]. When implanted in bone, CaP materials such as HA and β-tricalcium phosphate (β-TCP) interact with body fluids, cells, and tissues. It is generally accepted that CaP ceramics are bioactive and osteoconductive.

Bioactivity is a property of the ceramic surface that induces biological integration of living soft and hard tissues. The core mechanism of bioactivity is the partial dissolution and release of ionic products *in vivo*, elevating local concentrations of calcium and phosphate and precipitating a biological apatite on the surface of ceramics [8, 9]. This apatite layer formed *in vivo* contains various biological molecules and is colonized by osteoblastic cells producing the bone extracellular matrix. As the result of bioactivity, CaP bone substitutes support the bone healing process by guiding bone tissue over their surface by the process of *osteoconduction*. Such bioactive materials allow newly formed bone tissue to grow into any surface irregularities.

For more than three decades, CaPs in the form of HA and β-TCP ceramics have found clinical applications in orthopedic, spinal, and maxillofacial surgery as bone substitutes [10–13]. However, HA and β-TCP materials are sparingly soluble in body fluids, and there is no evidence of degradation by cellular activity, such as the action of macrophages or bone-resorbing cells such as osteoclasts. As a consequence, the biodegradation rate of bioceramics is much slower than bone ingrowth, and these materials are still present in the body several years after implantation [10, 12].

For this reason, biomimetic materials, which are not manufactured at the high temperatures used for bioceramics, are being developed worldwide. These

Table 2.1 Chemical compositions, Ca/P molar ratio, solubility, pH, and temperature stability range in aqueous solutions of some synthetic and biological calcium orthophosphates

Orthophosphate	Abbreviation	Chemical formula	Ca/P	Solubility $-\log(K_s)$[a]	pH and temperature (°C) stability
Monocalcium phosphate monohydrate	MCPM	$Ca(H_2PO_4)_2 . H_2O$	0.5	1.14	0.1–2.0 25°C
Monocalcium phosphate, anhydrous	MCPA	$Ca(H_2PO_4)_2$	0.5	1.14	0.1–2.0 > 80°C
Dicalcium phosphate dihydrate (brushite)	DCPD	$CaHPO_4 . 2H_2O$	1.00	6.59	2.0–5.5 25°C
Dicalcium phosphate, anhydrous (monetite)	DCPA	$CaHPO_4$	1.00	6.90	2.0–5.5 > 80°C
Octacalcium phosphate	OCP	$Ca_8(HPO_4)_2(PO_4)_4 . 5H_2O$	1.33	96.6	5.5–7.0 25°–37°C
Calcium-deficient apatite	CDA	$Ca_{10-x}\square_x(HPO_4)_x(PO_4)_{6-x}(OH)_{2-x}\square_x$[c] $(0 < x < 2)$	Variable 1.33–1.66	~85.1	6.5–9.5 25°–37°C
Amorphous calcium phosphate	ACP	$Ca_x(HPO_4)_y(PO_4)_z . nH_2O$ n = 3.0–4.5; 15–20 wt% H_2O	Variable 1.2–2.2	25.7–32.7	5–12 4°–37°C
β-Tricalcium phosphate	β-TCP	β-$Ca_3(PO_4)_2$	1.50	28.9	[b]
α-Tricalcium phosphate	α-TCP	α-$Ca_3(PO_4)_2$	1.50	25.5	[b]
Biphasic Calcium Phosphate	BCP	β-$Ca_3(PO_4)_2$ + $Ca_{10}(PO_4)_6(OH)_2$	Variable 1.55–1.65	ND	[b]

(continued)

Table 2.1 (continued)

Orthophosphate	Abbreviation	Chemical formula	Ca/P	Solubility $-\log(K_s)$[a]	pH and temperature (°C) stability
Hydroxyapatite	HA	$Ca_{10}(PO_4)_6(OH)_2$	1.67	116.8	9.5–12.0 > 80°C
Fluoroapatite	FA	$Ca_{10}(PO_4)_6F_2$	1.67	120.0	7–12 > 80°C
Tetracalcium phosphate	TTCP	$Ca_4(PO_4)_2O_2$	2.0	38–44	[b]

ND, not determined

[a] The solubility at 25°C in water is given as the logarithm of the ion product of the given formulas with concentrations in mol/l

[b] These compounds cannot be precipitated from aqueous solutions and form only at elevated temperatures (β-TCP > 800°C, α-TCP > 1125°C, TTCP > 1300°C)

[c] []represents a lacuna in the crystal lattice of hydroxyapatite

Table 2.2 Main infrared vibration bands and X-ray diffraction lines of some relevant calcium orthophosphate compounds

		IR peaks		XRD lines	
Compound	Chemical formula	υ (cm^{-1})	Assign.	2θ (°)[a]	Intensity (%)
DCPD	$CaHPO_4 .2H_2O$	3542	H_2O	11.681	100
		3490	intracrystal.	20.935	100
		1132	HPO_4	29.258	75
		1060		30.506	50
		984		34.156	50
		525		34.426	30
OCP	$Ca_8(HPO_4)_2(PO_4)_4.$ $5H_2O$	1105	HPO_4, PO_4	4.722	100
		1070		9.441	15
		1031		25.872	17
		954		26.002	20
		603		31.555	33
		530		31.704	32
β-TCP	β-$Ca_3(PO_4)_2$	1120	PO_4	17.005	20
		1043		25.803	25
		970		27.769	55
		943		31.027	100
		606		34.372	65
		551		52.946	25
HA	$Ca_{10}(PO_4)_6(OH)_2$	3562	OH	25.879	40
		1081	PO_4	31.774	100
		1030	OH	32.197	60
		954	PO_4	32.902	60
		631		34.049	25
		601		46.713	30
		570		49.469	40

IR, infrared; XRD, X-ray diffraction; DCPD, dicalcium phosphate dihydrate (brushite); OCP, octacalcium phosphate; β-TCTP, β-tricalcium phosphate; HA, hydroxyapatite

[a] XRD data are from JCPDS cards 9-0077 (DCPD), 26-1056 (OCP), 9-0169 (β-TCP), 9-0432 (HA). 2θ values are given for Cu Kα X-ray source ($\lambda = 1.54060$Å)

biomimetic materials attempt to resemble biological apatite in regard to their composition, crystallinity, and mechanical strength. Calcium phosphate cements (CPCs) are examples of biomimetic materials [14]. As found in other fields, CPCs set at ambient temperature by hydrolysis and acido-basic reactions. Upon mixing with aqueous solutions, initial CaP powders are dissolved and precipitated into less-soluble phases. During the precipitation reaction, new crystals grow and join particles, thus providing mechanical rigidity to the cement. Hardening occurs within dozen of minutes, yielding to a compressive strength of 20 to 60 MPa. The hardening rate is influenced by the powder/liquid ratio and the addition of chemicals. CPCs may be reinforced with biodegradable polymers to provide low elastic modulus to the composites. Despite the variability of formulations, the CPCs lead to only three end products: dicalcium phosphate dihydrate (brushite) (DCPD), calcium-deficient apatite (CDA), and octacalcium phosphate (OCP).

Another drawback of synthetic CaP bioceramics being used as bone substitutes is their poor mechanical properties, which do not allow them to be used in load-bearing areas. For this reason, the clinical applications of CaP materials are currently focused on coating dental implants and metallic prostheses or for filling bone defects in maxillofacial and orthopedic surgery in combination with metal plates and screws.

2.2 Properties and Structure of Calcium Phosphate Ceramics

Calcium orthophosphates have various chemical compositions, crystallographic structures, and solubilities in water (Tables 2.1, 2.2). Despite a large number of compounds, CaPs are easily distinguished using infrared (IR) spectroscopy and x-ray diffraction (XRD) (Table 2.2). Each compound is characterized by an IR spectrum or XRD pattern, which provides a “fingerprint” of their structure.

Hydroxyapatite and β-TCP bioceramics are usually manufactured starting from well characterized CaP powders, mixed with pore makers, and sintered at elevated temperatures (e.g., 1000°–1300°C) [3]. Research has primarily focused on both the formulation of appropriate bioceramic chemistry and optimization of the physical pore structure. Mastering the chemistry of CaP bioceramics is crucial for reproducible and controlled production processes as well as for ensuring the adequate biological response upon implantation in bone tissue [15]. There are numerous methods for precipitating CaP powders from aqueous solutions [2–5, 16–19]. As illustrated in Fig. 2.1, various CaP phases can be precipitated by neutralizing the successive acidity of phosphoric acid (H_3PO_4). Depending on several experimental conditions (pH, temperature) acidic, hydrated, or basic CaP phases with low or high crystallinity are precipitated. The most insoluble and thermodynamically stable phase is an apatitic CaP.

Monocalcium phosphate monohydrate (MCPM) is both the most acidic and water-soluble compound in the calcium orthophosphate family (Table 2.1, Fig. 2.1). It precipitates from highly acidic solutions. MCPM crystallizes into a triclinic structure with two formula units per cell. At temperatures above 80°C and under acidic conditions, the anhydrous form of monocalcium phosphate (MCPA) precipitates. Because of their high acidity and solubility, both MCPM and MCPA have never been found in biological calcifications such as bone and teeth mineral, and they are not capable of forming a direct bond with bone tissue. Nevertheless, MCPM is one of the components of several self-hardening CPCs [2,14].

Dicalcium phosphate dihydrate can be precipitated from aqueous solutions at pH ~4.0 to 5.5 and room temperature. It transforms into dicalcium

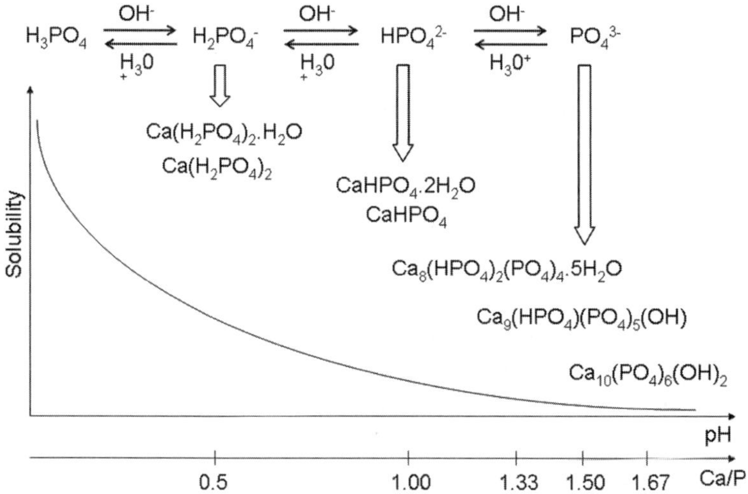

Fig. 2.1 Various calcium orthophosphate compounds obtained by neutralizing phosphoric acid. Calcium/phosphorus ratios (Ca/P) are reported in the figure. The solubility of calcium phosphates (CaPs) in water decreases drastically from left to right, hydroxyapatite being the most insoluble and stable phase

phosphate anhydrous (DCPA) at temperatures above 80°C. DCPD crystallizes into a monoclinic structure with four units per cell, whereas DCPA has a triclinic structure. DCPD is of biological importance because it is often found in pathological calcifications (i.e., dental calculi, urinary stones). It has been proposed as an intermediate phase of both bone mineralization and dissolution of enamel [4]. DCPD is used in the formulation of some CaP cements or in the synthesis of calcium-deficient apatite (CDA) by hydrolysis [5].

Octacalcium phosphate is often found as an intermediate compound during the precipitation of the thermodynamically more stable CDA. It plays an important role in the formation of apatitic biominerals [6]. Brown [7] first proposed that OCP is the initial phase in both enamel mineral formation and bone formation, and OCP subsequently hydrolyzes into CDA *in vivo*. Structurally, OCP consists of apatitic layers, with atomic arrangements of Ca and PO_4 similar to those of HA, separated by hydrated layers [4].

Calcium-deficient apatite can be easily prepared by dropwise titration of a saturated solution of $Ca(OH)_2$ with H_3PO_4 [17]. Another synthesis method developed by Heughebaert and Montel consisted of adding a calcium salt to a phosphate salt in basic media pH 11 buffered with ammonia (NH_4OH) [18]. After drying, the resulting powder was composed of CDA having the following chemical formula:

$$Ca_{10-x}\square_x(HPO_4)_x(PO_4)_{6-x}(OH)_{2-x}\square_x \quad \text{with } (0<x<2)$$

CDA crystals are poorly crystalline and of submicron dimensions. The precipitated powders have large specific surface areas, typically 25 to 100 m^2/g. Upon heating at 800° to 1000°C, a particular composition of CDA leads to a pure β-tricalcium phosphate [β-$Ca_3(PO_4)_2$] phase according to the chemical reaction:

$$Ca_9(HPO_4)(PO_4)_5(OH) \rightarrow 3\ \beta - Ca_3(PO_4)_2 + H_2O$$

In addition to this specific case, CDAs with various compositions can be precipitated in aqueous solution. Depending on its composition, the calcium-deficient apatite decomposes at around 800° to 1000°C, forming β-TCP and HA. A particularly relevant composition for bone substitutes is reached by heating a CDA having the following formula:

$$Ca_{9.5}\square_{0.5}(HPO_4)_{0.5}(PO_4)_{5.5}(OH)_{0.5}\square_{1.5}$$

At high temperature, this CDA with a Ca/P ratio of 1.58 leads to a mixture of HA and β-TCP in a weight ratio of 60:40, so-called biphasic calcium phosphate (BCP).

Amorphous calcium phosphate (ACP) is often encountered as a transient phase during the precipitation of CaPs in aqueous solutions. ACP formation is favored by rapidly mixing highly concentrated calcium and phosphate solutions at high pH and low temperature. ACP forms at the beginning of precipitation owing to a lower surface energy than that of OCP or HA. ACP crystallizes into a CDA by both internal hydrolysis and dissolution-reprecipitation. Its conversion to CDA is delayed by the presence of inhibitors of crystal growth, such magnesium, pyrophosphate, or carbonate [20]. The chemical arrangement of atoms in ACP preparations is still uncertain as many analytical methods do not provide accurate crystallographic information. X-ray patterns show a broad halo; infrared spectra exhibit featureless phosphate absorption bands; and electron microscopy shows spherical particles with diameters in the range 20 to 200 nm and diffraction rings [4, 5, 20]. Nevertheless, X-ray absorption spectroscopic data (RDF, EXAFS) and ab inito calculations support the hypothesis that the atomic arrangement in ACP is related to the HA structure [21–23]. As shown in Fig. 2.2, it has been proposed that the basic structural unit of ACP is a 0.95 nm diameter spherical cluster of ions with the composition $Ca_9(PO_4)_6$ [21]. A stepwise assembly of these clusters has been proposed to describe the crsytallization of HA and biological apatites [24].

Tricalcium phosphate cannot be precipitated from aqueous solution. β-TCP can be prepared only by heating CDA above 800°C or solid-state reactions. At temperatures above 1125°C, it transforms into the high temperature phase α-TCP. Although having exactly the same chemical composition, the two compounds differ by their crystal structure. As shown in Table 2.1, β-TCP is

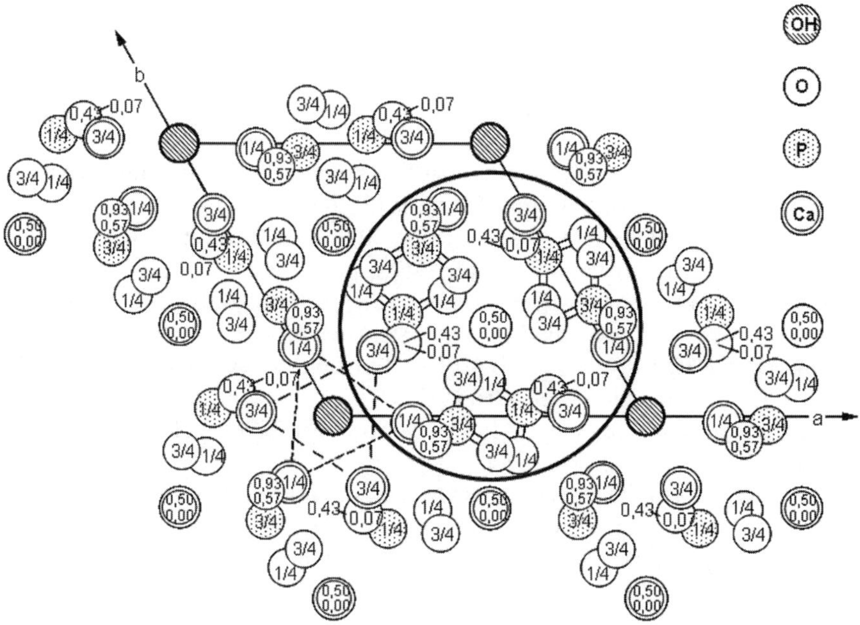

Fig. 2.2 Crystal structure of hydroxyapatite projected on the 001 plane of the hexagonal lattice with the space group $P6_3/m$. Note the OH ions located in the apatite channels. The *circle* shows the structural unit of amorphous calcium phosphate (ACP), a cluster of $Ca_9(PO_4)_6$ that is roughly spherical (0.95 nm in diameter). From [21], with permission of the publisher

less soluble in water than α-TCP, which is more reactive in aqueous systems. In contact with water or body fluids, α-TCP is rapidly hydrolyzed and reprecipitated as CDA; thus, it is incorporated in many CPCs.

Stoichiometric HA is the second most stable and least soluble CaP after fluoroapatite (FA) (Table 2.1). As shown in Fig. 2.2, the crystallographic structure of HA is hexagonal in the space group $P6_3/m$ [7]. The structure has tunnels in which hydroxyl ions are located. The preparation of pure HA from aqueous solutions is difficult owing to numerous ionic substitutions and possible lacunae in the crystal lattice. Some authors have reported its precipitation by slowly adding phosphate solution to the calcium solution and refluxing at 100°C for 1 hour [5, 25]. After filtration, the precipitate is washed, dried at 80°C, and heated at 800° to 1000°C to form a pure HA $Ca_{10}(PO_4)(OH)_2$ as evidenced by XRD and IR analysis (Table 2.2). A phenolphthalein test allowed detection of undesired traces of calcium oxide. HA powder or slurry can be mixed with polymer spacers and heated in the range 1000° to 1300°C to form macro porous ceramics [3, 26, 27].

Fluorapatite is the most insoluble phase in the CaP family. It crystallizes in the same crystallographic system as HA where hydroxyl ions are being substituted by fluoride ions in the apatite tunnels [4, 5]. FA easily forms solid solutions with HA, which are called fluorhydroxyapatites (FHA) and are described with the chemical formula:

$$Ca_{10}(PO_4)_6(OH)_{2-x}F_x \qquad \text{where } 0<x<2$$

It is relatively difficult to obtain pure FA by precipitation in aqueous solutions. Even high concentrations of fluoride ions leads to FHA owing to the formation of solid-state solutions being stabilized by hydrogen bonds between fluoride and hydroxyl ions in the apatite tunnels.

Tetracalcium phosphate (TTCP) cannot be precipitated from aqueous solutions. It can be prepared only by a solid-state reaction at temperatures above 1300°C. TTCP hydrolyzes rapidly to HA and calcium hydroxide. It is widely used for the preparation of self-setting CPCs.

Most of synthetic CaP compounds never occur in biological systems. In the skeleton, CaP is mainly present in the form of poorly crystallized calcium-deficient apatite. As the HA lattice may accommodate many ions, bone mineral contains traces of other elements, such as Mg, Na, Zn, CO_3 [4]. It is therefore impossible to give a precise chemical formula for the mineral of bone.

2.3 Dissolution and Formation of Calcium Phosphate Crystals

The solubility of CaP phases is mainly related to their chemical composition and crystal properties [2–5]. Different solubility product constants (K_s) have been reported for synthetic CaP compounds, as shown in Table 2.1. The solubilities are affected by cationic or anionic substitutions in the apatite lattice. For instance, carbonated or calcium-deficient apatite are more soluble than fluoroapatite (FA). Comparative dissolution in acetate buffer has given the following order of solubility: bone >> enamel >> β-TCP > HA. β-TCP has been found to dissolve faster than HA in physiological solutions. It also exhibits a greater rate of dissolution or degradation than HA upon implantation at heterotopic or ectopic sites. HA is the most stable phase under physiological conditions and has the slowest solubility and resorption kinetics in the human body. Implants made of sintered pure HA ceramics are present in bone defects many years after implantation. HA ceramics are thus considered nonresorbable, whereas β-TCP is resorbable based on the amount of implant left as a function of time. BCP ceramics made of a mixture of HA and β-TCP are preferable to the single compound for bone substitutes. Depending on the HA/β-TCP weight ratios, the solubility of BCP ceramics is closer to β-TCP or HA.

The dissolution of CaP ceramics is also affected by its porosity and particle size. Increasing the porosity greatly enhances the surface in contact with fluids and thus leads to a faster dissolution rate. As shown in Fig. 2.3, CaP ceramics exhibit macro pores with diameter sizes ranging from 200 to 600 μm. Because

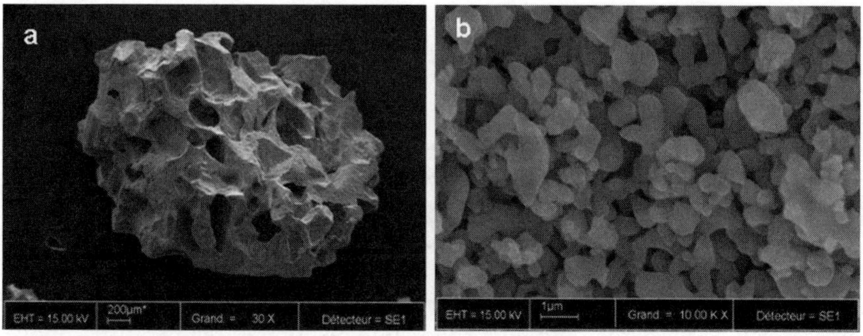

Fig. 2.3 Scanning electron microscopy (SEM) micrographs of macro/micro porous biphasic calcium phosphate (MBCP) ceramic granules. **a** Macropores 200–600 μm in diameter. **b** Micro porous surface

macro pores are well interconnected, they permit the percolation of fluids, cellsm and tissue within their structure [26, 27]. As illustrated in Fig. 2.3b, some ceramics exhibit a micro porous surface. Spherical CaP grains appear bounded by necks, leaving tiny pores about 0.1 to 1.0 μm. This remaining microporosity results from incomplete sintering of ceramics, especially when poorly crystalline precursor CaP powders and low sintering temperature and time (e.g., 1000°–1200°C for 1–10 hours) are used.

Hydroxyapatite, β-TCP, and BCP ceramics are considered bioactive materials because they partly dissolve in body fluids and precipitate on their surface a biological apatite that favors bone tissue apposition. This process of dissolution/reprecipitation of CaP ceramics implanted at ectopic or heterotopic sites has been studied in detail using transmission electron microscopy (TEM) [8, 9] As illustrated in Fig. 2.4, the BCP grains partly dissolve in body fluids, leading to the precipitation of tiny apatite crystals on their surface or between them. TEM studies have shown that these apatite crystals are similar to bone apatite in regard to size, shape, and electron diffraction patterns [8, 9]. BCP ceramics composed of a soluble β-TCP and insoluble HA phase compromise dissolution while providing a substrate for biological apatite deposition. The abundance of the apatite micro crystals associated with large grains of ceramics appeared to be directly related to the HA/β-TCP ratio of BCP ceramic implants. A larger amount of β-TCP gave a greater amount of precipitated apatite crystals. These microcrystals were identified as carbonate-containing apatites intimately associated with an organic matrix similar to that of bone apatite [8]. This surface precipitation may incorporate various proteins and growth factors present in the microenvironment, which subsequently may promote cell attachment and function. The bioactive ceramics are thus assumed to have a surface phase equivalent biologically to bone mineral. It is thought that osteoblastic cells are attracted to this layer and produce the bone extracellular matrix (ECM) leading to bone apposition (osteoconduction) rather than fibrous tissue encapsulation of ceramics.

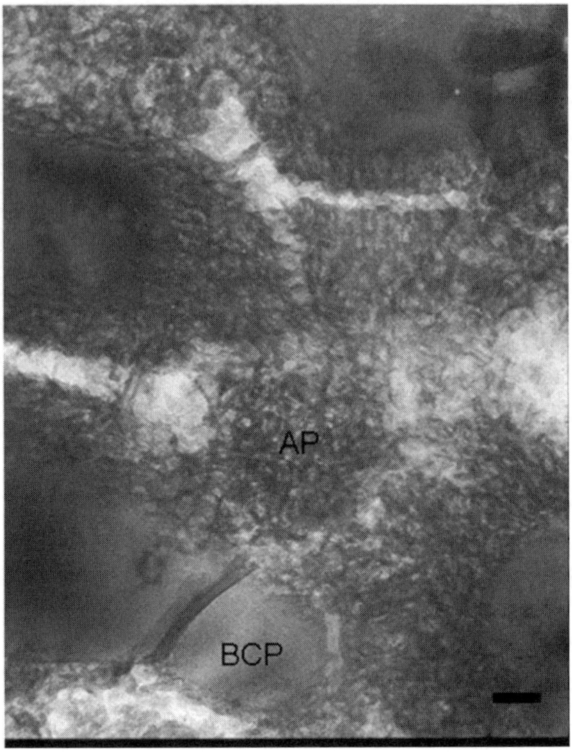

Fig. 2.4 Transmission electron microscopy micrograph of human biopsy harvested 1 year after spinal fusion with macro/micro porous biphasic calcium phosphate ceramic. The dissolution of calcium phosphate crystalline grains (*BCP*) and reprecipitation of nanometer-sized apatite crystals (*AP*) from body fluids between and in contact of BCP is shown. *Bar* = 200 nm

2.4 Biological Studies with Calcium Phosphate Bioceramics

Synthetic bone substitutes made of CaP ceramic have been used for various clinical indications because of their favorable bioactivity and osteoconductivity [3, 10–13]. The biological properties of these materials upon implantation in bone tissue are related to their physicochemical properties. CaP ceramics are more likely composed of β-TCP, HA, or mixtures (called BCP). As previously discussed, HA, β-TCP, and BCP ceramics exhibit bioactivity (i.e., the partial dissolution of ceramic and reprecipitation of biological apatite crystals). Bioactivity has been tuned by controlling both the chemical composition and crystallinity of ceramics. The precipitation of biological apatite onto the surface of bioceramics reduces its interfacial energy and favors the colonization of osteoblastic cells. These cells then produce the bone ECM; some bone-resorbing cells, the osteoclasts, degrade and remodel woven bone tissue into mechanically strong lamellar bone. Osteoclastic cells may also resorb the bioceramics, although its degradation in the body is more related to a physicochemical than a biological process. Consequently, bone tissue forms and grows at the expense of the synthetic filler. The difficulty lies in preparing bioceramics with a controlled degradation rate to match the kinetics of bone formation.

Several studies have shown that increasing the specific surface area and pore volume of bioceramics for bone repair might greatly accelerate the kinetic process of biological apatite deposition and therefore enhance the bioactivity and bone-bonding property. Pore-making agents are often introduced during the manufacturing process, leading to porosity in the CaP ceramics. Porous CaP ceramics allow rapid invasion of fluids, cells, and bone tissue growth. The precise control over porosity, pore size, and interconnection of bioceramics on different length scales is essential for understanding the structure–bioactivity relation and the rational design of better bone-bonding materials. Osteoblastic cells produced well mineralized, mature bone tissue in contact with bioceramics. Fig. 2.5 illustrates how bioceramics support bone tissue apposition on their surface. In this human biopsy specimen, macroporous biphasic calcium phosphate (MBCP) ceramics were used during spinal arthrodesis [10]. After 4 months and 1 year, biopsies were performed during the surgical removal of osteosynthetic materials and analyzed by histology. Polarized light micrography revealed mature bone tissue in direct contact with MBCP, demonstrating the osteoconductivity of bioceramics. *Ostoconductivity* is the ability to provide a scaffold for the formation of new bone on its surface by attachment, proliferation, and differentiation of bone-forming cells. As shown in Fig. 2.4, bone tissue in contact with the MBCP ceramic was well mineralized, exhibiting osteocytes, and Haversian systems. According to both observed and measured bone formation parameters, CaP bioceramics were ranked in order of bone-healing capacity. Low temperature-sintered BCP exhibited more favorable bioactivity and bone ingrowth properties than highly sintered β-TCP or HA bioceramics.

Although these synthetic fillers support the bone healing process, they generally lack osteoinductivity for regenerating bone tissue over large defects, where autologous bone grafts are preferred. Nevertheless, it has recently been shown that some porous CaP bioceramics induce ectopic bone formation after implantation into the muscles of large animals [28–35]. These biomaterials have demonstrated the ability to induce bone growth after 6 to 12 weeks in muscular

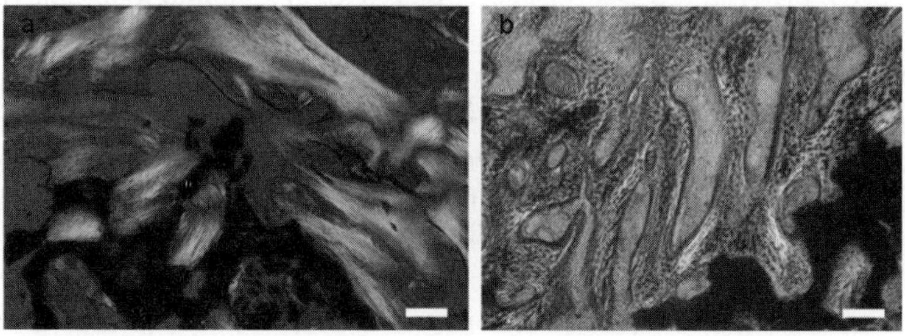

Fig. 2.5 Polarized light micrographs of human biopsy harvested (**a**) 4 months and (**b**) 1 year after spinal arthrodesis using macro/micro porous biphasic calcium phosphate (MBCP) ceramic. Lamellar bone with osteocytes and Haversian systems have formed in contact with the residual MBCP (*black areas*). *Bar* = 500 μm (*See* Color Insert)

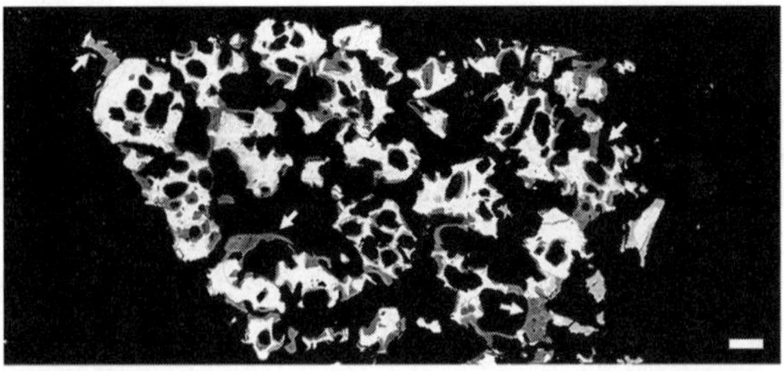

Fig. 2.6 Back-scattered SEM image of explants after 6 months of intramuscular implantation in sheep muscle. Mineralized bone containing osteocyte lacunae has formed ectopically (*arrows*) in contact with the MBCP granules (*white areas*) and inside the macropores. Non-mineralized tissue (muscle) appears in *black*. *Bar* = 1 mm

sites without the addition of osteogenic cells or bone growth factors prior to implantation. Fig. 2.6 illustrates this ectopic bone formation in contact with MBCP ceramics implanted in the dorsal muscles of sheep for 6 months. The MBCP ceramic was in the form of 1- to 2-mm granules composed of HA and β-TCP (60:40) with macropores of 450 μm and micropores of 0.43 μm, on average. After 6 months in the back muscles of sheep, the explants composed of MBCP granules were hard and encapsulated by normal muscle tissue. Ectopic bone formation with Haversian structures was observed in close contact with the MBCP granules. Back-scattered electron microscopy (Fig. 2.6) and micro computed tomography indicated that well mineralized bone with mature osteocytes had formed on or between the granules. The quantity of mineralized bone is approximately 10% of the implant volume. The ectopic bone showed trabeculae bridging the MBCP granules. Both the number and thickness of the trabeculae formed between the MBCP particles were comparable to those measured in trabecular bone [35].

Although bone induction by biomaterials has been described by many groups, it remains a subject of controversy, especially because the mechanisms are poorly understood. Recent *in vivo* studies have shown that materials should exhibit two features in order to induce ectopic bone: (1) a microporous surface and (2) a macroporous structure [32–35]. Because various bioceramic compositions demonstrated ectopic bone formation, osteoinduction does not, in fact, seem to be related to the chemistry of the material. Osteoinduction by biomaterials also seems to be animal-dependent; and so far it has been observed only in the muscles of large animals such as dogs, baboons, sheep, and goats. De Groot has proposed that CaP ceramics may concentrate bone growth factors from body fluids, which then trigger stem cells to form bone tissue [36]. Ripamonti postulated that the geometry of the material is a critical parameter in bone induction [32]. The osteoprogenitor cells might, in turn, recognize the bone-like apatite layer formed *in vivo* by dissolution-reprecipitation on the material and produce mineralized bone. Others have thought that low oxygen tension in the central region of the implants might provoke dedifferentiation of pericytes from blood microvessels into osteoblasts [37]. We thought that micro particles released from these incompletely sintered ceramics might provoke a specific inflammatory reaction leading to osteogenesis [35]. Circulating progenitor cells might differentiate into osteoblasts under stimulation of these inflammatory cytokines released by macrophages. The process might, in essence, be similar to the healing of bone fractures where debris and fragments of bone are present.

The cascade of biological events leading to material osteogenesis remains unclear for many investigators. In future, one can envision that this intriguing property will benefit synthetic bone substitutes. These advanced CaP bioceramics with superior bone-healing properties might replace biological bone-grafting materials such as autologous or demineralized bone.

Acknowledgments The authors acknowledge the company Biomatlante for providing biphasic calcium phosphate (MBCP^{TM}).

References

1. D.F. Williams. The Williams dictionary of biomaterials. Liverpool University Press (1999)
2. F.C.M. Driessens. Monographs in oral science. Vol. 10. Basel, Karger(1982)
3. K. De Groot. Bioceramics of calcium phosphate. CRC Press Inc.; Boca Raton, Florida (1983)
4. R.Z. Legeros. Calcium phosphates in oral biology and medicine. Monographs in Oral Science. Vol. 15. Basel, Karger (1991)
5. J.C. Elliot. Structures and Chemistry of the Apatites and Other Calcium Orthophosphates. Studies in Inorganic Chemistry 18. Elsevier; Amsterdam (1994)
6. L.C. Chow, E.D. Eanes. Octacalcium phosphate. Karger, Basel (2001)
7. W.E. Brown, *Nature* **196** (1962) 1048
8. G. Daculsi, R.Z. Legeros, B. Nery, K. Lynch and B. Kerebel. *J. Biomed. Mater. Res.* **23** (1983) 883
9. G. Daculsi, R.Z. Legeros. M. Heughebaert and Barbieux I. *Calcif. Tissue Int.* **46** (1990) 20
10. G. Daculsi and N. Passuti. *Biomaterials.* **11** (1990) 86
11. G. Daculsi, N. Passuti, S. Martin, C. Deudon. R.Z. Legeros and S. Raher. *J. Biomed. Mater. Res.* **24** (1990) 379
12. N. Passuti, G. Daculsi, J.M. Rogez, S. Martin and J.V. Bainvel. *Clin. Orthop. Relat. Res.* **248** (1989) 169
13. G. Daculsi, O. Laboux, O. Malard and P. Weiss. *J. Mater. Sci., Mater. Med.* **14** (2003) 95
14. B.R. Constantz, et al. *Science* **267** (1995) 1796.
15. L. Le Guehennec, E. Goyenvalle, E. Aguado, M. Houchmand-Cuny, B. Enkel, P. Pilet, G. Daculsi and P. Layrolle. *J. Biomed. Mater. Res. Appl. Biomater.* **72B** (2005) 69
16. P. Layrolle and A. Lebugle. *Chem. Mater.* **6** (1994) 1996
17. Y. Osaka, Y. Miura, K. Takeuchi, M. Asada and K. Takahashi. *J. Mater. Sci., Mater. Med.* **2** (1991) 51
18. J.C. Heughebaert and G. Montel. *Calcif. Tissue Int.* **34** (1982) 103
19. P. Layrolle, A. Ito and T. Tateishi. *J. Am. Ceram. Soc.* **81** (1998) 1421
20. E.D. Eanes, I.H. Gillesen and A.S. Posner. *Nature* **208** (1965) 365
21. A.S. Posner and F. Betts. *Acc. Chem. Res.* **8** (1975) 273

22. G. Treboux, P. Layrolle, N. Kanzaki, K. Onuma and A. Ito. *J. Phys. Chem.* A **104** (2000) 5111
23. G. Treboux, P. Layrolle, N. Kanzaki, K. Onuma and A. Ito . *J. Am. Chem. Soc.* **122** (2000) 8323
24. N. Kanzaki, G. Treboux, K. Onuma and A. Ito. *Biomaterials* **22** (2001) 2921
25. H. Yamasaki and H. Sakai. Biomaterials. **13** (1992) 308.
26. S.H. Li, J.R. De Wijn, P. Layrolle and K. De Groot. *J. Biomed. Mater. Res.* **61** (2002) 109
27. S.H. Li, J. De Wijn, P. Layrolle and K. De Groot .*J. Am. Ceram. Soc.* **86** (2003) 65
28. U. Ripamonti. *Biomaterials* **17** (1996) 31
29. C. Klein, K. De Groot, W. Chen, Y. Li and X. Zhang. *Biomaterials* **15** (1994) 31
30. Z. Yang, H. Yuan, W. Tong, P. Zou, W. Chen and X. Zhang. *Biomaterials* **17** (1996) 2131
31. H. Yuan, Z. Yang, Y. Li, X. Zhang, J.D. De Bruijn and K. De Groot. J. Mater. Sci.: Mater. Med. **9** (1998) 723
32. H. Yuan, Z. Yang, J.D. De Bruijn, K. De Groot and X. Zhang. Biomaterials. **22** (2001) 2617
33. H. Yuan, M. Van Den Doel, S. Li, C.A. Van Blitterswijk, K. De Groot and J.D. De Bruijn. J. Mater. Sci. Mater. Med. **13** (2002) 127
34. P. Habibovic, J. Li, C.M. Van Der Valk, G. Meijer, P. Layrolle, C.A. Van Blitterswijk and K. De Groot. *Biomaterials* **26** (2005) 23.
35. D. Le Nihouannen, G. Daculsi, A. Saffarzadeh, O. Gauthier, S. Delplace, P. Pilet and P. Layrolle. *Bone* **36** (2005) 1086
36. K. De Groot. *Tissue Eng.* **4** (1998) 337
37. L. Diaz-Flores, R. Gutierrez A. Lopez-Alonso, R. Gonzalez and H. Varela. *Clin. Orthop.* **275** (1992) 280

Chapter 3
Characterization of Thin Calcium Phosphate Coating

Bas Feddes, Pío González, Julia Serra, Juan Pou, Stefano Chiussi, Joop G. C. Wolke, and Christian Jäger

Abstract For the development and improvement of thin calcium phosphate (CaP) coatings, a thorough understanding of the compositional, structural, and mechanical aspects of the coatings is required. This chapter reports on the basic principles of the techniques and how to apply them for the characterization of (thin) CaP coatings. The advantages and limitations of the techniques are described; and at least one example of how the technique can be used to investigate CaP coatings is provided. The techniques include (1) those that are photon-based: Fourier transform infrared spectroscopy, Raman spectroscopy, x-ray photoelectron spectroscopy, x-ray diffraction; (2) microscopy techniques: scanning electron microscopy and transmission electron microscopy; (3) ion beam techniques: Rutherford back-scattering spectrometry, elastic recoil detection; (4) nuclear magnetic resonance; and (5) several mechanical characterization techniques.

3.1 Introduction

A thorough understanding of the compositional, structural, and mechanical aspects of thin calcium phosphate (CaP) coatings is required if these coatings are to be developed and improved. For the thick CaP coatings, traditionally infrared spectroscopy, x-ray diffraction, electron microscopy, and mechanical testing were already commonly used for the characterization of CaP coatings. Today, these techniques are still valuable for analyzing CaP coatings, but many other techniques have also proven to be powerful in the characterization of (thin) CaP coatings.

This chapter reports on the principles of the techniques and how to apply them to analysis of (thin) CaP coatings. It describes the advantages and limitations, and it always introduces at least one example to give the reader a flavor of how the technique can be used for the investigation of CaP coatings. The

B. Feddes (✉)
Philips Research, High Tech Campus 34, 5656 AE, Eindhoven, The Netherlands
e-mail: bas.feddes@tiscali.nl

B. León, J.A. Jansen (eds.), *Thin Calcium Phosphate Coatings for Medical Implants*,
DOI 10.1007/978-0-387-77718-4_3, © Springer Science+Business Media, LLC 2009

chapter is not a complete overview of all literature available for the application of analysis techniques on CaP coatings. In all cases, however, some reference is made to standard studies that can be consulted for more detailed information. First, some photon beam-based techniques are described: infrared, Raman, and x-ray photoelectron spectroscopy and x-ray diffraction. Then, some electron beam-based techniques, mostly microscopy, are discussed, followed by the techniques that make use of ion beams as a probing method. A not common, yet powerful technique for the analysis of CaP coatings is nuclear magnetic resonance, for which an extensive description follows. The chapter finishes with a section on mechanical testing of thin CaP coatings.

3.2 Infrared Spectroscopy

Infrared (IR) spectroscopy is a fast, simple chemical analysis technique based on the interaction of IR light with matter. This technique is sensitive to the presence of chemical functional groups in a sample, thereby allowing identification of structural fragments of the molecules.

Infrared spectroscopy [1] is based on the interaction of electromagnetic radiation with molecules. Two conditions need to be met for molecules to absorb IR light and cause absorption in the IR spectrum.

1. Molecules must possess functional groups with a permanent dipole moment, resulting from electric charge asymmetry of the molecule. The alternating electric field vector of the IR light induces vibration of the bond by the transfer of energy to the molecule. The absorption of the radiation intensity at certain frequency can be observed in the IR spectrum. Molecules without a permanent dipole moment can also interact with IR radiation, as the interaction of the electric field vector makes the charge of the molecule asymmetrical, leading to temporary formation of the so-called induced dipole moment.
2. The quantum theory implies that molecules can have only specifically allowed or quantized vibrational energies. As a result, a necessary condition for IR radiation absorption to occur is that the energy of the IR light impinging on a molecule must be equal to a vibrational energy level difference.

Most molecules have functional groups that absorb radiation in the mid-IR range, which is found between 4000 and 400 cm^{-1}. It should be mentioned that for spectroscopy the wavelength of the light is usually expressed in wave numbers (cm^{-1}), defined as the reciprocal of the wavelength.

Most of the intense features found in IR spectra can be ascribed to fundamental transitions of the molecule, and the correlation between these bands and the chemical structure is the basis of IR spectroscopy being a powerful tool for chemical analysis. For the identification of unknown molecules from their IR spectra, several characteristics of the absorption bands should be carefully considered (i.e., the position, intensity, and full width at half maximum).

Infrared spectroscopy also has certain limitations. First, it is not sensitive to single atomic entities, such as monatomic ions dissolved in water, noble gases, and homonuclear diatomic molecules (N≡N or O=O), due to their symmetry. Second, in case of the analysis of complex mixtures, interpretation of the spectra is difficult or ambiguous owing to overlapping of the IR bands.

3.2.1 Application Example

Figure 3.1 shows a typical IR spectrum of carbonated hydroxyapatite (HA) coatings. In Fig. 3.1 some of the typical vibration modes are represented at the corresponding measured vibrations. The main IR absorption bands can be attributed to the following functional groups [2–5].

1. Phosphate groups (PO_4^{3-}) exhibit a sharp peak located at 1031 to 1049 cm^{-1} (asymmetrical stretching vibration, n_3) with a shoulder at 1085 cm^{-1} and a weak band at 960 cm^{-1} with a shoulder (948 cm^{-1}) corresponding to the symmetrical stretching (n_1) vibration. Two well resolved peaks attributed to the asymmetrical bending (n_4) modes emerge at around 565 and 601 cm^{-1}.

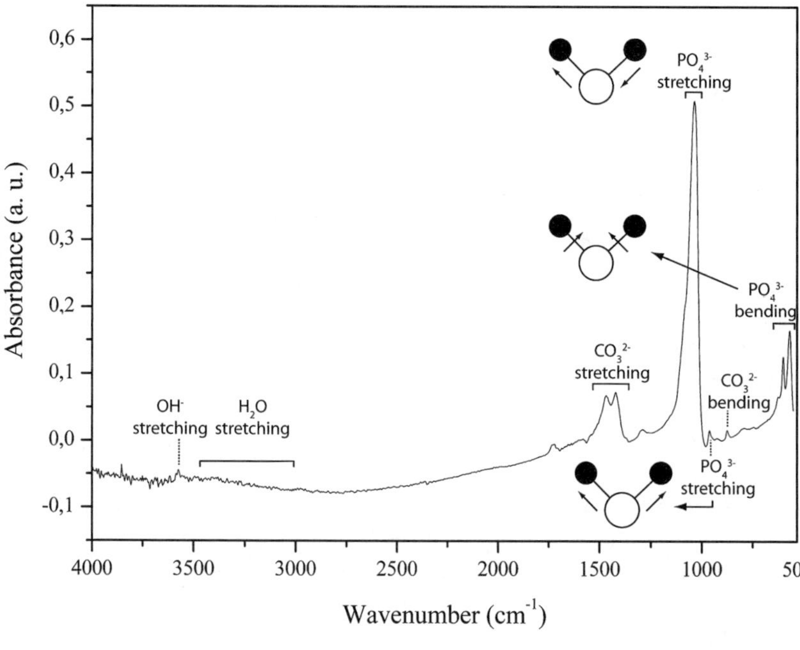

Fig. 3.1 Infrared spectrum of a carbonated hydroxyapatite (HA) coating recorded with a Fourier transform infrared (FTIR) spectrometer with a spectral resolution of 4 cm^{-1}. The film was grown by pulsed laser deposition (PLD) in H_2O vapor atmosphere with a substrate temperature of 460°C. Some of the vibration modes (symmetrical and asymmetrical stretching and asymmetrical bending) are indicated

Broadening, shifting, and lowering of the intensity of the bands are observed in films with low crystallinity grade or poor stoichiometry.

2. The main IR absorptions of carbonate groups (CO_3^{2-}) are well resolved at 1420 and 1467 cm^{-1}. These are associated with the asymmetrical stretching (n_3) modes and a weak band appearing at 875 cm^{-1} related to the asymmetrical bending (n_2) vibration. This vibration is characteristic of the substitution of CO_3^{2-} groups in the apatite lattice. The presence of nonresolved components in the range 1419 to 1513 cm^{-1} leads to broadening of the bands and shifting of the peaks.
3. The broad absorption band of adsorbed water (H_2O) can be observed in the range 3700 to 3000 cm^{-1} (water stretching vibration) and is the result of the hygroscopic character of the crystalline carbonated HA films [5]. Another peak at around 1600 cm^{-1} is attributed to water in the HA due to its hygroscopic character. These bands are absent in films grown or treated at high temperatures.
4. The hydroxyl group (OH^-) has a vibrational mode that appears at around 632 cm^{-1} as a shoulder of the main $n_4PO_4^{3-}$ band, and a stretching mode is located at 3571 cm^{-1} with a shoulder at 3550 cm^{-1}. The presence of an additional weak band at 3645 cm^{-1} is attributed to the OH^- vibration from a $Ca(OH)_2$ phase.

3.3 Raman Spectroscopy

After the invention of laser light sources during the early 1960s, Raman spectroscopy was found to be a useful tool for qualitative analysis, functional group identification, and molecular structure and conformational elucidation. A variety of fundamental and practical questions can be answered by Raman spectroscopy in a nondestructive way, namely on phases, material quality, composition, strain, effects of external perturbations (temperature, pressure, stress), and determination of thermodynamic and polarization properties.

Raman and Krishnan described the basics of Raman scattering in 1928. It was found that when a sample is irradiated by monochromatic light, some of the light scattered by molecules is wavelength-shifted relative to the incident radiation, and this frequency shift encodes information about the vibrational frequencies of the scattering molecules. The principle of the Raman effect [6–8] can be explained by a classic theory approach. When the electric field E of the exciting radiation with frequency v, $E = E_o \sin(2\pi vt)$, impinges on the molecule, an oscillating dipole moment 3–modulated with the frequency of the incident wave is induced

$$\mu = \alpha E = \alpha E_o \sin(2\pi vt)$$

where a is the polarizability of the molecule. It should be noted that the polarizability can be different for the three axis, leading to the formation of a distorted ellipsoid, which has a dimension similar to that of the molecular volume. As a result, the molecule radiates after light absorption a wave with the same frequency as the exciting light, the so-called Rayleigh radiation. If, in addition, the molecule undergoes some internal motion, such as vibration or rotation, the oscillating dipole will have superimposed on it vibrational or rotational oscillation. Then the polarizability becomes

$$\alpha = \alpha_o + \beta \sin(2\pi v_{vib} t)$$

where a_o is the polarizability in equilibrium, and b is the ratio of polarizability change with the vibration. The dipole moment is

$$\mu = \alpha E = (\alpha_o + \beta \sin(2\pi v_{vib} t) E_o \sin(2\pi v t))$$

and we find

$$\mu = \alpha_o E_o \sin(2\pi v t) + \tfrac{1}{2}\beta E_o (\cos 2\pi(v - v_{vib})t - \cos 2\pi(v + v_{vib})t)$$

where the first term corresponds to Rayleigh scattering, and the second term refers to Raman scattering, which contains some discrete number of frequencies with higher and lower values with respect to the incident radiation.

The scattered radiation analyzed by a spectrometer shows the central intense Rayleigh scattering peak and two sidebands for each vibration, shifted to higher and lower frequency values: the Raman lines. Ground-state molecules produce lines shifted to energies lower than the source, and lines at higher frequency are due to molecules in excited vibrational states. These lines, the result of the inelastic scattering of light by the sample, are called Stokes and anti-Stokes lines, respectively.

Raman vibrational spectra contain information about all aspects of the molecular structure. This information can be expressed as Raman frequencies, intensities, and depolarization factors. Complementary information can be obtained from IR spectroscopy, as Raman and IR spectra show many bands at practically the same frequency but with quite different intensities. As a general rule, a vibration is “IR active” when it modulates the dipole moment, and it is “Raman active” when the molecular polarizability is modulated. Symmetrical vibrations and bonds between identical atoms usually show strong Raman and weak IR bands. Raman spectroscopy has special advantages over IR spectroscopy when solutions in water or coatings on glass are investigated because water and glass emit only a weak Raman signal, leading to good quality spectra.

3.3.1 Application Example

The Raman spectrum of HA single crystals is dominated by a sharp peak at 960 cm^{-1}, which corresponds to the stretching mode (n_1) of phosphate groups, and three weak and broad bands around 1070 cm^{-1} (n_3, PO_4^{3-} stretching mode), 590 cm^{-1} (n_4, PO_4^{3-} bending mode), and 430 cm^{-1} (n_2, PO_4^{3-} stretching mode) [9]. These Raman emissions were also found for other CaP bulk materials and inorganic components of bone tissue but with different relative line intensities [10, 11].

Figure 3.2 shows the Stokes spectrum of an HA coating that was obtained using the near-IR (NIR) Fourier transform technique with YAG laser excitation. The dominant features in the spectrum are formed by a broad doublet at 770 and 702 cm^{-1} and smooth bands at higher frequencies (1152 and 1515–1582 cm^{-1}) [10, 11]. Because there were no corresponding bands in the anti-Stokes region, it is reasonable to assume that these bands may be produced by fluorescence emission, causing the band to emerge at 600 to 900 cm^{-1} and the corresponding overtone-like bands (1152 and 1515–1582 cm^{-1}) at higher frequency values [9]. These bands are artifacts of NIR Raman spectroscopy and should be disregarded in the normal Raman analysis. Nevertheless, useful information on the structure of multiphase CaP coatings [11–13], ranging from an amorphous CaP to a pure crystalline HA, can be obtained from careful

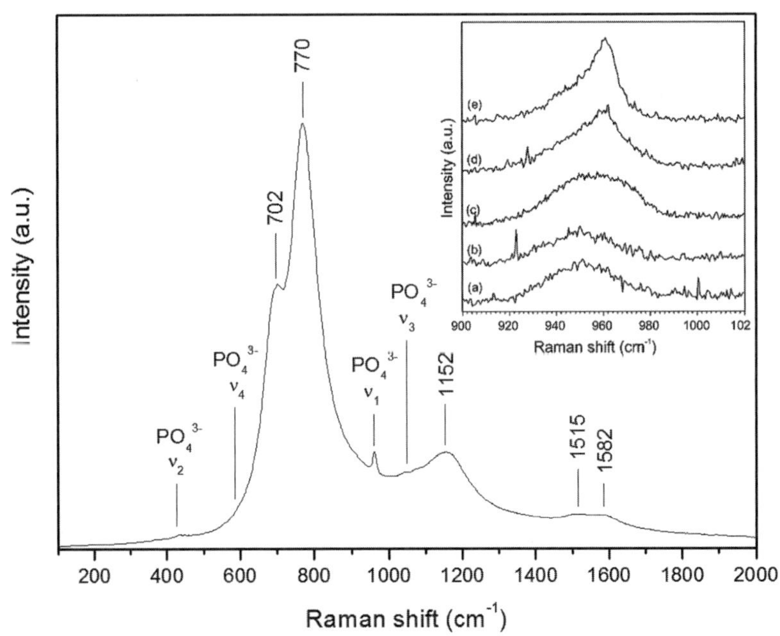

Fig. 3.2 Typical Raman spectrum of HA coating recorded with a Bruker RFS100 FT-Raman spectrometer equipped with an Nd:YAG laser (1064 nm) as an excitation source (4 cm^{-1} resolution, 512 scans, 1500 mW laser power). The HA film was grown on Ti substrate by electrophoretic deposition at room temperature. **Inset** Raman spectra of PLD coating deposited in a H_2O atmosphere at various substrate temperatures: *a*, 20°; *b*, 200°; *c*, 400°; *d*, 500°; *e*, 600°C. These spectra were recorded using the excitation wavelength of an Ar-ion laser (488 nm). From [12], with permission

analyses of the dominant Raman signal in the range between 900 and 1000 cm^{-1} (Fig. 3.2, inset).

- A sharp single line at 962 cm^{-1}, attributed to the symmetrical phosphate stretch, is characteristic of crystalline HA; the presence of a relatively small, almost indistinct shoulder toward lower wave numbers is attributable to a not well crystallized apatite structure (Fig. 3.2e).
- Additional bands at 947 and 970 cm^{-1} indicate the existence of β-TCP and α-TCP phases (Fig. 3.2c).
- A doublet at 941 and 947 cm^{-1} confirms the presence of tetracalcium phosphate (TTCP) phases in the coating.
- A broad band centered at 950 cm^{-1} is characteristic of an amorphous cap structure (Fig. 3.2a).

Although Raman spectroscopy is a powerful, nondestructive characterization procedure, the technique also has some disadvantages. The interpretation of Raman spectra of CaP coatings is a complicated task because the intensity of the Raman signals is weak compared to those of bulk materials. Additionally, precautions should be taken in the spectrum interpretation as fluorescence and resonance effects can be present. Normal Raman bands and fluorescence can be discriminated by observing the anti-Stokes and Stokes spectra [9].

3.4 X-ray Photoelectron Spectroscopy

X-ray photoelectron spectroscopy (XPS), also known as electron spectroscopy for chemical analysis (ESCA), is a powerful technique that provides qualitative and quantitative information on the type and amount of elements in the near surface region of a sample [14]. Some information on the chemical state or molecular environment can be extracted as well. The technique can be used for analyzing all elements, except hydrogen and helium, in the near surface region of 1 to 10 nm depth; and a controlled erosion by ion sputtering can be used for uncovering new "surface regions" when depth profile analysis of coatings is needed.

XPS is based on the phenomenon that atoms emit electrons when irradiated with photons of sufficient energy, also known as the photoelectric effect. Commercial XPS instruments typically use x-rays resulting from electron bombardment of Mg or Al targets, providing radiation of 1254 and 1487 eV, respectively. These x-ray photons have sufficient energy for exciting the inner core electrons of the elements near the sample surface, causing the emission of photoelectrons with a kinetic energy of

$$E_{kin} = h\nu - E_{bind} - \phi \tag{3.1}$$

where E_{kin} is the kinetic energy of the ejected photoelectron; $h\nu$ is the energy of the x-ray photon used; E_{bind} is the binding energy of the atomic orbital from which the photoelectron is originating; and φ is the spectrometer work function, the latter being the energy needed by the photoelectron to escape the sample in the direction of the detector.

3.4.1 Qualitatitive and Quantitative XPS

Because ϕ and $h\nu$ are known in a setup and the kinetic energy is measured using the XPS analyzer, E_{bind} can be calculated directly. A strongpoint of XPS is that all emitted electrons have binding energies that are specific for each element, so qualitative and quantitative determinations of the emitting elements are usually straightforward. In principle, the area under an XPS peak relates to the abundance of a species in the sample. However, the cross section for the photoelectric effect varies among the elements, and a correction factor must be applied to the measured peak to adjust the area and provide a quantitative result. This factor, also called the sensitivity factor, is usually derived from measuring thick stoichiometric reference samples. Caution should be practiced in simply copying these factors from system to system as they depend on the specific characteristics of the electron analyzer being used.

Another topic that complicates quantitative analysis to some extent but is often neglected is the varying escape depth, "attenuation length," of the electrons. Although ionization through absorption of the x-rays occurs to a depth of a few micrometers, only those electrons that are created within a few nanometers below the solid surface can potentially leave the sample to be detected. The attenuation length of electrons emitted from CaP coatings is known and depends on their kinetic energy [15], which is derived from the electron *binding* energies (Eq. 3.1) of the most significant species (Ca, P, O), in the sample. Imagine a thin film (~1–2 nm), for example, in an interface study of a CaP coating on a substrate. Most electrons that are emitted in the right direction escape the material. However, when the coating thickness is increased, the electrons with lower kinetic energies have a reduced chance of escaping. As a result, if no correction is made for varying attenuation lengths, an apparent gradient in coating composition can be measured that is not real. Also due to the same effect, a thin layer of (organic) contamination on top of the CaP coating (e.g., after cell culture experiments) influences the coating composition determination. The abundance of the species emitting electrons with low kinetic energy might be underestimated. Finally, caution should be practiced during quantification when the sample roughness has a considerable effect on the attenuation length of the electrons.

3.4.2 Chemical Shifts

The chemical environment of an atom influences the valence shell orbital, which in turn influences the binding energy of the core electrons. As a result, a shift in the kinetic energy of the photoelectrons can be measured that provides a tool for determining the chemical structure of the analyzed sample. During XPS analysis, insulating samples charge and the XPS peaks shift accordingly. A possible misinterpretation can be avoided by shifting all spectra such that a known reference material in or on top of the sample is at the expected position. Usually the position of the carbon contamination (which is virtually always present) on top of a sample is used; alternatively, one can use an additional element, such as gold, that has been deposited on the surface for this purpose. Unfortunately, there is some discrepancy in the literature regarding the reference value that should be used for the carbon reference; 284.6 eV and 285.0 eV are most widely used. In case of using binding energies found by other authors, it should be determined to which binding energies these values were measured.

3.4.3 Application Example

Figure 3.3A depicts an example of carbon C(1 s) spectra of polystyrene (PS) with and without 2 nm CaP that were measured in an interface study of CaP on

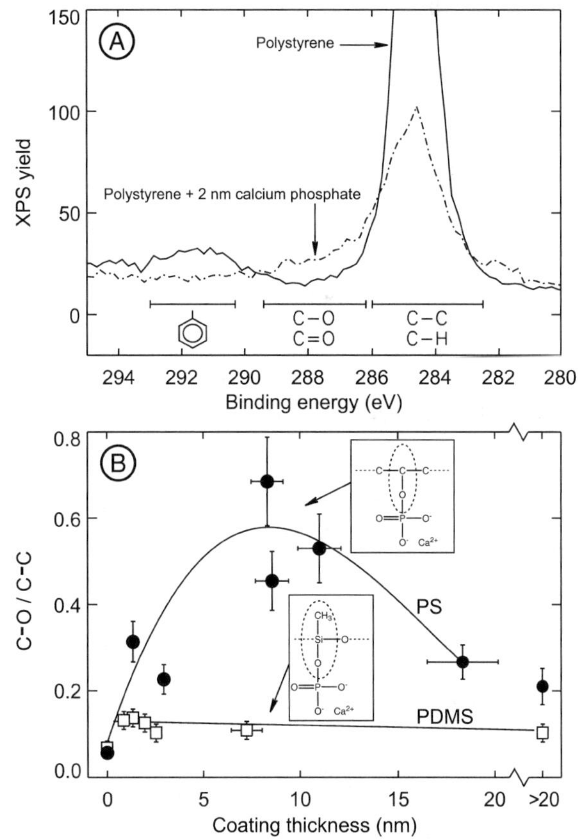

Fig. 3.3 **A** X-ray photoelectron spectroscopy (XPS) spectra of polystyrene (*PS*) with and without 2 nm of CaP (CaP). **B** C–O/C–C ratio as a function of CaP coating thickness for PS and polyydimethylsiloxane (*PDMS*). **Insets** Likely configurations of the initial bonding of CaP to PS and PDMS

polymers for better understanding coating adhesion. The CaP coatings of varying thickness were deposited by radiofrequency (RF) magnetron sputter deposition. The charging during XPS analysis was corrected for by shifting the main C–C peak to 284.6 eV.

The untreated PS shows two peaks, the main one representing the C–C/C–H bonds (further abbreviated as C–C) and a weak peak around 292 eV associated with the aromatic group of PS (not further considered here). When a 2 nm CaP coating is deposited, there is a strong decrease of the C–C peak, a result of the PS getting out of probing depth. At 288 eV, a clear side peak appears that is originated by different carbon-oxygen configurations (further abbreviated as C–O). This experiment was performed for varying CaP thickness using both PS and polydimethylsiloxane (PDMS) (silicone rubber) as substrate. The derived C–O/C–C ratios are plotted in Fig. 3.3B, revealing that for PS the C–O/C–C ratio increases with coating thickness from about zero to 0.6 for a 9 nm thick coating, decreasing again with increasing thickness. Obviously, many C–O bonds are formed during deposition of the CaP coating on PS, and the decrease of the C–O/C–C ratio is caused by the fact that the interface is getting out of probing reach. Further supported by the observation that P enrichment was found near the interface [16], these results proved that the CaP coating established a bond to the carbon chains of the PS via the phosphate groups (Fig. 3.3B, inset). Interestingly, when the same experiment is performed on PDMS, the C–O/C–C ratio remains low (Fig. 3.3B), and the relative P abundance near the interface was again found to be high [17]. This result indicates that no direct bond between the C of the PDMS and the phosphate groups is established now and that the carbon side groups of the PDMS are removed (Fig. 3.3B, inset), implying that a direct bond between Si of the PDMS and the phosphate groups has been formed. This example clearly shows how powerful XPS can be in studying thin layers of CaP (e.g., in an interface study).

3.4.4 Depth Information

The previous example suggests that XPS is suitable only for studying extremely thin layers or interfaces of CaP. This is certainly not the case. First, when the top few nanometers of a CaP coating is representative of the whole coating, XPS can of course be used to study coating composition. A rather sophisticated method to influence the probing depth during the analysis is to vary the angle between the sample surface and the analyzer in a technique called angle-resolved XPS. Of course, the analyzed region still never exceeds ~10 nm as the attenuation lengths of the electrons are limited. Deeper regions of a sample can only be analyzed using controlled erosion of the surface by ion sputtering. Which kind of ions is used for this purpose depends on the type of specimen and the desired depth profile characteristic. Soft erosion might be most suitable for determining sharp interfaces, and strong sputtering is more suitable for analyzing regions deeper in the material. However, during such a depth profile analysis, one should be aware of the risk of preferential sputtering of the weaker bonded species, as this process might lead to erroneous quantification. Moreover, the impact of the ions on the sample can charge its surface and modify the energy of the emitted photoelectrons as well as enhance the roughness of the surface. Furthermore, the measured composition of the sample can be misinterpreted owing to the "knock-on" effect (the process of the sputtering ion "knocking" an element deeper into the sample). In addition to depth profiling, the sputtering effect is widely used to gently clean the surface of a sample to remove ambient contamination prior to XPS analysis.

3.5 Auger Electron Spectroscopy

In addition to the photoelectrons induced by x-rays, Auger electrons are emitted when electrons with lower binding energies drop into the core vacancy level produced by the photoelectron emission; the Auger electrons release energy, causing ejection of the outer electrons. This process can also be induced by using electrons as the primary beam in a process called Auger electron spectroscopy (AES). However, as the exposure of an electrically insulating coating to the beam of electrons causes severe charging, AES is usually not applied in studies on CaP coatings, except in cases where a conducting substrate is analyzed prior to CaP coating deposition [18, 19].

3.6 X-ray Diffraction

X-ray diffraction refers to a nondestructive analytical technique that uses the diffracted intensity of a monochromatic x-ray beam as a function of the incident and exit angle. Information can be derived about the crystallographic structure, chemical composition, and physical properties of materials and thin films. In addition, it can be used to calculate precise lattice parameters, crystallite size, preferred orientation, and lattice stress.

When monochromatic x-rays impinge on a sample, the x-rays are scattered ("diffracted") by atoms in the material. If the atoms in the material are arranged in a crystalline structure, this scattering results in maxima and minima in the diffracted intensity distribution. The signal maxima follow Bragg's law

$$n\lambda = 2d\sin\theta$$

in which n is an integer, λ is the x-ray wavelength, d is the distance between crystal lattice planes, and θ is the diffraction angle. Thus, for each lattice spacing d, Bragg's law predicts a maximum at a characteristic diffraction angle θ. When the intensity of the detected x-rays is plotted as a function of the angle θ, an XRD pattern is obtained that is characteristic for the sample material [20].

The conventional Bragg-Brentano (also called θ–2θ) XRD geometry is not useful for the study of thin, graded composition and multilayered thin films because of poor sensitivity and the presence of interfering effects from the substrate. To increase performance, a slight change has to be made to the geometry by choosing a fixed low angle of incidence of the x-rays (for θ, typically 0.5°–3.0°). With such geometry the x-rays pass through a slit system and fall on the sample at a grazing angle while the detector scans the XRD pattern. Because the grazing-incidence angle is fixed, the sample is analyzed by moving the detector only; and, unlike Bragg-Brentano geometry, a focusing circle is not maintained. Thin-film XRD is a nonfocusing geometric arrangement that makes use of parallel, rather than divergent, x-rays diffracted from suitably oriented crystallographic planes. An attachment placed between the diffracting planes and detector slit absorbs converging and diverging diffracted X-rays and allows only parallel x-rays to pass. The advantage of this thin film configuration is the strong reduction of the penetration depth to as little as a few micrometers, by which it becomes possible to investigate thin films (polycrystalline, monocrystalline, textured, and epitaxially grown thin films) without caring about the presence of the substrate.

3.6.1 Application Example

In the case of CaP coatings, phase recognition can usually be performed quite easily. The absence of crystalline peaks usually indicates an amorphous coating. As an example for the application of XRD, three samples prepared by RF magnetron sputter deposition are compared. Ti-6Al-4 V was used for the substrate. The target in the RF magnetron sputter deposition system consisted of a thick plasma-sprayed HA layer on top of a copper disk. The substrates were coated while fixed on a substrate holder. The substrates were either positioned statically above the HA sputter target or rotated, thereby moving over the target part of the time. The following samples were prepared.

- Stationary sputtered coating with a thickness of 3.5 to 4.0 μm
- Rotated sputtered coating with a thickness of 3.5 to 4.0 μm
- Rotated sputtered coating with a thickness of 3.5 to 4.0 μm and heat-treated for 1 hour at 650°C

The crystal structure and the residual stress of each film was determined by thin-film XRD using a Philips diffractometer utilizing CuKα radiation (Fig. 3.4). The XRD pattern of a stationary deposited sputter coating showed a crystalline apatite structure with a preferred (002) crystallographic orientation. The apatite (002), (102), (112), and (202) reflections are at angles of 25.9°, 28.1°, 32.4°, and 34.0°, respectively. A coating deposited with a rotating substrate holder showed an amorphous structure without sharp reflection lines. The broad peak around

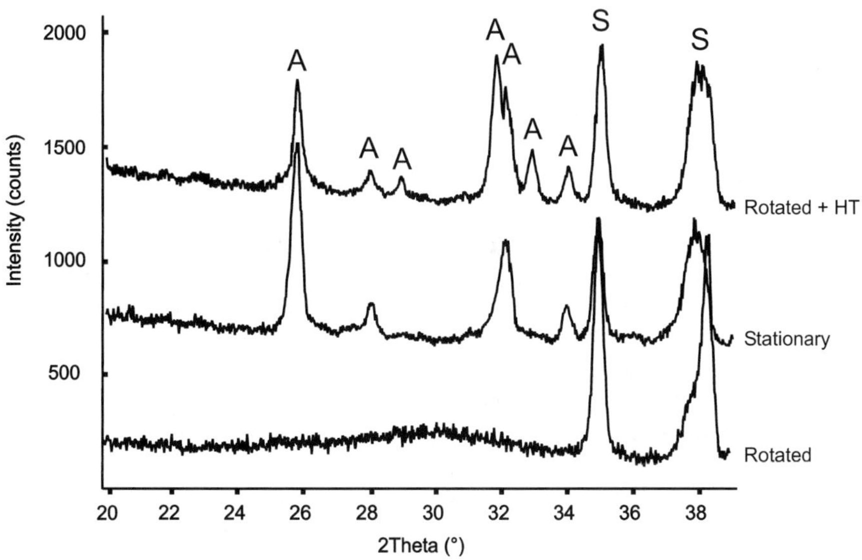

Fig. 3.4 X-ray diffraction (XRD) patterns of sputtered CaP coatings. *A*, positions of apatite reflections; *S*, reflections due to the substrates

30° degrees is indicative for an amorphous CaP coating. A heat treatment for 1 hour at 650°C changed the amorphous structure into a more randomly oriented apatite structure, comparable to the standard XRD pattern of HA powder (JCPDS #9-0432) [21, 22].

Interestingly, the residual stress state in a film can also be determined by XRD by measuring the *d* spacing of a given reflection along several directions in the sample [23]. If the unstressed lattice spacing d_c is known, the measured lattice spacing can be used to calculate the strain components ε of the film, and the stress σ can be calculated. For this calculation, Young's modulus E and the Poisson ratio v must be known. This way of determining the stress was also used for the CaP coatings of Fig. 3.4. An internal standard of silicon powder was dispersed on the sputtered films to correct the observed diffraction angles for errors caused by small sample displacement. It was found that the coating conditions (rotary or stationary substrate holder) influenced the residual stress in the coating. Stationary sputtered coatings had a crystalline structure directly, but the deposited coating showed the presence of compressive stresses. In contrast, the heat treatment of the amorphous coating resulted in a crystalline coating that was free of stress. Obviously, choosing the right deposition conditions can optimize the residual stress in the coating.

XRD is a powerful tool for the characterization of CaP coatings. In addition to phase recognition, it can be used to estimate the stress in the coating. By choosing a suitable geometry, XRD analysis can even be performed on coatings less than 0.1 μm.

3.7 Electron Microscopy Techniques

Accelerated electrons can be used as "ionizing radiation," which is the general term given to radiation capable of removing electrons from the attractive field of the nucleus. The main advantage of this type of ionizing radiation is that it produces a wide range of secondary signals from the specimen [24], as summarized in Fig. 3.5.

The electrons in the beam can be elastically or inelastically scattered by the atoms of the sample. The *elastic scattering* is defined as a process that does not significantly change the electron energy but appreciably changes the direction of the electron passing the specimen. This frequent effect is important in electron microscopy because it provides a sufficient amount of deflected electrons for producing diffraction patters on the basis of Bragg's law. *Inelastic scattering*, in contrast, refers to any process that causes the incident electron to lose a detectable amount of energy. There are many processes that could cause such an energy loss of the electron. The inelastic scattering processes involve transfer of the impinging electron energy to the electrons or atoms of the specimen and are eventually responsible for trapping an electron in a solid. In general, almost all of the kinetic energy of the incident electron heats the specimen, and a small part of the energy may escape as x-rays or secondary electrons, which are both extremely useful for chemical analysis and imaging of the specimen, as described below.

When the electron beam penetrates a specimen, some of the electrons interact with the nuclei of the atoms. The negatively charged electrons are attracted to the positive nuclei; some of them, instead of being captured by the "gravitational pull" of the nuclei, circle them and are back-scattered without slowing down. Because all the elements have different-sized nuclei, the number of these back-scattered electrons (BSEs) changes with the atomic number; and as a consequence an image with compositional information can be obtained.

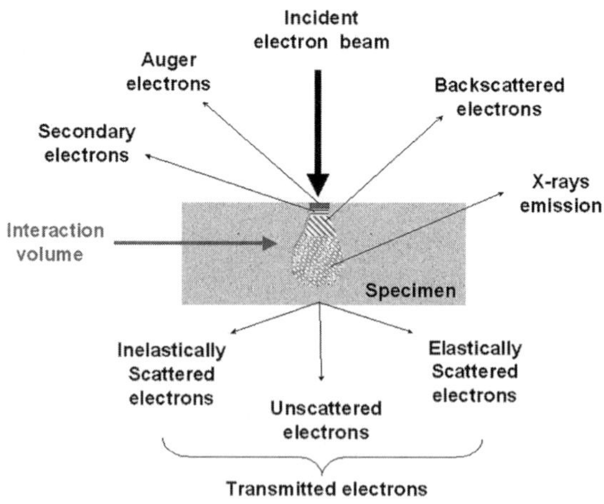

Fig. 3.5 Various signals generated when an electron beam interacts with a specimen

On the other hand, the incident electrons can also interact with the electrons of the specimen. As a result of this interaction, some electrons are expelled and exit the sample surface. The production of such *secondary electrons* with only low kinetic energy is strongly related to topography because only those that are close to the surface can exit the sample and thus be detected.

If the impinging electrons knock a core electron from its position, the electron from an outer shell filling this vacancy releases energy to relax. This release of energy can cause the emission of high energy radiation in the x-ray range or be transferred to another electron, which is then ejected from the atom, the so-called Auger electron. The energy of these x-rays especially, characteristic of the particular atomic species, is often used in SEM to identify the material and establish x-ray microanalysis. Filling outer shell vacancies, on the other hand, causes emission of photons in the visible range, an effect known as *cathodoluminescence*, which is often used to determine band structures of nonmetallic specimens.

The main concept used to define the quality of a microscope is the resolution. In the broadest sense, the resolution is simply defined in terms of its ability to discriminate between two discrete objects. The ultimate resolution of the electron microscope is always given by an expression of the form

$$d = AC_s^{1/4}\lambda^{3/4}$$

in which A is a constant, C_s is the spherical aberration, and λ is the wavelength.

3.7.1 Scanning Electron Microscopy

The development of the scanning electron microscopy (SEM) during the early 1950s opened new research areas in the medical and physical sciences because it allowed imaging of a great variety of specimens. With SEM, an incident electron beam produced by an electron gun, accelerated by high voltage, and focused on the specimen surface by a series of electromagnetic lenses scans the surface of the specimen by means of a series of deflection coils and synchronized with a cathode-ray tube (CRT). The signals produced as a result of the beam interaction with the specimen surface are collected by an appropriate detector, amplified, and displayed on the CRT.

The classic SEM [24, 25] is based on two signals: secondary electrons (SEs) and back-scattered electrons (BSEs). The SEs allow high resolution imaging of the surface morphology because the orientation of the surface features influences the number of electrons reaching the detector, thus causing variations in image contrast that represent the sample surface topography. The BSEs provide images of elemental composition variation as well as surface topography. Because high-energy BSE can escape from much deeper regions than secondary electrons, surface topography is not as accurately resolved as through SE.

The great advantage of BSE imaging is that the efficiency of BSE production is proportional to the mean atomic number of the sample materials, which results in image contrast as a function of composition. Thus, elements with a high atomic number appear brighter than elements with a low atomic number.

The bombardment of the surface with accelerated electrons generates not only the above-mentioned beneficial effects that are used for specimen characterization but also considerably increased negative charge on the surface. If no measures are taken, this charge buildup becomes rapidly strong enough to reject the incoming primary electrons and deviate them, causing a distorted image. In the case of isolating samples such as ceramics (including CaP), polymers, and biological materials, the specimens are therefore usually coated with a thin (~10 nm) conducting layer of carbon or gold for minimizing charging effects.

Moreover, when performing conventional SEM, any interactions of the electrons before reaching the specimen surface must be avoided. This implies that the electron beam as well as the specimen must be under high vacuum conditions and that, particularly in the case of biological specimens, water, solvents, or other materials that could vaporize in the vacuum must be previously removed. Nowadays, a specially designed SEM called environmental SEM (ESEM) is available that can be used to view even wet samples, allowing examination of specimens surrounded by a gaseous environment. This new technology exploits the collisions between BSEs or SEs and the gas molecules for producing more electrons and ionizing the gas molecules. This increase in the number of electrons effectively amplifies the original electron signal. The generated positive gas ions are attracted to the negatively biased specimen neutralizing the charging effects.

In the literature, several authors have studied the influence of the deposition and postdeposition parameters regarding the morphology and structure of biocompatible CaP coatings produced by various techniques [26–35]. SEM analysis was the main tool to study the behavior of the coatings during *in vitro* tests, for example to follow the dissolution process in simulated physiological solutions, cellular adhesion and proliferation, and biomimetic processes [31, 36–41].

Figure 3.6 shows a typical SEM image of a homogeneous CaP coating, including a cross section of the columnar structure of the coating produced by

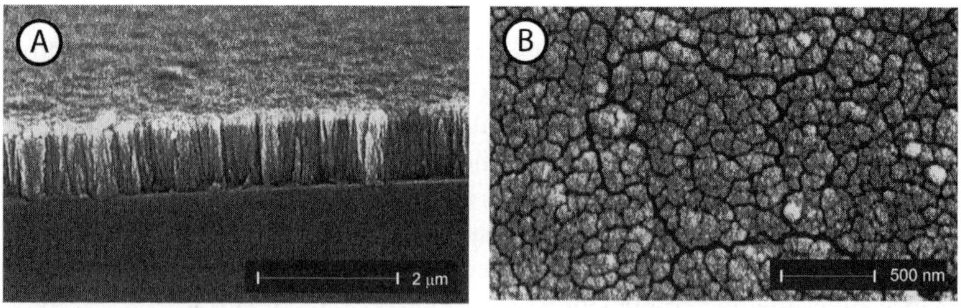

Fig. 3.6 Typical scanning electron micrograph of the CaP coatings grown by PLD. **A** Cross section. **B** Surface morphology

laser ablation, and high magnification view of the surface morphology revealing the fine structure of the material.

3.7.2 *Energy Dispersive X-ray Spectroscopy*

When a high energy electron penetrates a solid, most of its energy is initially lost through ionization of the atoms in the specimen resulting in the ejection of electrons from their energy levels, as explained in the introductory part of this chapter. To stabilize the atom, electrons from higher energetic levels fall immediately into the vacancies, releasing their excess energy by emitting x-ray photons, having energies corresponding to the difference between the two specific shell energies.

With x-ray microanalysis [42], these photons are detected and analyzed, either by energy dispersion—energy dispersive x-ray spectroscopy/energy dispersive x-ray spectroscopy/energy dispersive x-ray analysis (EDS/EDX/EDAX)—or wavelength dispersion (WDS), providing a rapid qualitative method for determining the elements in the imaged region. Depending on the required information, the complexity of such measurements can be quite different. The simplest analysis is the study of the relative distribution of elements across a specimen surface without regard to absolute concentrations. In the case of a thick specimen the concentrations can be derived easily, but for thin specimens the thickness, substrate type, penetration depth of the electron beam, and escape depth of the generated x-rays must be taken into account. If absolute concentrations are required for providing at least semiquantitative analysis, standards have to be used (i.e., samples with known concentrations of an element) for comparing them with the obtained results using a procedure known as ZAF (atomic number absorption fluorescence) analysis [24].

3.7.3 *Transmission Electron Microscopy*

The main principles of transmission electron microscopy (TEM) [43] are based on diffraction of the accelerated electron beam with the atomic potential. The resulting diffracted electron beams can form diffraction spots but can also be recombined to form an image of the specimen. The use of electromagnetic lenses allows diffracted electrons to be focused into a regular arrangement of diffraction spots that are projected and recorded as the electron diffraction pattern. The space where the diffraction pattern is formed is called *reciprocal space*, and the space at the image plane or at a specimen is called *real space*. The transformation from the real space to the reciprocal space is mathematically given by the Fourier transform. The great advantage of TEM is its ability to observe, by adjusting the electromagnetic lenses, both electron microscope images (information in real space) and diffraction patterns (information in reciprocal space) for the same region. As a result of numerous advances in optics and microscope design, modern TEM microscopes are capable of a resolution of < 0.1 nm, which allows imaging of individual atoms.

By inserting a selected area aperture and using parallel incident beam illumination, one can easily obtain a diffraction pattern from a specific area as small as 100 nm in diameter. Moreover, the recently developed micro-diffraction method, where incident electrons are converged on a specimen, can be used to obtain diffraction patterns from an even smaller area of only a few nanometers in diameter. Because such selected area diffraction patterns can be recorded from almost every grain in a polycrystalline material, reciprocal lattices and mutual crystal orientation relations can be easily determined. Thus, single crystal structural information can be obtained for many materials with single crystals of sizes that are not suitable for x-ray or neutron diffraction. Such materials include metastable or unstable phases, products of low temperature phase transitions, fine precipitates, and nanosized particles, among others.

To acquire an electron microscope image, the electron diffraction pattern must first be obtained. By passing the transmitted beam or one of the diffracted beams through a small objective aperture (positioned in the back focal plane) and changing lenses to the imaging mode, an image with enhanced contrast can be produced. If only the transmitted beam is used, the observation mode is called the *brightfield* method; and if one single diffracted beam is selected, it is called *darkfield* method. If more than two diffracted beams are selected on the back focal plane using a large objective aperture, an observation mode called high resolution TEM (HRTEM) is obtained. The image resulting from a multiple beam interference is called the *phase contrast* image. For a thin specimen and under aberration-compensating conditions of a microscope, the phase contrast corresponds closely to the projected potential of a structure.

The crystallinity of a CaP coating determines the dissolution rate of the coating in "*in vivo*" conditions. Therefore, TEM has been used by various groups to study the crystalline structure of the coatings and, combined with other techniques such as x-ray diffraction (XRD), to distinguish octacalcium phosphate (OCP) from HA and other CaPs [34, 44]. TEM analysis has also been used to study the intermediate layers at the interface between the coating and substrate. A graded nanograin microstructure can be obtained at this interface by controlling the experimental parameters of the deposition process. Figure 3.7 is a TEM image of a CaP coating. It consists of a functionally graded HA (FGHA) coating processed on silicon substrates using ion beam-assisted deposition [45].

The main drawback of TEM is that the preparation of the specimens is time-consuming. Moreover, although the specimen should obviously be thin, the method depends on the sample type and information that is sought [43]. The general thinning protocol for preparation from "bulk" material involves the following stages.

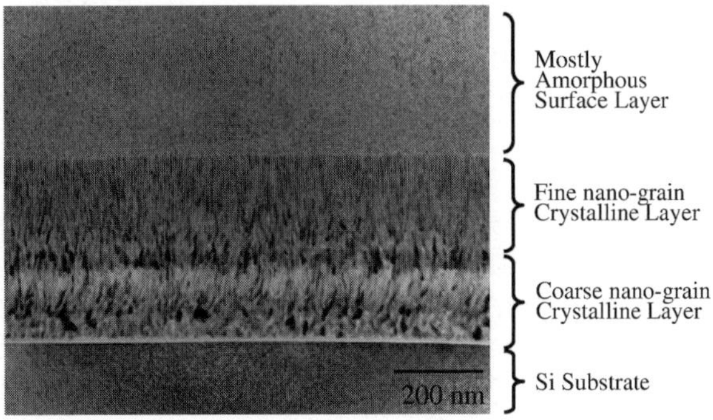

Fig. 3.7 Cross-sectional transmission electron microscopy image of FGHA coating processed on silicon substrates using ion beam assisted deposition. From [45], with permission

1. Create a thin slice, 100 to 200 μm thick, of the bulk sample.
2. Cut a 3 mm disk from the slice.
3. Pre-thin the central region of the disk to a few micrometers (generally this stage is referred to as "dimpling"). The aim of this process is to thin the center of the disk while minimizing damage to the sample surface.
4. Perform final thinning of the disk. Two techniques are generally used for this last stage: electro-polishing/chemical polishing and ion/atom milling.

Engqvist et al. [46] described the combined use of focused ion beam (FIB) microscopy and high resolution electron microscopy for the first successful preparation and analysis of an intact metal–bone interface.

3.8 Ion Beam Techniques

Ion beam analysis (IBA) techniques can be used to obtain concentration depth profiles of the elements in a material. Samples are brought into a vacuum setup, and a beam of primary mono-energetic ions from an MV accelerator impinges on the material. Depth profiles can be derived from the back-scattered ions or the atoms that are knocked out of the sample. IBA techniques are suitable for the investigation of thin CaP coatings, as the techniques are quantitative and sensitive up to ~1 μm depth.

3.8.1 Rutherford Back-Scattering Spectrometry

The most common form of IBA is Rutherford back-scattering spectrometry (RBS) in which the material under investigation is exposed to a beam of ions, typically 1 to 3 MeV He^+, and the energy of the back-scattered He ions are measured by a solid-state silicon-based detector. The primary ions are scattered upon collision with the atoms in the material. Most of the back-scattered ions collide only once with a target atom. The energy fraction with which the primary ions return after such a single collision, kinematic factor K, is given by:

$$K = \frac{E_1}{E_0} = \left(\frac{\sqrt{M_2^2 - M_1^2 \sin^2\theta} + M_1 \cos\theta}{M_1 + M_2} \right)^2 \qquad (3.2)$$

In this equation, E_0 is the energy of the incoming ion, E_1 is the energy of the back-scattered ion after collision, M_1 is the mass of the incoming particle, M_2 is the mass of the target atom, and θ is the back-scattering angle relative to the ongoing beam (Fig. 3.8, inset).

An RBS spectrum is obtained when the yield, the number of ions, within a certain energy interval is plotted. An example of an RBS spectrum of a thin CaP coating on polystyrene (PS) is given in Fig. 3.8. From Eq. 3.2 it can be seen that the energy of the back-scattered He ion increases with the mass of the target atom. Thus, the mass differences of Ca, P, and O result in three clearly distinguishable peaks, which can be observed in Fig. 3.8. The carbon in the PS substrate, being lighter than oxygen, appears well below the oxygen signal from the CaP coating; and hydrogen does not appear in the spectrum, as the helium cannot back-scatter from an element equal or lower in mass.

In RBS, quantification is easy and accurate. The yield of ions scattered from an element x of a thin film (Y_x, the area under the peak) is given by

$$Y_x = \frac{Q\Omega\sigma_x N_x}{\sin\alpha} \qquad (3.3)$$

in which Q is the number of incoming ions, Ω is the solid angle of the detector, N_x is the coverage of the element (number of atoms per unit area), σ_x is the cross section for the scattering event, and the angle α is defined in Fig. 3.8. The full

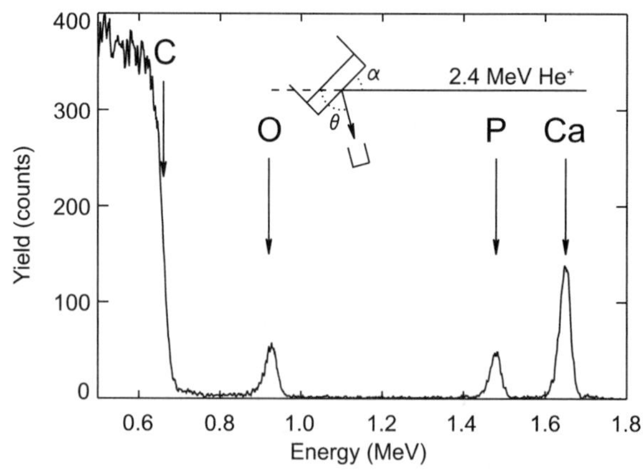

Fig. 3.8 Rutherford back-scattering spectrometry (RBS) spectrum of a thin CaP coating on PS. **Inset** Configuration used for the measurement

equation for the scattering cross section can be found elsewhere [47]. An important property of this equation is that for constant scattering geometry, σ_x is proportional to the square of the Z number of the target atom (Z_x). Because Q, Ω, and α are all constant within one measurement, the ratio of two elements (x and y) in the coating can be found using:

$$\frac{N_x}{N_y} = \frac{Y_x}{Y_y}\frac{\sigma_y}{\sigma_x} \tag{3.4}$$

This equation is also valid for thick films of constant composition. If all components of the coating are separately visible in the RBS spectrum, the total coating *composition* can accurately be found. The coating *coverage* can be found by either comparing the measured yields to that of a known reference sample or by comparing the measured yield to the height of the signal from the known substrate material. A convenient way to deduce coating coverage and composition is to simulate the RBS spectrum using software such as RUMP [48] or NDF [49]. It is important to realize that with RBS the coating coverage (the number of atoms per unit area) is determined, not the coating thickness. However, when the density of the deposited coating is known, coverage can easily be transformed into coating thickness.

An MeV ion traverses a material in an almost straight line, ionizing neighboring target atoms. Chances of a head-on collision are extremely small as a material mostly consists of empty space, MeV ions can penetrate it up to several microns before being completely stopped. This does not imply that ions can travel through material without any loss of energy. Interactions with electrons and weak interactions with nuclei cause deceleration of the ions in a process called *electronic* and *nuclear stopping*. In Fig. 3.8, He scattered from the carbon of the polymer near the interface with the CaP coating leaves with the energy given by Eq. 3.2, but with deeper penetration of the PS substrate some energy is lost. Ions that back-scatter from deeper inside the material return with lower energy and as a result end up at lower energies in the RBS spectrum. Although this effect might seem to complicate the analysis, it bears important information that can be used to deduce depth profiles of the various elements in the coating and/or substrate. As useful empirical relations exist that predict stopping in materials of any composition, it is possible, using the previously mentioned software packages, to derive depth profiles from the measured RBS spectra. Some ambiguity cannot always be avoided. However, using prior knowledge of the sample (e.g., the materials that are present) or other approaches (e.g., taking spectra at different angles α or θ), the actual concentration depth profiles can be reconstructed.

Figure 3.9 gives an application of RBS in a study of the behavior of CaP coatings in simulated body fluid (SBF) [50]. The virgin CaP coatings were deposited on silicon substrates. The Ca/P ratios were varied between 0.6 and 4.7 by varying the deposition parameters. This variation is clearly visible from the Ca and P peak areas in the "virgin" spectra in Fig. 3.9. The

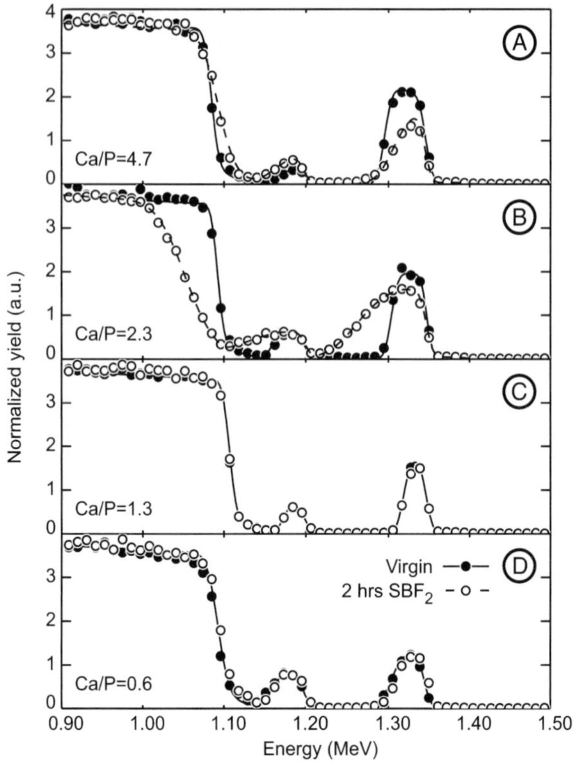

Fig. 3.9 RBS spectra of CaP coatings on a silicon substrate before and after immersion in simulated body fluid (*SBF*). The varying Ca/P ratios of the virgin coatings show different reactivity upon SBF immersion. From [50], with permission

samples were annealed to induce crystallization and subsequently immersed in SBF (twice the Ca and PO_4 concentrations) for 2 hours to study the effect of coating composition on nucleation behavior. The coatings with Ca/P ratios 0.6 and 1.3 remained inert. After 2 hours there were no signs of coating growth or dissolution as the RBS spectra remained equal. On the coating with a Ca/P ratio of 2.3, nucleation of a CaP precipitate clearly occurred and the average Ca/P ratio of the coating and precipitate decreased. The slopes of the Ca and P peaks were not as steep anymore, indicating considerable roughness in the coating. The CaP coating with a Ca/P ratio of 4.7 behaved quite differently. Upon immersion in SBF the coating partially dissolved, preferably the Ca, leading to a lower Ca/P ratio after immersion.

This example shows several of the attractive features of RBS: Spectra are relatively easy to interpret; ratios of elements can be often estimated directly from the raw spectra; and the availability of spectrum simulation software allows absolute quantification of the coating composition and coverage for complicated spectra. As mentioned, the analysis can be further refined by taking several spectra of the same specimen under different angles α or θ (Fig. 3.8, inset). By varying α, the effective travel distance through the coating is influenced, allowing the choice of a greater probing depth or better resolution in the near-surface region of the coating. It was shown that some information on sample roughness could be extracted from the spectra. The drawback of a rough sample, however, is that it usually complicates accurate analysis of RBS spectra considerably.

In RBS measurements, He^+ ions are used that are typically accelerated to energies of 1 to 3 MeV. The probing depth of the analysis can be influenced by varying the energy of the ions. Scientists have some good reasons to use this quite limited energy range for standard RBS measurements. As stated before, the scattering cross section is proportional to the Z numbers of the target atoms. However, deviations from this ideal behavior become apparent when higher energies are used because of nuclear interactions that occur resulting from the closer ion–target nucleus approach. Deviations in scattering cross sections can easily reach an order of magnitude or more, making quantification—one of the strong points of RBS—less straightforward. On the other hand, the strongly increased cross section can also be used to its advantage to increase sensitivity for specific elements (e.g., oxygen in CaP) [51]. Care has to be taken with low ($<$ 1 MeV) energy levels because the primary ions do not fully penetrate the electron clouds of the target atoms at these levels. The partial shielding of the nuclear charge by the electrons causes deviations from ideal cross section behavior, again complicating analysis. He^+ ions are, by far, the most often used as the primary beam. Hydrogen beams can be attractive in some cases for their greater probing depth potential. Ions heavier than He can also be used. They provide better mass separation in the analysis but are nevertheless not often used, especially because many accelerators are not able to produce such beams.

3.8.2 Elastic Recoil Detection

During the high-energy collision between the primary ion and the target atom, not only the back-scattered ions but also some of the target atoms, the *recoils*, are ejected from the target and can be used for analysis. The ratio of the energy of the incoming ion transferred to the recoil is given by

$$\frac{E_2}{E_0} = \frac{4M_1M_2}{(M_1+M_2)^2}\cos^2\phi \tag{3.5}$$

The angle ϕ is the angle under which the recoil is scattered relative to the original direction of the incoming primary ion. If the energy of the recoils is detected instead of the primary ions, the technique is called elastic recoil detection (ERD), also known as elastic recoil detection analysis (ERDA) or forward recoil spectrometry (FRS).

In its simplest form, also possible with a He beam, ERD is used only for determining the hydrogen depth profile of a sample, something that is not possible using RBS because a back-scattering event is possible only when the primary ion is lighter than the target atom. To be able to determine the hydrogen depth profile, the energy of the hydrogen recoils of the sample have to be measured. The sample is placed at a grazing angle, and the detector is placed in a forward direction. To avoid the scattered primary (helium) ions from entering the detector, a foil, often made of Mylar, is placed between the sensor and the detector. The small hydrogen ions penetrate all the way through the foil, whereas the heavier particles (He or heavier recoils) are brought to a full stop. The hydrogen depth profile can be calculated from the hydrogen energy spectrum, as was also shown for CaPs [52, 53].

Elastic recoil detection can also be performed in a more advanced way by mass separation of the recoils using a transmission and a stop detector. Obviously, this is not possible in the case of RBS because all back-scattered atoms have the same mass (e.g., He), whereas the recoils in ERD have a different stopping power because of their different masses. Figure 3.10 shows a two-dimensional ERD spectrum of a CaP coating on a silicon substrate [54]. A gas detector was used that has two plates (Fig. 3.10, inset). All recoils pass the first detector part, losing some of their energy, proportional to the recoil mass. This effectively allows mass separation of the recoils. The remaining energy of the recoils is detected in the second part of the detector. The separation on the mass allows background-free detection and therefore a background-free depth profile of some of the mass up to a certain depth. C, N, O, and F can all be detected without background in the spectrum of Fig. 3.10. This technique was used, for example, to determine accurately and background-free the oxygen content of CaP coatings before and after incubation in a cell culture [55].

In Fig. 3.10 the heavier masses (Ca, P, Si) are not well separated. This situation can sometimes be improved to a certain extent by choosing a different gas pressure in the detector and a different primary ion and ion energy. However, RBS is usually a more suitable technique for heavier masses. RBS and ERD are

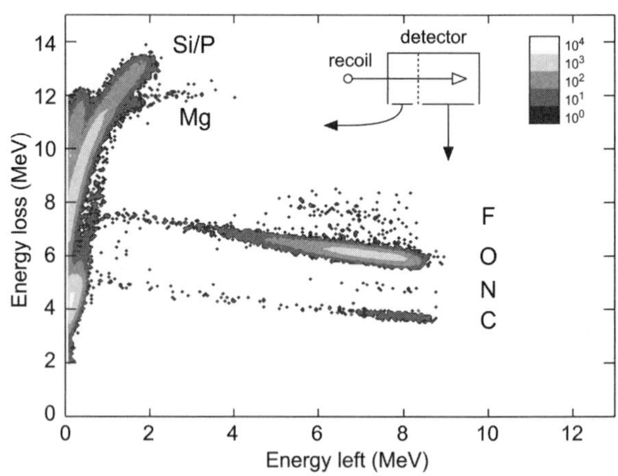

Fig. 3.10 Two-dimensional elastic recoil detection (ERD) spectrum of a CaP coating on a silicon substrate. **Inset** Energy loss in the first part of the detector (vertical axis); the horizontal axis shows the remaining energy that is lost in the second part of the detector. The elements with lower masses (*C*, *N*, *O*, *F*) can be detected background-free. From [54], with permission of the author

therefore two complementary techniques. RBS is most useful for analyzing the heavier target atoms in a matrix (Ca and P in CaP coatings), and ERD is powerful in determining the depth profiles of lighter elements (e.g., H, C, N, O, F).

3.8.3 Low Energy Ion Scattering

Low energy ion scattering (LEIS) is capable of analyzing the outermost layer of a material. Primary ions, of which the typical energy is in the kiloelectron volt (keV) range, are immediately neutralized upon entering the sample. As only the ions are detected in LEIS, effectively only the outermost layer is probed. Obviously, this technique is extremely sensitive to surface contamination, which can be gently removed from a sample by sputter cleaning. The technique is not yet common in the analysis of CaP coatings but has shown its usefulness in an absorption study on the outermost layer of a CaP coating [56].

3.8.4 Proton-Induced X-ray Emission

Exposing a sample to a megaelectron volt (MeV) proton beam causes inner shell ionizations of atoms in the sample. When the outer shell electrons fill the vacancies, the excess of energy is emitted as an x-ray photon. A detector measures the x-ray energies that are highly specific for the emitting element. Compared to EDS, proton-induced x-ray emission (PIXE) offers a better signal/noise ratio, allowing good sensitivity to trace elements, sometimes reaching the parts per million level. However, PIXE can also be used to determine the composition of thicker CaP coatings [51, 52, 57], although no depth information is obtained by this technique. PIXE can also be performed using micro beams of proton, allowing lateral mapping of trace element distributions.

3.8.5 Secondary Ion Mass Spectrometry

Secondary ion mass spectrometry (SIMS) is a technique in which a surface is bombarded by 5 to 25 keV primary ions. The masses of positive and negative ionized species (both ions and charged clusters) that are sputtered from the surface are measured. From these measurements, information on clusters can be revealed on atomic arrangements. The technique is also suitable for detecting low concentrations of species in CaPs. When a small number of bombarding ions is used ($< 10^{13}$ atoms/cm^2 per measurement), the measured surface is almost undamaged. This region is called the "static" regime. Static SIMS was used, for example, to discriminate between different CaP phases [58, 59] by detecting the ratio of PO_2^- and PO_3^- clusters.

SIMS is extremely surface sensitive. However, when information from deeper layers is required, SIMS can also be performed in combination with sputter depth profiling, similar as for AES and XPS, in a technique called "dynamic SIMS."

3.9 Nuclear Magnetic Resonance

Structural elucidation of thin CaP layers (< 10 μm thick) on a molecular level are difficult for a number of reasons: (1) the coating deposition processes undergo highly nonequilibrium conditions; (2) other cations or anions may be inserted into the structure deliberately (specific ion exchange for designed properties such as dissolution rates); and (3) their high surface/volume ratio. In all three cases, disordered chemical structures may form in the coatings. The first reason can be easily understood: If the system is not given sufficient time to relax (i.e., to crystallize) during the growth process (e.g., lower target temperature, thermal conduction properties, deposition time), amorphous network regions will be present in addition to crystalline parts. Similarly, different ionic radii of substituted ions will lead to internal stress as well as modified chemical compositions and even changed electric charges. Finally, if the coatings become increasingly thinner, the relative surface layer "volume"—in which stress, strain, and disorder of the structure occurs—may become comparable in size to the crystalline bulk part. This is particularly important for nano-scale coatings and crystals and is considered in the section on solid-state nuclear magnetic resonance (NMR).

This section focuses on NMR and its use for characterizing CaP coatings. Two aims are pursued here: The first section is a brief overview on NMR, focusing on practical aspects. The second part is a short review of NMR studies of (1) crystalline calcium (ortho- and hydrogen) phosphates; (2) CaP coatings; and (3) nanocrystalline HA and the mineral phase in bone.

As thin coatings are meant to provide conduction of bone formation, one is faced with the challenge of studying not only the "bulk structure" of the coatings but, more importantly, their surface regions and structures and the chemical interactions with molecules as the final target.

3.9.1 Relevant NMR Basics

NMR is a most suitable spectroscopic tool for clarifying the structures of liquids and solids. It is not intended here to describe the resonance effect in detail but only its basics for the purpose of understanding in which cases NMR can be applied. The reader is referred to standard textbooks for details [60, 61].

NMR requires the presence of nuclear spins I in the sample with which a magnetic dipole momentum μ is connected. These magnetic dipoles interact with a strong, static, homogeneous magnetic field B_0 generated by a superconducting solenoid. For a given spin number I, quantum mechanics allows the existence of only 2I + 1 energy levels over which the macroscopic large number of nuclear spins of the sample thermodynamically distribute (Boltzmann distribution), leading to a net magnetization M_0.

The energy difference (or resonance condition) between two energy levels is given by:

$$\Delta E = \hbar\omega = \hbar\gamma B_0$$

or in frequency units

$$\Delta \upsilon = \gamma B_0 \tag{3.6}$$

These nuclear spins can absorb energy from the magnetic field component of an applied radiofrequency field, with a frequency given by the resonance condition in Eq. 3.6. At constant B_0 field strength, the resonance frequency is controlled by the gyromagnetic ratio γ. In other words, different types of nuclear spins resonate at different frequencies, as shown in Table 3.1 for typical atoms present in CaPs.

In other words, the NMR spectra of different nuclei (^1H or ^{31}P) can be measured totally separated from each other. Their spectra do not overlap in one experiment. This can be an advantage, as it acts as a kind of information filter: ^1H NMR yields the proton proximity (e.g., H_2O molecules, OH^- units, HPO_4^{2-}). ^{31}P NMR, in turn, identifies the first and second coordination shells around the phosphorus atoms only (e.g., ortho- and di- polyphosphates, cation identification included). Hence, the structural interpretation can be easier. For comparison, the Fourier transform infrared (FTIR) spectrum contains all types of vibrations, including overtones of all molecular units in the sample; and one of the challenges is to assign all bands to the various vibrations of different units

Table 3.1 Resonance frequencies for typical atoms present in CaP at two B_0 field strengths

	^1H	^{31}P	^{43}Ca	^{17}O	^{23}Na	^{39}K
B_0	I = ½	I = ½	I = 7/2	I = 5/2	I = 3/2	I = 3/2
field strength	99.8%	100%	0.145%	0.0037%	100%	93.1%
9.3950 T	400	161.923	26.913	54.227	105.805	18.666
14.0926 T	600	242.884	40.368	81.340	158.706	27.998

Results are in megahertz (MHz)

The top row displays the spin number and natural abundance of the isotopes. Usually ^1H and ^{31}P nuclear magnetic resonance (NMR) spectra are acquired for coatings because of their high natural abundance. ^{43}Ca NMR is difficult because of its extremely low natural abundance and the low NMR frequency (as is the case for ^{39}K). No systematic investigations have been published so far. ^{17}O NMR is possible but requires isotopic enrichment for solids. ^{43}Ca, ^{17}O, ^{23}Na, and ^{39}K have spin numbers larger than ½. They represent so-called quadrupole nuclei, which require special NMR experiments [67] for obtaining good quality NMR spectra at once, which can be quite difficult. This is one of the major differences between the two spectroscopic tools.

However, the actual resonance frequency depends on internal interactions within the sample, such as the dipole interaction between the nuclear spins, or the so-called chemical shift. The *chemical shift* describes a frequency shift of the resonance line from the pure Larmor frequency caused by the electron density distribution as result of the chemical bonding scenarios in the sample; hence, it is the desired direct monitor for the molecular units in a sample. The chemical shift is proportional to the applied external field B_0. Therefore, it is given in parts per million (ppm) units (10^{-6})—i.e., frequency shifts divided by the NMR Larmor frequency such that the results are independent from the B_0 field.

Signals of water molecules, OH^- units, and hydrogen phosphate groups can be distinguished in an ^{1}H NMR spectrum. Similarly, phosphate and hydrogen phosphate units as possible molecular groups in CaPs can be found by ^{31}P NMR. Figure 3.11 displays the ^{1}H and ^{31}P NMR spectra of crystalline and nanocrystalline HA. The ^{1}H NMR line at 0 ppm is caused by the hydroxyl protons of HA. For crystalline HA, this line is narrow and there is also only a single ^{31}P resonance. For nanocrystalline HA, the ^{1}H signal has the same position but it is somewhat broader. Furthermore, the spectrum displays a water signal at 5 ppm and a broad component between 17 ppm and about 4 ppm caused by protons of hydrogen phosphate units in an amorphous state [62]. The ^{31}P NMR line is highly asymmetrical, and it looks as if it consists of a broad asymmetrical pattern and a narrower component on top of it, in contrast to the narrow line at 2.3 ppm for crystalline HA.

For such complicated situations, NMR offers various possibilities to gain further insight to the bonding scenario in the samples. Two-dimensional (2D) NMR [61] is an important tools. In such a 2D heteronuclear correlation spectrum (HETCOR) one can correlate, for example, ^{1}H with ^{31}P signals of neighboring phosphate units. A simple application example is explained below. Such 2D techniques require a polarization transfer step, where ^{1}H

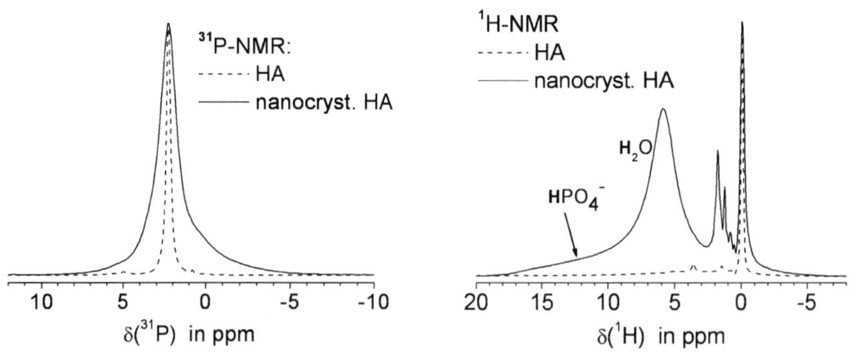

Fig. 3.11 ^{31}P and ^{1}H NMR line shapes of crystalline and nanocrystalline HA (*nanocryst. HA*)

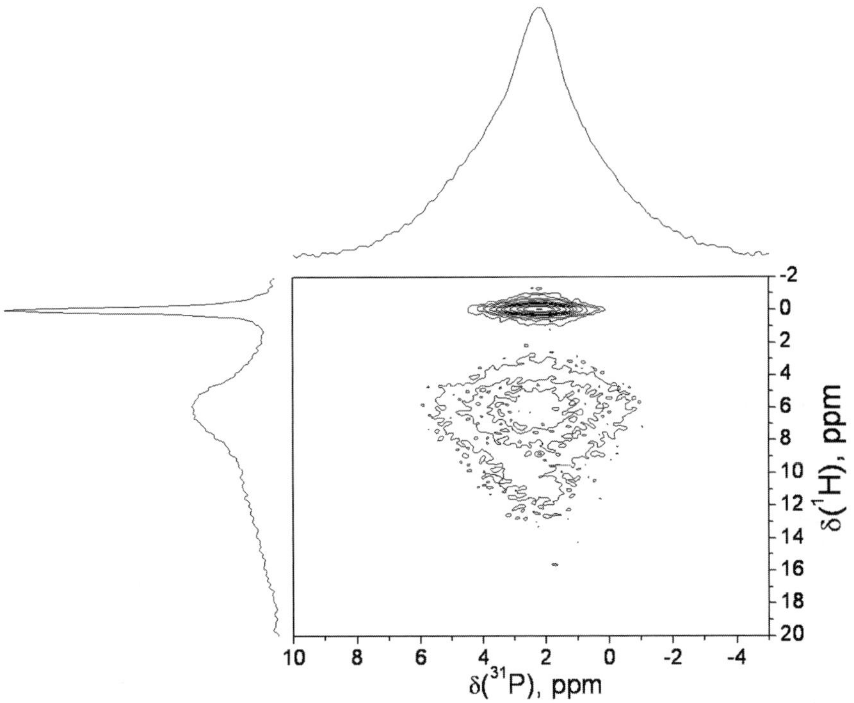

Fig. 3.12 Two-dimensional ^{1}H-^{31}P HETCOR NMR spectrum of nanocrystalline HA with the skyline projections on the ^{1}H axis (*left*) and the ^{31}P axis (*top*)

magnetization is transferred to the ^{31}P spins. One possibility is the so-called cross-polarization (CP) transfer process [63]. Figure 3.12 displays the 2D ^{1}H–^{31}P HETCOR spectrum of nanocrystalline HA. The 2D contour plot shows two distinct signals: the OH^{-} protons in close proximity to the phosphate groups in the crystalline HA core of nanocrystalline HA (top part of the 2D contour plot) and the broad correlation signals of water (5 ppm) and the protons of the hydrogen phosphate unit (4–17 ppm) with the phosphorus nucleus of the same hydrogen phosphate group (for more details see [62]).

The NMR spectra of solid samples are usually measured using magic angle sample spinning (MAS). The sample is filled in a small cylindrical container rotating around the "magic" angle of 54.7° with respect to the external B_0. The rotation frequency can reach 18 kHz (4 mm rotor) or 35 kHz (2.5 mm system). Under these circumstances, the dipole interaction can be averaged and does not broaden the NMR line. Simultaneously, the anisotropic (orientation dependent) parts of the chemical shift are averaged but conserve the isotropic chemical shift. The NMR spectrum consists of a narrow line at the isotropic chemical shift position. In addition, so-called MAS spinning sidebands spaced by the rotor frequency are present if the chemical shift anisotropy is comparable to or larger than the MAS frequency. This isotropic chemical shift position is used for the structural assignments shown and explained in Fig. 3.11 and 12.

Last but not least, it must be mentioned that NMR enables quantitative measurements. The signal area is directly proportional to the number of nuclei giving rise to this particular NMR signal. Hence, the relative number of atoms in the respective structural units can be determined unambiguously by integrating the corresponding NMR lines; no additional calibration is needed. This holds true even for amorphous materials and explains why NMR is a suitable tool to study the short and medium range order of glasses or any other disordered solid [64]. For example, it is possible to distinguish quantitatively between ortho-, di- and poly-/metaphosphate units even in the amorphous state (Q^0, Q^1, and Q^2 groups, respectively; Q^n nomenclature, with *n* being the number of bridging oxygen atoms to adjacent phosphate groups).

3.9.2 Application Examples

A brief review on NMR investigations of CaPs comprises this section. Crystallinity of phosphates is not only a question of the crystal size alone. Crystal growth kinetics is an important parameter, and therefore the time and temperature conditions of the deposition processes control the result. Three examples are given regarding results of NMR studies of crystalline (bulky) phosphates, plasma-sprayed layers, and synthetic nanocrystalline HA and the mineral phase in bone.

3.9.2.1 Characterization of Crystalline CaPs

The data collection here is restricted to typical crystalline calcium containing orthophosphates because higher condensed phosphates have not yet been observed in CaP coatings. A comprehensive description of the structure of crystalline apatites and orthophosphates, including their analysis, can be found in the monograph by Elliott [65] and in various other articles (e.g., [66–70]).

Stoichiometric HA displays a single narrow ^1H and ^{31}P NMR line at ~0.1 ppm and 2.3 ppm, respectively. The typical error is ± 0.1 ppm. Monetite ($CaHPO_4$) shows ^1H peaks at 13.6 ppm and 16.2 ppm for the protons of the three crystallographic distinct hydrogen phosphate groups in the crystal structure. ^{31}P peaks appear at ~0 ppm and –1.5 ppm. For brushite ($CaHPO_4 \bullet 2H_2O$), the water signal is found at 6.4 ppm, and an acidic proton resonance occurs at 10.4 ppm; the ^{31}P resonances are at 1.3 ppm and 1.7 ppm. For further information the reader is referred to the numerous original publications in the literature.

Tricalcium phosphate (TCP)—α-$Ca_3(PO_4)_2$ and β-$Ca_3(PO_4)_2$—must be mentioned as well. Their ^{31}P NMR line shapes are somewhat surprising, as

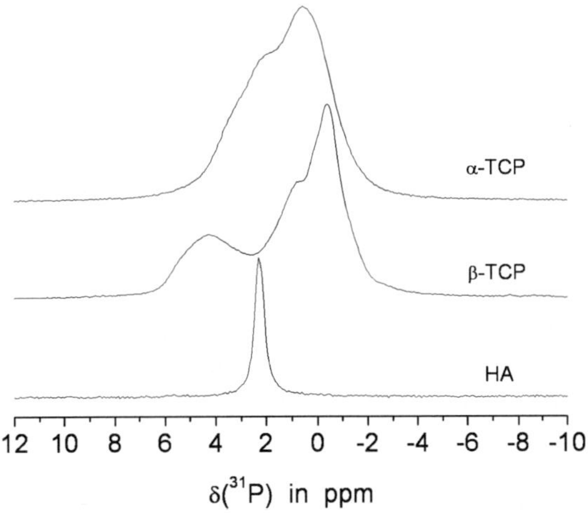

Fig. 3.13 ^{31}P spectra of α-triCaP (*α-TCP*) and *β-TCP* [$Ca_3(PO_4)_2$] in comparison to HA

shown in Fig. 3.13. In contrast to the narrow HA resonance, rather broad lines are found. Most importantly, their line widths increase linearly with larger B_0 fields. The structural origin of this unusual behavior is not yet clear.

3.9.2.2 NMR of Plasma-Sprayed Coatings

Although NMR is a highly useful tool, one of its drawbacks is certainly related to the fact that at least some milligrams of materials must be available for an experiment. This sample amount must be scratched off the substrate, especially when the substrate is metallic.

To our knowledge, only two articles have been published so far dealing with NMR investigation of layers. Hartmann et al. [70] studied the structure of plasma-sprayed HA using FTIR, XRD, and ^{1}H and ^{31}P NMR. Apart from a small HA signal, the ^{31}P NMR spectrum shows three additional resonances at 6.0, 3.1, and 1.0 ppm. None of them corresponds to crystalline structures of stoichiometric calcium orthophosphates or hydrogen phosphates. Similarly, the ^{1}H spectrum displays four further resonances in addition to a small HA signal at 0 ppm. This suggests that HA plays only a minor role in the coatings and that nonequilibrium structures have been formed during the plasma-spraying process and remain in the coating. To gain more insight about the local structure, ^{1}H-^{31}P HETCOR experiments were carried out. They showed that various nondistorted and differently distorted PO_4 groups exist with and without nearby OH^- groups. Furthermore, the authors showed that the NMR spectra of the plasma-sprayed coatings are similar to those occurring in heat-treated HA powder at certain temperatures and times. To this end, IR and NMR spectra of heat-treated crystalline HA powder (as a function of the temperature with constant time and as a function of time at constant temperature) were acquired. It was concluded that partially dehydrated HA (also named oxyhydroxyapatite, oxyHAp [71]) structures determine the complex local structure of the plasma-sprayed coating.

In a subsequent study, the same authors investigated the structure and phase composition of HA coatings deposited on Ti6Al4V coupons [71] using atmospheric plasma spraying. The investigated samples comprised coatings with and without a TiO_2 bond coat as well as coatings incubated for various times (up to 12 weeks) in SBFs under physiological conditions. It was found that coatings in the presence of the TiO_2 bond coat obtained a substantially increased proportion of crystalline (well ordered) HA at the expense of disordered structures such as oxyHAp. Similarly, upon thermal decomposition, these coating contain more crystalline degradation products such as TCP and TTCP and less amorphous CaP. Furthermore, incubation of these TiO_2-assisted coatings in SBF promotes formation of a larger amount of HA as the disordered structures, the thermal decomposition products, and the ACP exhibit substantially higher solubility.

Meanwhile the sensitivity of modern NMR spectrometers has been improved considerably. Some recent data (unpublished) show that NMR measurements are feasible using the sample amount scratched from 20 cm^2 with a coating thickness of about 5 μm.

3.9.2.3 NMR Studies of Nano-crystalline HA and of Bone

Calcium phosphate is the inorganic component of many biological hard tissues, the most prominent ones being bone and teeth [72–74]. Platelet-like CaP crystals exist in bone having typical dimensions of the order of a few nanometers in thickness and some tens of nanometers in length. The preparation and study of synthetic nanoparticles prepared *in vitro* [75] is also interesting for two reasons: We can learn more about the process of formation of this biomineral *in vivo*, and we can prepare materials for medical purposes that closely resemble the natural model (e.g., for repairing lost bone in clinical medicine) [76].

The interesting point is that both the mineral phase in bone and artificial nanocrystalline HA have nonstoichiometric compositions, assuming that HA is the dominating crystal phase. Nanocrystalline HA particles may have grain sizes in the range of 10 to 100 nm, and Ca^{2+} deficiency is a common feature [75, 77]. Typical Ca/P ratios of about 1.50 to 1.57 are reported, in contrast to 1.67 for stoichiometric HA [$Ca_{10}(PO_4)_6(OH)_2$]. Finally, OH^- depletion is reported in the mineral phase of bone and has been confirmed by various methods including titration, FTIR, NMR, neutron scattering, and Raman spectroscopy [78–81]. Cho et al. were the first to determine the OH^- content in a bone sample using NMR and found only 20% of the expected value for HA [82].

It is interesting to note that in the "material synthesis community" Ca^2 deficiency is used to describe the nonstoichiometry of the nanocrystals, whereas OH^- depletion is used for bone. In our view, it reflects only different ways of describing the same structural phenomenon.

Obviously, the nonstoichiometry of HA nanocrystals is a common feature, and this type of material has been studied extensively using NMR [83, 84]. Unfortunately, in none of these studies was the structural origin of the Ca^{2+} deficiency discovered; although detailed information on the local structure was available from the NMR experiments. For example, the presence of hydrogen phosphate groups was concluded from the NMR spectra, and water molecules were found. By exploiting different relaxation behaviors, it was also possible to distinguish ordered and disordered HA regions on nanoparticles synthesized by a wet mechanochemical reaction [84].

The structural origin of the nonstoichiometry of nanocrystalline HA produced via a precipitation route [75] has been solved using 2D NMR [62]. It was shown that elongated HA nanoparticles with a typical size of $10 \times 10 \times 40\ nm^3$ consist of a crystalline core composed of stoichiometric HA covered with an approximately 1 nm thick amorphous layer having an overall chemical composition close to that of OCP. Only about 45% of the total phosphate content is contained in the crystalline HA core. The Ca/P ratio estimated from the NMR spectra yields a value of 1.52, which is very close to the 1.51 obtained by wet chemical analysis.

3.9.3 Outlook

The detailed structural elucidation of thin CaP coatings is a real challenge and by no means an easy task. The thickness of layers on the order of about 10 μm is presumably not the main problem. The key issue is that a wide variety of molecular structures—even amorphous ones—form during growth of the coating structure. Indeed, NMR reveals the presence of various structural motives in thin coatings: crystalline HA parts; different kinds of hydroxyl unit, some of them grouped together; and various hydrogen phosphate and phosphate anions. This problem of multiple and disordered structural motives becomes even more important if the dimensions of the crystals or coatings become smaller and smaller. Clearly, internal stress appears in the network region just below the surface such that small bonding angle and bond length variations result. This broadens Bragg peaks in XRD analyses, absorption bands in IR spectroscopy, and NMR signals. If, in addition, the surfaces of these crystal have a changed chemical composition compared with the bulk (e.g., different frozen-in nonequilibrium structures formed during the process of fast cooling in plasma or hydrogen phosphate groups formed in bone or nanocrystalline HA), it is clear that such altered surface regions can be analyzed only with difficulty. The only successful approach is to use all available methods and spectroscopic tools together. NMR can play an important role because it does not suffer strongly from the effects of nanoscopic particle sizes and amorphous structures. Although much detailed structural information can be gained using NMR, our knowledge of the structure of thin CaP coating is still limited. However, it is an important issue for understanding structure–property relations and to improve the design of biomaterials.

3.10 Mechanical Testing of Thin CaP Coatings

3.10.1 Adhesion Testing

Adhesion to the substrate is one of the main properties of a coating and is probably the most important reason for the development of thin CaP coatings. Adhesion between two bodies can be defined as the state in which the surfaces in contact remain joined by means of forces of a different nature: Van der Waals forces, electrostatic forces, and forces related to the different types of chemical bonding. An ideal adhesion test method should measure only coating adhesion, but the experimental methods available give an adhesion value that is, as a general rule, less than the real value due to the residual stresses of the coating and the intrinsic error of the test method [85].

Several methods have been developed to evaluate adhesion of a thin coating to a substrate: pressure-sensitive tape test, acceleration test, electromagnetic stressing, shock wave test, tensile and shear test, laser spallation, acoustic imaging, indentation testing, scratch test. Among them only the tensile test (pull-off) and the scratch test have been widely used to measure adhesion of thin CaP coatings to their substrates.

3.10.1.1 Tensile Test

The tensile test consists of subjecting a specimen assembly composed of one coated and one uncoated component to a tensile load, as shown in Fig. 3.14. The components to be tested must be bonded together by a polymeric adhesive. The adhesive may be in film form or bulk form, but it must have a

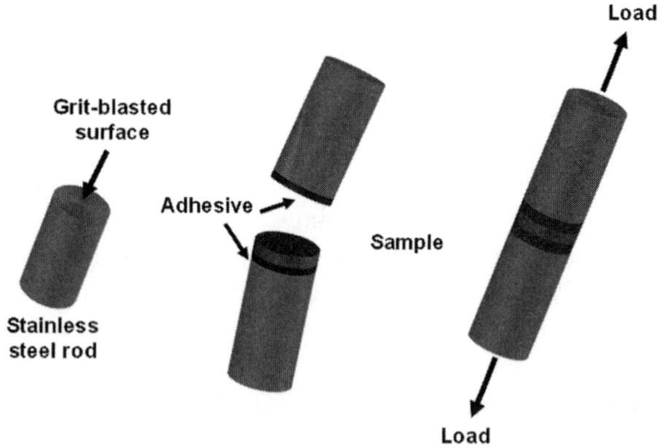

Fig. 3.14 ASTM-F1501-94 procedure for evaluating the adhesion of CaP coating

minimum bulk tensile strength as high as the minimum required adhesion or cohesion strength of the coating. The tensile load must be applied normally to the plane of the coating utilizing a tension machine, which is capable of determining the maximum strength of the coating or interface. It is important that the loading is purely normal and that no bending moments are applied at the interface. The results are given in terms of adhesion strength, which is the maximum load (i.e., the record peak load) over the substrate area on which the coating is applied. A standard test method to perform this adhesion measurement has been adopted [86].

Special precaution must be taken when interpreting the results if the coating has some degree of porosity or has developed cracks. In these cases, the adhesive used when preparing specimens for this test may have inadvertently penetrated the coating, reaching the substrate and leading to misleading high strength [87]. The main advantage of this method is that it gives absolute numbers, thereby allowing direct comparison between coatings produced by different methods [88].

3.10.1.2 Scratch Test

The scratch test has seen widespread use for measuring the adhesion of thin CaP coatings. The test consists of a stylus that is drawn over the sample surface under a normal force that is increased either stepwise or continuously until the coating detaches. The normal force at the moment of coating detachment is called the critical load (L_c) and gives a comparative value of coating adhesion.

Complete detachment of the coating is not always observed even when the coating fails [89]. It has been found that coatings fail in several ways when subjected to scratch testing [90, 91]. Common failure modes include spalling, buckling, chipping, conformal cracking, and tensile cracking, among others. An exhaustive atlas of thin coating failure under the scratch test is available to identify the type of coating failure [92]. Figure 3.15B shows two thin CaP coatings tested by the scratch method and exhibiting different failure modes [93]: lateral flaking and ductile lateral delamination, respectively. Coating failure during scratch testing can also be detected by other means, such as measurement of high frequency vibrations using acoustical emission transducers, friction force measurements, observation of the track under an optical microscope, or observation of the track by SEM and EDS.

Three scratching procedures are currently employed, depending on the information sought and the apparatus available [92]: (1) With the progressive load scratch test (PLST), the load of the indenter increases linearly as the indenter moves across the test surface at a constant speed. (2) With the constant load scratch test (CLST), the normal load is increased in increments between successive scratches carried out under a constant load at different locations on the sample surface until failure occurs. (3) With the multi-pass scratch test (MPST), the testing mode consists of repeated scratching in the same scratch track under a constant subcritical load.

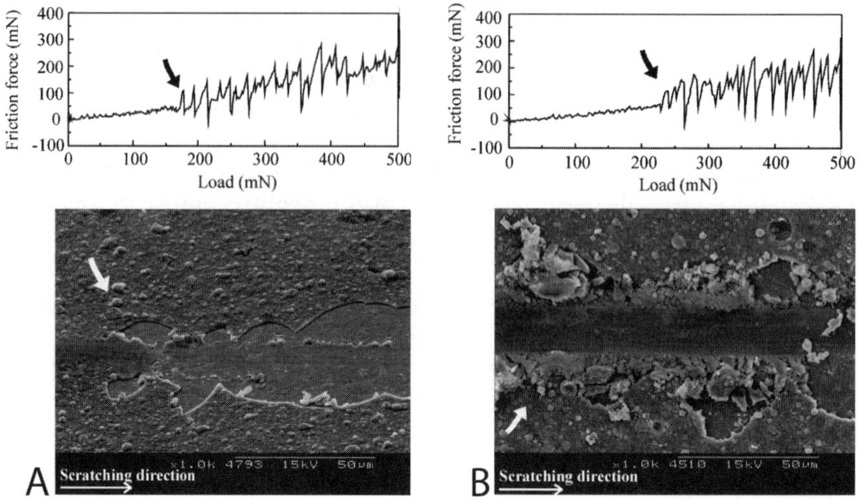

Fig. 3.15 Two thin CaP coatings deposited by PLD under different conditions exhibiting different failure modes. **A** Lateral flaking. **B** Ductile lateral delamination. From [93], with permission

In general, the PLST mode is used as a first-order assessment of critical loads corresponding to major coating damage and failure, whereas the CLST mode allows statistical damage analysis of coatings along their surface. The MPST mode subjects the coated surface to a low cycle fatigue-type contact.

The adhesion value given by the scratch test method is affected by a number of factors that can be classified into the following groups [94, 95].

- Intrinsic factors: loading rate, scratching speed, indenter tip radius, indenter hardness, indenter tip wear.
- Extrinsic factors: substrate hardness, coating thickness, coating roughness, substrate roughness prior to coating, friction force, friction coefficient, among others. As a general rule, an increase in substrate hardness and/or coating thickness promotes an increase in the critical load given by the scratch test.

Therefore, some test parameters have been widely accepted to standardize the method, such as the use of a diamond Rockwell C stylus (usually with a tip radius of 200 mm).

Owing to the many variable parameters involved in the scratch test, no single relation between the critical load and other parameters can be used. Rather, individual tests are well suited to relative comparison of the same film–substrate combination prepared under different conditions.

3.10.2 Nanoindentation

Indentation testing with an appropriate device is one of the simplest ways to measure the mechanical properties of a material. It is performed by deforming the material and measuring the indentation made. In the case of a thin film, it is necessary to deform the material on a small scale; thus, the indentation is made at the nanometer level, and the procedure is known as nanoindentation [96].

Nanoindentation has become popular due to the ease with which a wide variety of mechanical properties can be measured without removing the film from the substrate. Another advantage is its ability to obtain maps of properties by probing at several points of the coating.

The thin film properties most frequently measured in nanoindentation experiments are the elastic modulus (E) and the hardness (H) [97]. The most common method for measuring hardness and modulus using nanoindentation involves making a small indentation in the film, usually with a diamond Berkovich indenter, while continuously recording the indentation load and the displacement during one complete cycle of loading and unloading (Fig. 3.16). A typical load/displacement graph during a complete nanoindentation cycle is shown in Fig. 3.16 (inset) in which F_{max} is the peak load, h_{max} is the displacement at peak load, $S = dF/dh$ is the initial contact stiffness (i.e., the slope of the initial portion of the unloading curve), and h_r is the displacement found by linearly extrapolating the initial portion of the unloading curve to zero load.

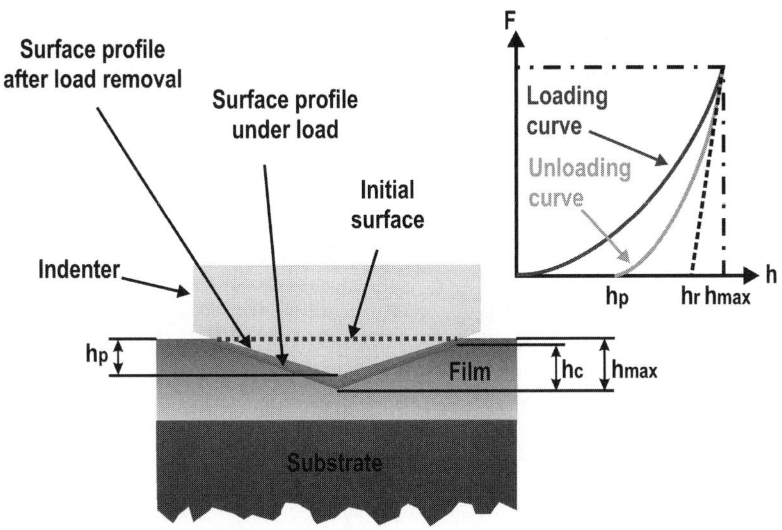

Fig. 3.16 Nanoindentation procedure to accomplish a thin CaP coating on a substrate. **Inset** Typical load/displacement graph obtained during a nanoindentation measurement. The *dotted line* is tangential to the initial part of the unloading curve. *F*, force; *h*, indentation depth; h_p, indentation depth after unloading; h_c, contact depth; h_{max}, maximum indentation depth; hr, intersection of the tangential line to the unloading curve at F_{max} with the displacement axis

According to the ISO 14577 standard [98], Martens hardness (HM), or universal hardness, is defined as the maximum applied load, F_{max}, divided by the contact area $A_s(h)$ at that load:

$$HM = \frac{F_{max}}{A_s(h)} = \frac{F_{max}}{26.43 \times h^2} \tag{3.7}$$

where

$$A_s(h) = \frac{3\sqrt{3}\tan(\alpha)}{\cos(\alpha)} h^2 \tag{3.8}$$

in which the parameter α refers to the face angle of the indenter. In the case of the Berkovich indenter, which is a three-sided pyramidal indenter, $\alpha = 65.03°$.

To ensure that the substrate is not affecting the measurement of the coating properties, the size of the contact impression must be small compared to the film thickness. A conservative rule is that the depth of the contact should not exceed 10% of the total thickness of the coating.

Excluding the size of the imprint and the load applied during the indentation, the main difference between nanoindentation and conventional microhardness testing is that the latter is unable to give elastic modulus measurements. This is due to the fact that the measurements are made after the load has been removed from the specimen (therefore, the elastic deformation is not taken into account), whereas with nanoindentation by recording the complete cycle of loading and unloading both the elastic and the plastic behavior of the film are included in the measurement [99]. The elastic modulus of the coating obtained by nanoindentation, E_{IT}, is given by:

$$E_{IT} = \frac{1-(\nu_s)^2}{\frac{1}{E_r} - \frac{1-(\nu_i)^2}{E_i}} \tag{3.9}$$

where ν_s is Poisson's ratio of the coating, E_r is the reduced modulus, ν_i is Poisson's ratio of the indenter (0.07 for diamond), and E_i is the elastic modulus of the indenter (1141 GPa for diamond). The reduced modulus can be calculated from the indentation data according to the expression

$$E_r = \frac{S\sqrt{\pi}}{2\sqrt{A_p(h_c)}} \tag{3.10}$$

where $A_p(h_c)$ is the projected contact area, which for a Berkovich indenter is given by

$$A_p(h_c) = 23.96 \times h_c^2 \tag{3.11}$$

Therefore, the hardness and the elastic modulus of the coatings can be obtained directly from the complete load–displacement curve.

Acknowledgments The authors thank the following persons for helpful comments and useful discussions: Frank Malz, Sergey Maltsev, Mario Fichera, Edwin van der Wal, Eugenio Solla, Lourdes Rial, and Antonio Riveiro.

References

1. B. Smith. In: Infrared Spectral Interpretation. (CRC Press, Boca Raton, FL, 1999), p. 3.
2. R.V. Santos, R.N. Clayton, American Mineralogist 80 (1995) 336.
3. Posset, E. Löcklin, R. Thull, W. Kiefer. J. Biomed. Mater. Res. 40 (1998) 640.
4. J.L. Arias, F.J. García-Sanz, M.B. Mayor, S. Chiussi, J. Pou, B. León, M. Pérez-Amor. Biomaterials 19 (1998) 883.
5. B. Mayor, J. Arias, S. Chiussi, F. García, J. Pou, B. León and M. Pérez-Amor, Thin Solid Films 317 (1998) 363.
6. N.B. Colthup, L.H. Daly, S.E. Wiberley. In: Introduction to Infrared and Raman Spectroscopy. (Academic Press, San Diego, 1990), p. 60.
7. C.N. Banwell. In: Fundamentals of Molecular Spectroscopy. (McGraw-Hill, London, 1994).
8. B. Schader. In: Practical Fourier Transform Infrared Spectroscopy. (Academic Press, San Diego, 1990), p. 167.
9. H. Tsuda, J. Arias, B. Leon, J. Arends. Appl. Spectrosc. 52 (1998) 1122.
10. R. Smith, I. Rehman. J. Mat. Sci: Mat. Med. 5 (1995) 775.
11. U. Posset, E. Löcklin, R. Thull, W. Kiefer, J. Biomed. Mater. Res. 40 (1998) 640.
12. J.M. Fernández-Pradas, L. Clèries, E. Martínez, G. Sardin, J. Esteve, J.L. Morenza. Appl. Phys. A 71 (2000) 37.
13. L. Clèries, J.M. Fernández-Pradas, G. Sardin, J.L. Morenza. Biomaterials 19 (1998) 1483.
14. D. Briggs, M.P. Seah. In: Practical Surface Analysis. Vol. 1. Auger and X-ray Photoelectron Spectroscopy. (Wiley, New York, 1990).
15. B. Feddes, A.M. Vredenberg, J.G.C. Wolke, J.A. Jansen. Surf. Inter. Anal. 35 (2003) 287.
16. B. Feddes, J.G.C. Wolke, J.A. Jansen, A.M. Vredenberg. J. Vac. Sci. Technol. A 21 (2003) 363.
17. B. Feddes, A.M. Vredenberg, J.G.C. Wolke, J.A. Jansen. Biomaterials 25 (2004) 633.
18. K.E. Hwang, C.S. Kim. Mat. Sci. Eng. C 23 (2003) 401.
19. M. Manso, M. Langlet, M. Fernández, L. Vázques, J.M. Martínez-Duart. Mat. Sci. Eng. C 23 (2003) 451.
20. H.P. Klug, L.E. Alexander. In: X-ray Diffraction Procedures, 2nd edition. (Wiley, New York, 1974).
21. J.G.C.Wolke, K. van Dijk, H.G. Schaeken, K. de Groot, J.A. Jansen. J. Biomed. Mat. Res. 28 (1994) 1477.
22. J.C. Elliot. In: Structure and Chemistry of the Apatites and Other CaPs. (Elsevier, Amsterdam, 1994).
23. E.L. Haase. In: Proceedings of the International Conference on Advanced Methods in X-ray and Neutron Analysis of Materials. (Plenum, New York, 1988).
24. P.J. Goodhew, F.J. Humphreys. In: Electron Microscopy and Analysis. (Taylor & Francis, London, 1988).

25. S.K. Chapman. In: Working with a Scanning Electron Microscope. (Lodgemark Press, Orpington, Kent, UK, 1986).
26. J.M. Fernández-Pradas, L. Clèries, G. Sardin, J.L. Morenza, Biomaterials 23 (2002) 1989.
27. L. Clèries, E. Martinez, J.M. Fernández-Pradas, G. Sardin, J. Esteve, J.L. Morenza. Biomaterials 21 (2000) 967.
28. J.M. Fernández-Pradas, G. Sardin, J.L. Morenza, Appl. Phys. A 76 (2003) 251.
29. F. Lusquiños, J. Pou, J.L. Arias, M. Boutinguiza, B. León, M. Pérez-Amor, F.C.M. Driessens, J.C. Merry, I. Gibson, S. Best, W. Bonfield, J. Appl. Phys. 90 (2001) 4231.
30. M. Vallet-Regí, J. Peña, I. Izquierdo-Barba, Solid State Ionics 172 (2004) 445.
31. S.C.G. Leeuwenburgh, J.G.C. Wolke, M.C. Siebers, J. Schoonman, J.A. Jansen. Biomaterials 27 (2006) 3368.
32. F.J. Garcia-Sanz, M.B. Mayor, J.L. Arias, J. Pou, B. León, M. Pérez-Amor, J. Mater. Sci. Mater Med. 8 (1997) 861.
33. J.L. Arias, M.B. Mayor, J. Pou, B. León, M. Pérez-Amor. Appl. Surf. Sci. 186 (2002) 448.
34. Q. Zhang, Y. Leng, R. Xin. Biomaterials 26 (2005) 2857.
35. J.G.C. Wolke, J.P.C.M. Van Der Waerden, K. De Groot, J.A. Jansen. Biomaterials 18 (1987) 483.
36. N. Moritz, M. Jokinen, T. Peltola, S. Areva, A. Yli-Urpo. J. Biomed. Mater. Res. Part A. 65 (2003) 9.
37. M.C. Kuo, S.K. Yen. J. Mater. Sci. 39 (2004) 2357.
38. L. Clèries, J.M. Fernández-Pradas, G. Sardin, J.L. Morenza. Biomaterials 19 (1998) 1483.
39. L. Clèries, J.M. Fernández-Pradas, J.L. Morenza. J. Biomed. Mater. Res. 49 (2000) 43.
40. M.C. Siebers, X.F. Walboomers, S.C.G. Leeuwenburgh, J.G.C. Wolke, J.A. Jansen. Biomaterials 25 (2004) 2019.
41. H.S. Azevedo, I.B. Leonor, C.M. Alves, R.L. Reis. Mater. Sci. Eng. C 25 (2005) 169.
42. J.A. Chandler, A.M. Glauert. In: X-ray Microanalysis in the Electron Microscope. (North-Holland, Amsterdam, 1987).
43. D.B. Williams, C.B. Carter. In: Transmission Electron Microscopy. (Plenum, New York, 1996).
44. R. Xin, Y. Leng, N. Wang. J. Crystal Growth 289 (2006) 339.
45. T. Blalock, X. Bai, A. Rabiei. Surf. Coat. Technol. 201 (2007) 5850.
46. H. Engqvist, G.A. Botton, M. Couillard, S. Mohammadi, J. Malmström, L. Emanuelsson, L. Hermansson, M.W. Phaneuf, P. Thomsen. J. Biomedical. Mater. Res. Part A 78 (2006) 20.
47. L.C. Feldman, J.W. Mayer. In: Fundamentals of Surface and Thin Film Analysis. (Elsevier, Amsterdam, 1986), p. 26.
48. L.R. Doolittle. Nucl. Instrum. Meth. Phys. Res. B 9 (1985) 344.
49. N.P. Barradas, C. Jeynes, R.P. Webb. Appl. Phys. Lett. 71 (1997) 291.
50. E. van der Wal, J.G.C. Wolke, J.A. Jansen, A.M. Vredenberg. Appl. Surf. Sci. 246 (2005) 183.
51. A.M. Ektessabi. Nucl. Instrum. Meth. Phys. Res. B 127/128 (1997) 1008.
52. A.M. Ektessabi, M. Hamdi. Surf. Coat. Technol. 153 (2002) 10.
53. K. van Dijk, C.H.M. Maree, J. Verhoeven, F.H.P.M. Habraken, J.A. Jansen, J. Biomed. Mat. Res. 42 (1998) 266.
54. E. van der Wal. In: Bioactivity and Surface Reactivity of RF-sputtered CaP Thin Films. PhD thesis, University of Utrecht, ISBN 90-393-3491-9.
55. E. van der Wal, A.M. Vredenberg, P.J. Ter Brugge, J.G.C. Wolke, J.A. Jansen. Biomaterials 27 (2006) 1333.
56. E. van der Wal, S.J. Oldenburg, T. Heij, A.W. Denier van der Gon, H.H. Brongersma, J.G.C. Wolke, J.A. Jansen, A.M. Vredenberg. Appl. Surf. Sci. 252 (2006) 3843.

57. M. Jelínek, V. Olšan, L. Jastrabík, V. Studnička, V. Hnatowicz, J. Kvítek, V. Havránek, T. Dostálová, I. Zergioti, A. Petrakis, E. Hontzopoulos, C. Fotakis. Thin Solid Films 257 (1995) 125.
58. C.C. Chusuei, D.W. Goodman, M.J. van Stipdonk, D.R. Justes, E.A. Schweikert. Anal. Chem. 71 (1999) 149.
59. H.B. Lu, C.T. Campbell, D.J. Graham, B.R. Ratner. Anal. Chem. 72 (2000) 2886.
60. R. Freeman. In: A Handbook of Nuclear Magnetic Resonance. (Bath Press, Avon, UK, 1987).
61. K. Schmidt-Rohr, H.W. Spiess. In: Multidimensional Solid-State NMR and Polymers. (Academic Press, San Diego, 1994).
62. C. Jäger, T. Welzel, W. Meyer-Zaika, M. Epple, Magn. Reson. Chem. 44 (2006) 573.
63. A. Pines, M.G. Gibby, J.S. Waugh. J. Chem. Phys. 59 (1973) 569.
64. C. Jäger. In: Analysis of the Composition and Structure of Glass and Glass Ceramics. (Springer, New York, 1999), p. 197–232.
65. J.C. Elliott. Structure and Chemistry of the Apatites and Other Calcium Orthophosphate. (Elsevier, Amsterdam, 1994).
66. J.P. Yesinowski, H. Eckert. J. Am. Chem. Soc. 109 (1987) 6274.
67. P.S. Belton, R.K. Harris, P.J. Wilkes. J. Phys. Chem. Solids 49 (1988) 21.
68. W.P. Rothwell, J.S. Waugh, J.P. Yesinowski. J. Am. Chem. Soc. 102 (1980) 2637.
69. L.M. Rodriguez-Lorenzo. J. Mater. Sci. Mat. Med. 16 (2005) 393.
70. P. Hartmann, C. Jäger, S. Barth, J. Vogel, K. Meyer, J. Solid State Chem 160 (2001) 460.
71. R.B. Heimann, H.V. Tran, P. Hartmann. Mat.-wiss. u.Werkstofftech. 34 (2003) 1163.
72. H.A. Lowenstam, S. Weiner. In: On Biomineralization. (Oxford University Press, Oxford, UK, 1989).
73. S. Mann. In: Biomineralization. (Oxford University Press, Oxford, UK, 2002).
74. S. Weiner, H.D. Wagner. Rev. Mater. Sci. 28 (1998) 271.
75. T. Welzel, W. Meyer-Zayka, M. Epple. Chem. Commun. 10 (2004) 1204.
76. J.L. Miquel, L. Facchini, A.P. Legrand, X. Marchandise, P. Lecouffe, M. Chanavaz, M. Donazzan, C. Rey, J. Lemaitre. Clin. Mater. 5 (1990) 115.
77. R.M. Wilson, J.C. Elliott, S.E.P. Dowker, L.M. Rodriguez-Lorenzo. Biomaterials 26 (2005) 1317.
78. J.D. Termine, D.R. Lundy. Calcif. Tissue Res. 13 (1973) 73.
79. C. Rey, J.L. Miguel, L. Facchini, A.P. Legrand, M.J. Glimcher. Bone 16 (1995) 583.
80. J.E. Roberts, L.C. Bonar, R.G. Griffin, M.J. Glimcher. Calcif. Tissue Int. 50 (1992) 42.
81. C.K. Loong, C. Rey, L.T. Kuhn, C. Combes, Y. Wu, S.H. Chen, M.J. Glimcher, Bone 26 (2000) 599.
82. G. Cho, Y. Wu, J.L. Ackerman. Science 300 (2003) 1123.
83. R.N. Panda, M.F. Hsieh, R.J. Chung, T.S. Chin. J. Phys. Chem. Solids 64 (2003) 193.
84. T. Isobe, S. Nakamura, R. Nemoto, M. Senna, H. Sfihi. J. Phys. Chem. B 106 (2002) 5169.
85. J. Valli, U. Makela, A. Matthews. Surf. Eng. 2 (1986) 49.
86. ASTM F1501. Standard test method for tension testing of CaP coating.
87. Y.C. Tsui, C. Doyle, T.W. Clyne. Biomaterials 19 (1998) 2015.
88. F.J. García-Sanz, M.B. Mayor, J.L. Arias, J. Pou, B. León, M. Pérez-Amor. J. Mater. Sci. Mater. Med. 8 (1997) 861.
89. A.J. Perry. Thin Solid Films 78 (1981) 77.
90. P.J. Burnett, D.S. Rickerby. Thin Solid Films 154 (1987) 403.
91. V. Bellido-González, N. Stefanopoulos, F. Deguilhen. Surf. Coat. Technol. 74–75 (1995) 884.
92. EN 1071-3. Advanced Technical Ceramics Methods of Test for Ceramic Coatings. Part 3. Determination of Adhesion and Other Mechanical Failure Modes by a Scratch Test.
93. L. Clèries, E. Martínez, J.M. Fernández-Pradas, G. Sardin, J. Esteve, J.L. Morenza. Biomaterials 21 (2000) 967.
94. J. Valli. J. Vac. Sci. Technol. A 4 (1986) 3007.

95. P.A. Steinmann, Y. Tardy, H.E. Hintermann. Thin Solid Films 154 (1987) 333.
96. G.M. Pharr, W.C. Oliver. MRS Bull 17 (1992) 28.
97. W.C. Oliver, G.M. Pharr. J. Mater. Res. 7 (1992) 1564.
98. ISO 14577-1:2002. Metallic Materials: Instrumented Indentation Test for Hardness and Materials Parameters.
99. M.F. Doerner, W.D. Nix. J. Mater. Res. 1 (1986) 601.

Chapter 4
In Vitro and *In Vivo* Evaluation of Thin Calcium Phosphate Coatings

Ulrich M. Gross and Dirk Lassner

Abstract This chapter starts with general considerations on wound healing; the main cells and their structures and functions; and methods of *in vitro* and *in vivo* evaluation. Implants with thin calcium phosphate (CaP) coatings can enhance or inhibit wound healing mechanisms on various levels of gene expression and protein production. Therefore, some techniques to elucidate the material and tissue interactions are mentioned. Bone development, the various types of bone, and bone fracture healing are presented. Thin CaP coatings of implant material can be investigated in *in vitro* test systems using primary cells or cell lines in culture. More reliable results can be expected from *in vivo* investigations with animal models. Important results of such investigations are presented. The prediction of the clinical performance of thin CaP coatings on the basis of *in vitro* and *in vivo* models is limited. Therefore, retrieval studies of surgically explanted or postmortem uncovered implants should be obligatory.

4.1 Introduction

Biomedical materials development and application in human medicine is a research area dating back only some four to five decennials. It entails an interdisciplinary approach where materials science meets biology and medicine. Practically every discipline in the medical field is involved, including surgery, orthopedics, dentistry, internal medicine, and dermatology, among others. This fact implies that a wide range of specialties have to work together to find a common language where necessary and to profit from the achievements of foreign disciplines to reach solutions for medical problems. The pertinent field of thin coatings is related to improved implant fixation, for example of metallic or ceramic materials in bone, connective tissue, oral mucosa, or skin.

U.M. Gross (✉)
Institute of Pathology, Free University of Berlin, Campus Benjamin Franklin, Hindenburgdamm 30, D 12200 Berlin, Germany
e-mail: ugross@zedat.fu-berlin.de, and Institute of Cardiac Diagnostics and Therapy (IKDT), Moltkestrasse 31, D 12203 Berlin, Germany
e-mail: ugross@zedat.fu-berlin.de

B. León, J.A. Jansen (eds.), *Thin Calcium Phosphate Coatings for Medical Implants*, DOI 10.1007/978-0-387-77718-4_4,

Materials' structures and properties interacting with biological structures in bone are the main focus. The whole body of knowledge comprising surgical indications and techniques and wound healing in bone and adjacent soft tissues cannot be explained in detail in this chapter. Therefore, readers who are interested in more detailed information are directed to standard textbooks of pathology, biomaterials evaluation, biomaterials science, and bone engineering [1–4].

Because every surgical act to insert or implant a device in tissue must be connected to an incision, any implantation must coincide with the dissection of epithelium and adjacent tissue, whether soft tissue or mineralized tissue (i.e. connective tissue, bone, or cartilage). The result is a wound that heals in a number of stages. The basic processes of would healing imply trauma, injury, reaction, cellular migration, extracellular matrix (ECM) organization and remodeling, and cell proliferation [1].

There is already considerable knowledge regarding the various cell types involved in the early phase after surgical trauma. Immediately after injury, rupture of vessels, blood extravasation, and blood clot formation predominate (Fig. 4.1). Blood clots contain platelets that release factors to influence the reaction, such as platelet-derived growth factor (PDGF). In the next stage,

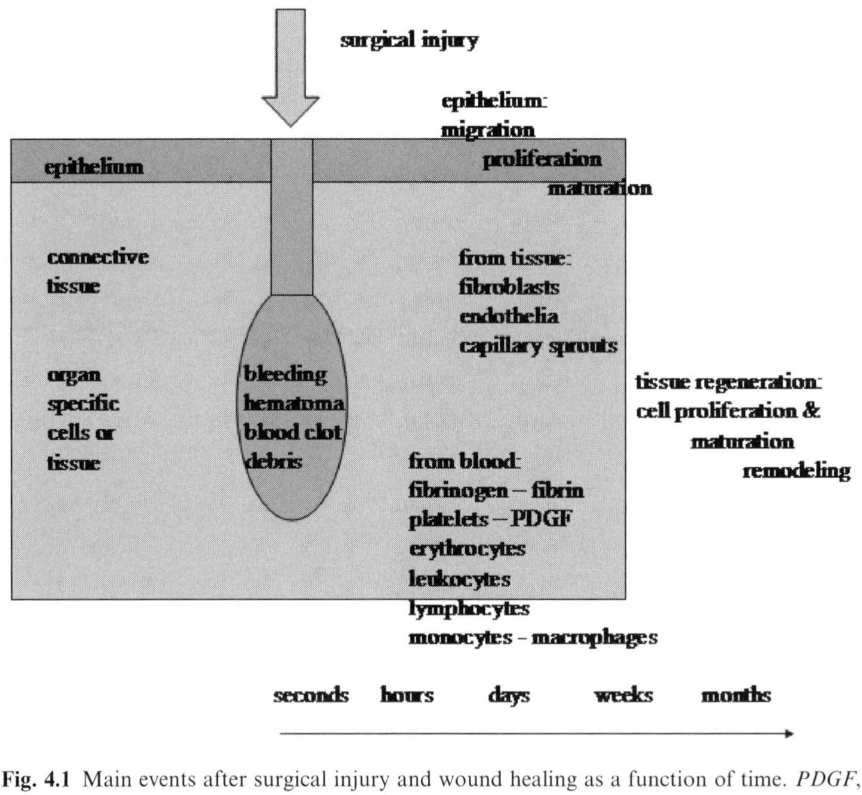

Fig. 4.1 Main events after surgical injury and wound healing as a function of time. *PDGF*, platelet-derived growth factor (*See* Color Insert)

mostly at 1 to 3 days, when cell necrosis occurs, the recruited polymorphnuclear leukocytes (PMNs), macrophages, fibroblasts, and endothelia are present to remove cell and tissue debris and to begin to repair the ECM. At the same time, epithelia migrate and proliferate to coat surfaces where basal lamina allows it.

Circulating cells in blood attach to areas in the microvasculature around the site of injury and migrate to the extracellular space (e.g., PMNs and monocytes, among others). The monocytes differentiate to macrophages once in the site of injury. They play an important role in phagocytosis of cells and tissue debris. They also produce molecules that influence lymphocytes; that is, the immunological response of antibody-secreting B cells and their counterparts the T cells, which have specific functions in cell-mediated immunological reactions. They interact with local fibroblasts and other local cells (e.g., capillary endothelia, fibroblasts, pericytes).

The epithelia, whether at the external surface, the skin, or at internal surfaces such as mucosa, also react. They are able to glide on the basal lamina surface and proliferate to coat denuded surfaces.

The highly complex interrelations of the mentioned cell types is realized via molecules that are produced by individual cells, secreted, and taken up by target cells. These molecules usually have receptors that activate the cell metabolism in a specific way. More and more receptors, their intracellular signal transduction, and the activation of genes have become known over the years. Wound healing is a very old process in species development and deeply rooted in the ability of cells and tissues to react and also in the regeneration of cells and tissues.

Thin CaP coatings can be considered attempts to overcome the drawbacks of the first-generation biomedical materials that are, by definition, inert (i.e., unreactive) materials used to replace diseased or missing parts of a patient [5]. Second-generation biomedical materials should elicit a controlled action or reaction in the physiological environment. The first materials following this intention were systematically designed and made as bioactive glasses—composed of Na_2O-CaO-P_2O_5-SiO_2—by Hench et al. in 1971 [6]. These materials relied on a concept opposite to that for inert materials. They are bioactive and display mechanisms of controlled dissolution and stepwise ion exchange at the surface, resulting finally in a cascade of steps. They lead to the deposition of carbonated hydroxyapatite (HA) at the implant surface and the development of a bond to collagen fibers and mineralized tissue in the ECM. The leading phenomenon of these bioactive glasses and glass ceramics is the strong bond between the implanted material and the surrounding tissue (i.e., the mineralized or unmineralized ECM).

There were other groups taking up this concept, including Brömer et al. in Germany in 1975 [7] and Kokubo and Yamamuro in Japan in 1985 [8]. An important point in the concept of bioactive materials is that the absorbable material is ultimately replaced by the regenerating tissue of the patient.

Third-generation biomaterials are cell- and gene-activating materials (e.g., consisting of an absorbable scaffold that is loaded with specific gene-activating chemical substances). These materials should induce cell and tissue regeneration in a given implantation site and then dissolve and disappear totally after they have fulfilled their function [5]. It was shown that bioactive glasses can up-regulate families of genes within 48 hours of exposure to primary human osteoblasts. Activated genes can induce the production of numerous proteins that influence proliferation and differentiation of osteoblasts; transcription factors; cell-cycle regulators; signal transduction molecules; proteins involved in DNA synthesis, repair, and recombination; growth factors; and cytokines. The factors influence the inflammatory response to materials, cell-surface antigens and receptors, ECM components, and apoptosis regulators [5].

This situation requires an outline of some principles of cell physiology and biochemistry regarding genomics, transcriptomics, and proteomics [9–15]. For maintaining individuals and species, the information about structure and function is found within the genomic DNA that is packaged in chromosomes located in the nucleus of a cell (Fig. 4.2). It is known that the human genome contains 3 billion nucleotides, which are encoding roughly 30,000 genes. Only a

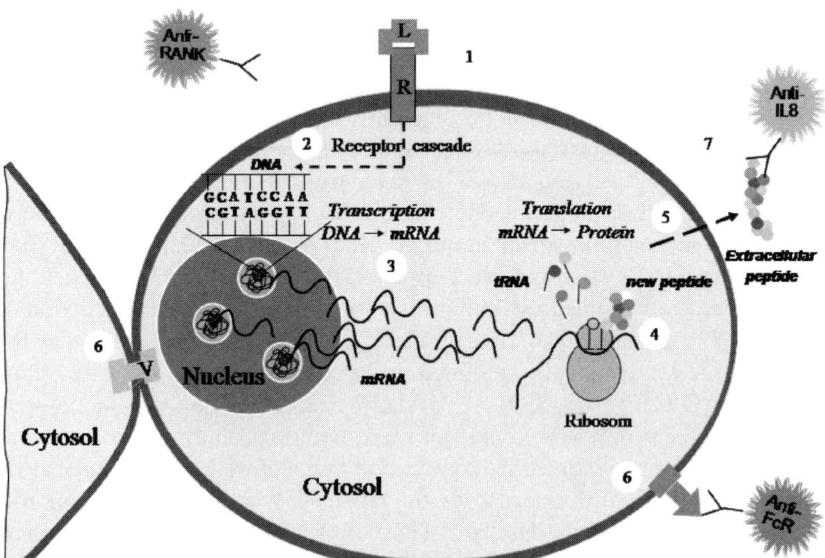

Fig. 4.2 (*1*) Cell with transmembrane receptor (e.g., RANK). (*2*) Receptor cascade for intracellular signal transduction with molecules such as TRAF6, c-Src, NF-κB, ERK, and MAPK traveling into the nucleus. (*3*) Molecules such as FOS, JUN, TRAP, and NFATs activate DNA transcription to mRNA. (*4*) Thereafter, mRNA leaves the nucleus through pores and goes into the cytosol, where it is taken up by ribosomes where the mRNA template is translated to proteins or polypeptides. Transfer RNA (tRNA) picks up amino acids, which are composed as determined by the mRNA template. (*5*) The new proteins or peptides are controlled by chaperones and are bonded by ubiquitin and destroyed in proteasomes (not shown), used intracellularly, or secreted. Alternatively, they can be used to build receptors (*6*) (e.g., FcR) or extracellular peptides and proteins (*7*). Molecules such as vinculin (*V*) and integrins attach the cell membrane to other cells (*See* Color Insert)

small portion of all genes is expressed temporarily. In one cell type there exists only a relatively small subset of proteins. The sum of proteins made or expressed in one cell is called the *proteome*. There are a number of genes encoding for proteins that are essential for normal cell structure and function (e.g., cell membrane, nucleus, nuclear membrane, cytoskeleton, signal pathways, energy metabolism, cell-cycle functions, and production of secretory proteins). These secreted substances build ECM, membranes (e.g., basal laminae), and tissues such as vessels, fasciae, nerves, skin, skeletal components including bones, cartilage, ligaments, and teeth. Cells and ECM can develop cooperating units.

Transcription is the process of copying the nucleotide sequence of single-stranded DNA segments into mRNA (Fig. 4.2). This process is located in the nucleus. The mRNA molecules leave the nucleus via its pores and reach ribosomes in the cytosol. There, triplet codons encode for definite amino acids. The sequence of amino acids in polypeptides and proteins differs according to information in the mRNA. Ribosomes are structures located outside the nucleus in the cytoplasm and at the endoplasmic reticulum (ergastoplasm). They build up peptides and proteins with the help of tRNA coupling with amino acids. Peptide or protein synthesis with the help of mRNA is termed *translation*. Mistakes in the sequence of amino acids and folding are controlled by chaperones. Wrongly composed or folded proteins are bonded by ubiquitin; they are split into proteasomes and deleted. Modern molecular biological analysis of physiological or pathological situations should include the simultaneous examination of genomic DNA sequences, gene expression studies by analysis of mRNA, and detection of existing proteins.

Analytical procedures are comparable for all three biological classes: screening to get an overview of the actual state or examination of individual candidates, which are known as *responsive markers*. For genome-wide screening on both nucleic acids (DNA, RNA), microarray technology (e.g., Affymetrix, FEBIT) [14, 15] or the more recent serial analysis of gene expression (SAGE) procedure [16] is used. Microarrays have become a standard tool in molecular biology has and have revolutionized genomics research. Microarrays are used extensively for profiling gene expression in many applications, including the discovery of gene function, drug evaluation and pathway dissection, classification of clinical samples, exon mapping, and investigation of splicing events. Arrays may be produced by deposition of presynthesized material or by in situ oligonucleotide synthesis [17]. Microarrays allow parallel analysis of up to 1 million target sequences in a single test. Microarrays are used for comparative studies.

Variations in DNA are mainly based on mutated sites or disease-relevant single-point mutations (SNPs). SNPs are detected by direct sequencing, a hybridization assay with solid phase arrays (DNA chips, blots), or an amplification test such as a real-time polymerase chain reaction (PCR) (TaqMan).

Differential gene expression is detected as down-regulation or up-regulation. Identification of differences in gene expression must be confirmed by single-marker tests. Confirmation of differential mRNA expression and turnover should be shown by simultaneous measurement of corresponding protein fractions. Proteomics examine the protein composition of cells and tissues or of body fluids such as blood or liquor. There are structural or viral proteins. Otherwise functional components such as antibodies or enzymes can also be determined by their specific reaction activity or function.

Peptidomics is study of the composition of short-length peptides in examined biological material; it is closely correlated to surrounding proteomics. Peptides by themselves are messengers like cytokines, hormones, or growth factors. Additionally, in a controlled manner, proteases degrade proteins to peptides in regulatory processes (prohormones) or for degradation and thereby produce traces of former proteosomes, which represent specific metabolic events in the cells or tissues. Applied methods for proteomics and peptidomics are comparable, with intrinsic advantages and drawbacks in both approaches.

In proteomics, the Western blot test (protein electrophoresis and subsequent blotting), immunoassays, and immunohistology are relevant techniques. The latter is used to identify a specific protein in a determined position (e.g., in an organ, tissue, or cell) or the adjacent ECM. For broad-band identification of proteins in patient samples (serum, liquor), protein or antibody arrays are used [18–22]. Antibody arrays are based on specific antibodies coupled to a solid phase. Studied protein preparations are incubated with these arrays, and immobilized antibodies bind complementary antigens. Subsequent binding of a second labeled antibody or direct labeling of protein in advance enables the final analysis of these arrays by a fluorescence scanner. The location of antibody–protein complexes identifies a specific protein that is bound to a known antibody. Such microarrays allow parallel analysis of up to 15,000 target proteins in one test. Microarrays are used for comparative studies.

The most interesting question regarding the interaction of bioactive materials with tissues and vice versa is related to released ions or particles from the implant surface and the change in the material by chemical species from the tissues. The role of these released chemical or physical species can be investigated to some extent by analysis of genomics, transcriptomics, and proteomics. The tools for this analysis are of a biochemical nature, as previously described. Apart from this biochemical analysis, determining the site in cells and tissue where the mentioned structures and processes are present is of utmost interest for a deeper understanding of the biomaterial's behavior. Conventional histological or cytological description of the substances and processes in cells and tissues is not enough. Structures and functions need to be quantified (e.g., using morphometry or other quantitative methods). Therefore, quantified morphological features with histology, including immunohistology, in situ hybridization, scanning electron microscopy (SEM), and transmission electron microscopy (TEM) increase our knowledge of cell and tissue behavior and contribute to the reliability of implanted biomaterials and devices. Some examples are given in the following sections. Detailed descriptions of conventional morphological methods for *in vitro* and *in vivo* evaluations applicable to thin CaP coatings are not described in this chapter because there are excellent publications on this subject [1–4].

4.2 Development of Bone Under Physiological Conditions Including Various Types of Bone

Normal embryonal and fetal development of bones follow a pattern during which stem cells are recruited and influenced by signaling pathways to differentiate and to express certain potentials hidden in the genome [23]. In this process, the human species uses some patterns of gene activation that are similarly operative in related mamalian species (Figs. 4.2, 4.3). The detection of these mechanisms comprises several levels: gene determination, gene activation, transcription of information into mRNA, translation of this message to the composition of proteins, quality control of protein structure, secretion of proteins, modification of secreted proteins extracellularly to form bone-specific ECM, and control the mechanisms of mineralization in highly specific areas of the ECM prepared to be mineralized [23, 24]. Some part of these processes can be observed by light microscopy. Changes in the surface structure can be detected by SEM [25]. Some more detailed structural information can be visualized by TEM [26]. Newer techniques allow visualization of highly specific changes in the phenotype of cells—e.g., in situ hybridization using complementary DNA [27, 28], immunohistochemistry using specific antibodies to identify specific proteins, electrophysiological techniques to identify transport mechanisms and the influence of cells on the way to developing into bone cells (i.e., osteoblasts and osteocytes) [29]. It is noteworthy that the development of bone (i.e., the skeleton) is influenced by systemic regulation of the body as well as by influences coming from the outside world (e.g., gravity, external load of the body including deformation). Influences come also from an internally regulated

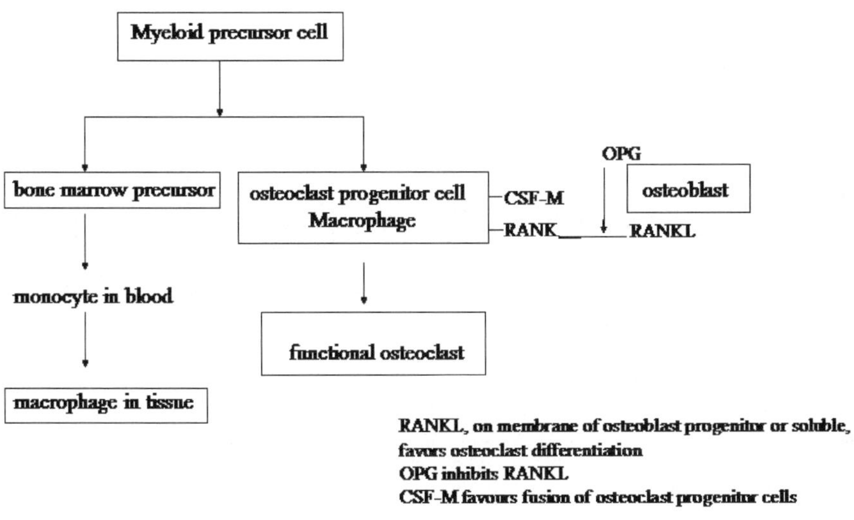

Fig. 4.3 Development of precursor cells to macrophages and osteoclasts

load (i.e., activity of muscles) and an artificial load, such as by implant systems. In the latter case, there is often an unusual and unphysiological load [30]. The regulation of bone structure and function is strongly influenced by the above-mentioned mechanisms and perhaps by unknown additional mechanisms.

4.2.1 Enchondral Ossification or Secondary Bone

The morphology of developing bone is described here because under pathological conditions (such as bone fracture or other bone injuries including surgical trauma) bone repair in some ways follows the patterns encountered during bone development [31]. Certain features of bone structure can be understood only when the developmental history of bone is known [32].

Early during embryonic development of an individual, bone anlagen display a phenotype of cells and ECM that are similar to cartilage, as depicted in Fig. 4.4, taken from embryo or fetus (body length not determinable because the material

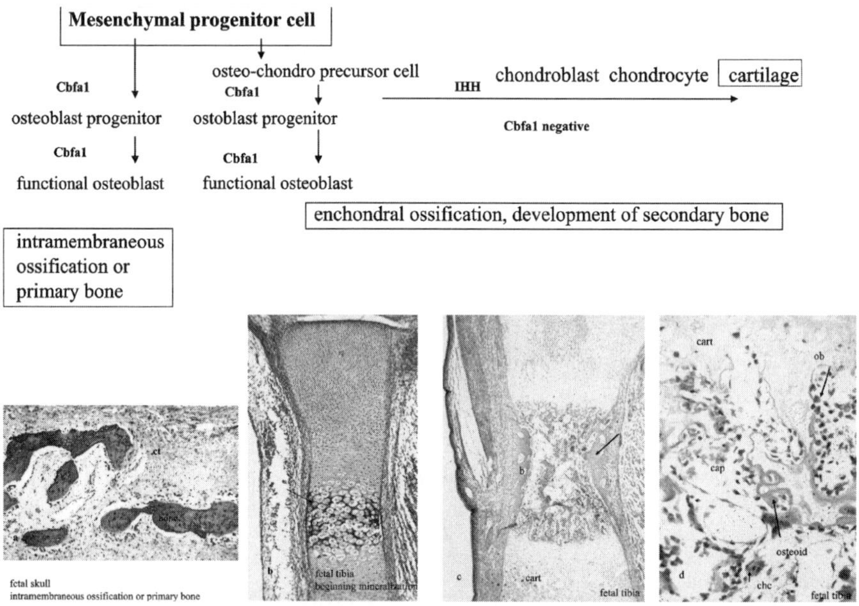

Fig. 4.4 Development of intramembraneous ossification, enchondral ossification, and cartilage. **a** Trabecular bone in connective tissue (*ct*) of the fetal skull. **b–d** Enchondral ossification of the fetal tibia. **b** In the middle of the tibia there is mineralized cartilage and bone (*b*) development. Later stages are seen in **c** and **d** with mineralized cartilage (*cart*), chondroclasts (*chc*), capillaries (*cap*), and osteoid covered by osteoblasts (*ob*). The various stages of bone and connective tissue differentiation can be observed during healing of fractured or surgically injured bone. Sections of tissue were formaldehyde-fixed, decalcified by EDTA, and stained with hemalaumn and eosin (*See* Color Insert)

was from abortions). Outside this bone anlagen there are anlagen of muscles, nerves, and other structures that are not dealt with in this study. At the edge of the bone anlage, the cells show another structure and other orientation as does the ECM. There, periosteal cells are not round but oval. In the center of the bone anlage, osteoblast precursors are more rounded and surrounded by cells resembling each other. In limb buds, this type of prebone structure can be observed some time longer than in the more centrally located bones of extremities (e.g., femur, tibia, humerus, radius, ulna). At a later stage, the mineralization of ECM between bone cell precursors can be seen beginning in the middle of these long bones and under a structure with elongated cells (periosteal cells) being oriented in parallel to the surface (Fig. 4.4b,c). The next step demonstrates sprouts of capillaries in and through the periosteal layer invading spaces in the mineralized part of the chondrocytic prebone, where these chondrocytes undergo apoptosis and dissolution, leaving spaces into which the capillaries develop (Fig. 4.4c,d). This setup of cell development and tissue formation continues in such a way that by the seventh to eighth week the center of the long bones is replaced by tissue with blood sinuses, increasing orientation of bone trabeculae in the compartment that is surrounded by cortical bone. Osteoblast progenitor cells and osteoblasts express the molecule Cbfa 1. Chondroblasts and chondrocytes do not express Cbfa 1.

Cartilage is still present in the proximal and distal ends of the long bones. Later, there are centers of bone development with trabecular bone structures in the proximal and distal epiphyses. Between these bone structures and the marrow cavity, a layer of cartilage is maintained. The proximal part contains proliferating chondroblasts that are arranged in columns displaying, from proximal to distal, increased differentation (i.e., growth of chondrocytes to big cell forms). Finally, these cells undergo apoptosis and autolysis, leaving some space whose walls are mineralized and into which capillaries sprout and osteoclasts and osteoblasts move in to build a highly ordered bone structure. This area represents the growth plate responsible for the growth of long bones in length and width. In the distal area above the epiphysis, there is another growth plate, with a proliferation zone facing the epiphysis; and below this cell layer are the above-mentioned zones of chondrocyte maturation and replacement by bone and bone marrow, as noted for the proximal zone.

4.2.2 *Intramembranous Ossification, Primary Bone, or Woven Bone*

The development of flat bones (e.g., in the skull) is, in principle, quite different. Mesenchymal cells, as precursors of osteoblasts, proliferate and transform into osteoblasts. They produce ECM that is characteristic for primary bone (i.e., collagen fibers in a woven arrangement). These fibers and the ECM between the fibers and osteoblasts are mineralized with the help of matrix vesicles. Matrix

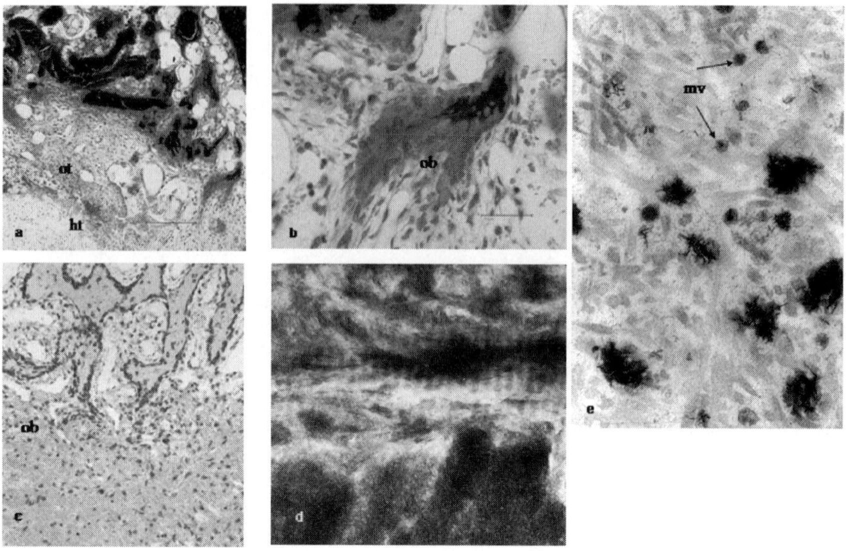

Fig. 4.5 Early stage of bone healing. **a** Seven days after operation, the edge of a drill hole, diameter 4 mm, is seen sagittally in the distal femur epiphysis of a Chinchilla rabbit with bone trabeculae; there are fragments of lamellar bone and new primary bone with the beginning of mineralization (*black areas*). Adjacent to the left lower corner is organization tissue (*ot*) with new capillaries in young fibrous tissue with macrophages degrading erythrocytes from the hematoma (*ht*). **b** At the same time, osteoblasts (*ob*) and some fibroblasts proliferate and mineralize the extracellular matrix (*ECM*) (*black areas*). **c** They express collagen Iα1 transcripts stained red (*dark areas*) by in situ hybridization and cover new bone trabeculae. These osteoblasts are derived from undifferentiated cells that are able to mineralize their ECM with the help of matrix vesicles (*mv*) shown in **e**. **d** Mineralized bone matrix is in continuity with compacted nanometer-sized apatite (organoapatite on the bottom) demonstrating bone bonding to artificial apatite, seen by TEM. Collagen spacing is 65 nm. **a, b** von Kossa & Paragon stain. **c** In situ hybridization with cDNA probe to detect collagen I α1. **d, e** TEM (*See* Color Insert)

vesicles are derived from osteoblasts, display a trilaminar membrane. and are filled during maturation with amorphous material—calcium—and at the inner part of the membrane with phosphate $[(PO_4)^{2-}]$ to form CaP crystals. The CaP crystals perforate the vesicular membrane and build clusters of apatite [33] (Fig. 4.5). The latter tend to coalesce to form calcifying fronts and thus represent the mineralized part of the primary bone.

Bone remodeling is the permanent reorganization (i.e., resorption and apposition according to the actual local biomechanical needs and under control of systemic hormonal and nutritional control) (Figs. 4.3, 4.5, 4.6) [34–36]. The process is primarily driven by osteoblasts, which are stimulated by parathyroid hormone (PTH). Activated osteoblasts express RANKL stimulating RANK receptors at the surface of osteoclast progenitor cells and macrophages for confluence to make functional osteoclasts. The inhibitory molecule for RANKL is osteoprotegerin

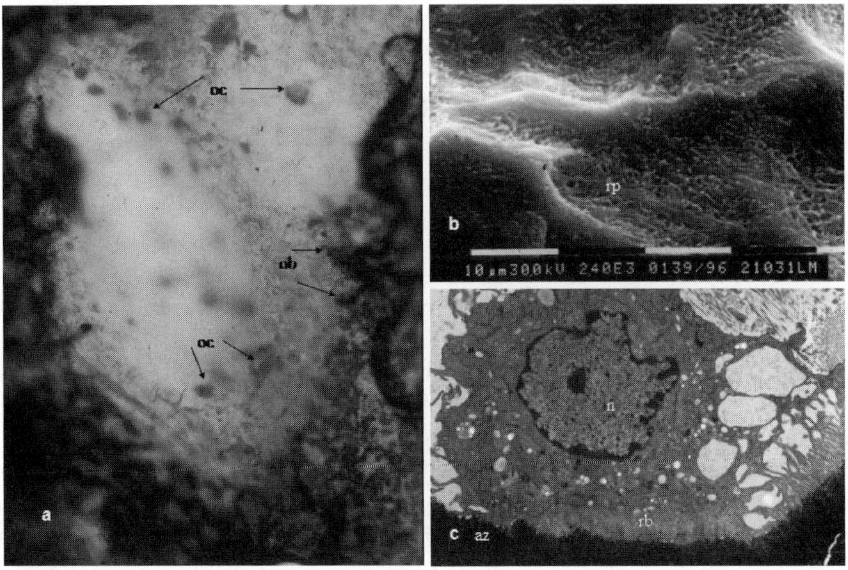

Fig. 4.6 **a** Internal surface of a Chinchilla rabbit humerus midshaft with a large resorption zone in the center and top of the bright area in which dot-like TRAP-positive cells, osteoclasts (*oc*), display projections contacting each other. In the right and left periphery and at the bottom, the black dotted area with osteoblasts (*ob*) positive for collagen Iα1 transcripts that were visualized using a radioactive method that shows black silver particles. Only a few areas are in focus owing to the curved surface of the diaphysis. The diameter of osteoclasts ranges up to 60 μm. **b** SEM view of the surface of the resorption zone with remnants of fibers interrupted by collagenase digestion in resorption pits (*rp*), indicating the surface morphology to which osteoblasts usually stick when they begin to attach for deposition of ECM of (lamellar) bone. **c** TEM view of a section through an osteoclast on top of organoapatite. At the periphery of the mineralized material is a zone of attachment (*az*) to the right lamellar structure of the ruffled border (*rb*), where the low pH of secreted protons dissolve mineral. At the center is one nucleus (*n*) and vacuoles (*See* Color Insert)

(OPG). Colony-stimulating factor for macrophages (CSF-M) plays a role in the fusion of macrophages to osteoclasts. The balance between bone apposition and bone resorption can be changed by various local and systemic factors that are described elsewhere [1–4]. Regarding implants, it is important to understand that unused (i.e., unloaded) bone is resorbed and disappears. Overloaded bone densifies owing to bone apposition to some extent.

When a fracture occurs (e.g., by massive unphysiological load or overload) or when the surgeon creates a defect in which to insert an implant, the continuity of bone is interrupted. At the fracture or operation site at least two fragments are found; and between them, owing to rupture of vessels and bleeding a hematoma develops (Fig. 4.5). Therefore, there are substances that are not supposed to be at the fracture site, especially blood components (e.g., platelets, erythrocytes, leukocytes, other blood cells). A description of all events at a fracture site is not possible here, but it can be understood that the various components influence the reaction at the fracture site. The unphysiological surfaces are covered by highly active cells, macrophages and osteoclasts, that can secrete or produce substances able to attract other cells. They prepare the fractured surfaces for osteoclastic resorption and bone apposition by osteoblasts. Apart from the possiblility that cells of mesenchymal origin develop into osteoblasts to form woven or primary bone, there is also the possibility that cartilage-like precursor of bone is developed from mesenchymal (stem) cells. This phenomenon is comparable to embryonic and fetal bone development in the various stages of secondary bone development. Bone surfaces and fragments of bone with living or dead osteocytes play an important role insofar as precursors of osteoblasts prefer to settle at these surfaces and to differentiate into osteoblasts and osteocytes. This differentiation is mediated by substances that are liberated at the exposed fractured surfaces and are attributed to bone matrix proteins, as first described by Reddi [37].

Morphologically comparable phenomena can be seen at surfaces of implanted materials (e.g., bioglasses and glass ceramics) (Fig. 4.7), calcium phosphates, calcium carbonates, and other implant materials that are known

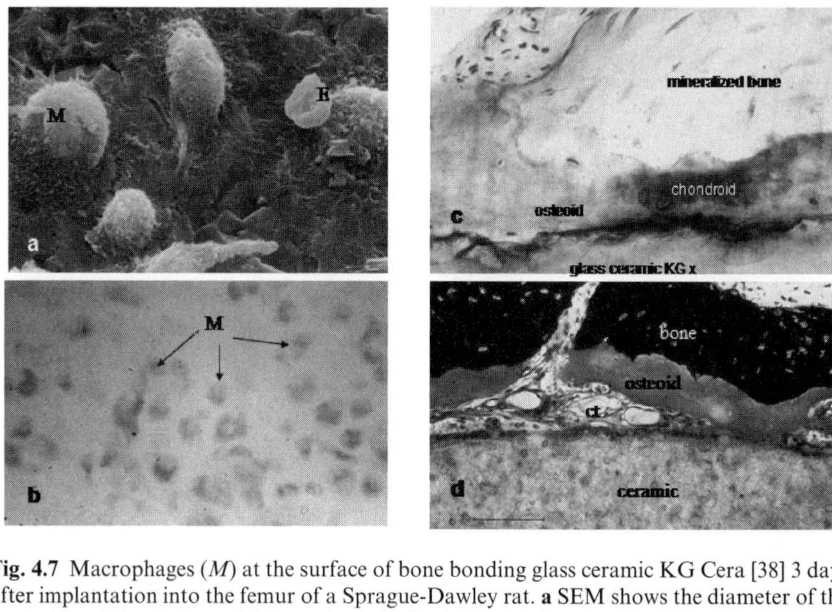

Fig. 4.7 Macrophages (*M*) at the surface of bone bonding glass ceramic KG Cera [38] 3 days after implantation into the femur of a Sprague-Dawley rat. **a** SEM shows the diameter of the erythrocyte (*E*) to be 7 μm. **b** Macrophages stained for acid phosphatase with red signal (*dark*). Macrophage diameters are 10–20 μm. **c** Inhibition of mineralization at the interface of glass ceramic KGx 245 days after implantation in the diaphysis of the rat femur. KGx contains (in wt%) SiO_2 34, $Ca(PO_3)_2$ 12, Na_2O 3.5, CaO 23, Al_2O_3 15, Ta_2O_5 12.5 [38]. Sawn section. Giemsa stain. **d** Inhibition of mineralization with a broad zone of osteoid and connective tissue (*ct*) at the surface and surrounding calcium zirconium phosphate [$CaTi_xZr_{4-x}(PO_4)_6$ with $x = 0$–4] 84 days after implantation into the distal Chinchilla femur epiphysis. Sawn section. Von Kossa & Paragon stain. *Bar* = 100 μm (*See* Color Insert)

to be biocompatible and osteoconductive [38–40]. Furthermore, it was demonstrated that some compositions are able to induce bone in nonosseous sites (e.g., in muscle). The surface structure of these materials plays a key role [41] in this bone induction.

It was demonstrated how the microstructure of resorption pits is organized [35] and that the structure itself (Fig. 4.6b) is able to influence osteocyte precursors to attach, differentiate, and secrete specific noncollagenous proteins and collagen. It was furthermore demonstrated that it can alleviate mineralization of the fibers and the interfiber space with apatite. The mineralization of ECM was taken as a template for the development of simulated body fluid [42].

Molecular biology provides methods, findings, and explanations that have to be applied to the interpretation of cellular and tissue reactions as known from histology and cytology. It is expected that these new methods can contribute to better interpretation of existing implants and their outcome. It is also expected that they can help predict thc behavior of new materials intended to be used as biomaterials for implantation and in extracorporeal devices.

There have been attempts (1) to analyze gene activation (i.e., DNA up- or-down-regulation using a microarray technique); (2) follow the path of transcription and analyze mRNA (transcriptome) after reverse transcription for production of cDNA (complementary DNA); and (3) control translation (i.e., the structure and function of proteins—proteome— intracellularly and extracellularly). There have also been studies of cluster analysis and gene expression profiles using cDNA microarray systems. An example compares human dental pulp stem cells with human mesenchymal stem cells for tissue engineering and for understanding biomaterials' interactions [43].

4.3 *In Vitro* Evaluation of CaP Coatings

The *in vitro* testing of biomaterial surfaces using cell culture systems renders some information that mostly presents highly specific answers. Because there are no generally accepted standards regarding the biological potential of cells, their status (e.g., number of passages), and other parameters, the results are hardly comparable. Nevertheless, some conclusions can be drawn from such experiments, as shown in Table 4.1.

Investigations exist with cell lines that can be considered to give more reliable results than using primary cells. However, cell lines usually are cell systems derived from tumors or represent immortalized cells that have gained some defects in the control of cell cycles, cell multiplication, regulation of metabolism, and potential to differentiate. Therefore, even with good and statistically convincing results, investigations with tumor cell lines must be interpreted with caution.

Usually the proliferation of cells in culture and on the surface of biomaterials is interpreted as something good and convincing in favor of a working

Table 4.1 Selected *in vitro* studies on calcium phosphate coatings

In vitro cell culture conditions, cell line, material	Objectives	Results	Reference
Mouse preosteoblast MC3T3-E1. Wet chemical precipitation, poorly crystalline calcium phosphate apatite crystals (PCA) on TCPS or glass	Cell proliferation, cell cycle, cell attachment, cell signaling pathway	Decreased cell proliferation, entry in S-phase of cell cycle delayed, reduced cell attachment, impaired signal transduction	Lee et al. Biomaterials, 27, 2006, 3738–3744
Human osteoblast-like cells from patients. Magnetron co-sputtering of silicon containing hydroxyapatite (HA), as deposited or heat-treated to increase crystallinity on titanium	Cell attachment, cell growth up to 56 days	Highest cell growth and mineralization on heat treated Si-HA films	Thian et al. Biomaterials, 26, 2005, 2947–2956
Human primary osteoblasts on octacalcium phosphate (OCP) and Mn-doped carbonate HA Mn-CHA) on titanium substrate by pulsed laser deposition (PLD)	Proliferation, viability, alkaline phosphatase activity, TGFß	Good proliferation, and viability, alkaline phosphatase higher than in control Ti, TGFß low at 3 and 7 days but higher at 14 and 21 days	Bigi et al. Biomaterials, 26, 2005, 2381–2389
Human fetal osteoblast cell line (hfob), and fibroblasts, on octacalcium phosphate thin film by pulsed UV laser deposition (PLD)	Cell proliferation, DNA replication, apoptosis, cell morphology, cell adhesion	Fibroblasts and osteoblasts adhere, normal morphology and proliferation, no signs of toxicity	Socol et al. Biomaterials, 25, 2004, 2539–2545
Osteoblasts cell line MC3T3-E1 or primary rat calvarial osteoblasts on poorly crystalline calcium phosphate apatite crystals (PCA) wet chemical from supersaturated solution on TCPS	Osteoblastic cells adhesion, proliferation, expression of gene markers, calcification	Attachment, proliferation, expression of gene markers, calcified matrix present	Hong et al. Biomaterials, 24, 2003, 2977–2984

(continued)

Table 4.1 (continued)

In vitro cell culture conditions, cell line, material	Objectives	Results	Reference
C3T3-E1 preosteoblasts on conventional apatite, precursor apatite spheres, large plate-like apatite (LPA), Small plate-like apatite (SPA), TCPS, biomimetic from SBF 1×, 1.5×, and 5×	Different apatite in microenvironment on preosteoblast spreading, viability, proliferation, gene expression	After 4 or 14 days TCPS was best for cell proliferation; apatite inhibited cell growth. LPA was best for osteocalcin, bone sialoprotein, and osteopontin expression	Chou et al. Biomaterials, 26 (2005) 285–295
Rat bone marrow cells. Calcium phosphate on Ti6Al4V by electrostatic spray deposition (ESD) or radiofrequency magnetron sputter coating (rf-msc). Thickness of coatings 2 μm each	Two experiments with sixfold samples. Cell proliferation 4, 8, and 14 days, ng DNA for proliferation, alkaline phosphatase, osteocalcin, RT-PCR mRNA collagen I and osteocalcin—SEM	Cell proliferation different in 1st and 2nd run. Cells confluent on both substrates with ECM and mineralized globules. Slight differences for alkaline phosphatase and osteocalcin between coatings	Siebers et al. Biomaterials 25 (2004) 2019–2027

TGFβ, transforming growth factor-β; UV, ultraviolet; TCPS, tissue culture polystyrene; Si-HA, silicon-substituted hydroxyapatite; RT-PCR, reverse transcription polymerase chain reaction; ECM, extracellular matrix; SEM, scanning electron microscopy hypothesis. Nevertheless, it must be pointed out that this positive outcome is a small nail to pin down a working hypothesis. Because *in vivo* there are many cell types cooperating in certain environments and at a determined time, the predictions can be erroneous. Furthermore, *in vivo* the turnover of the interstitial fluid plays an important role for the accumulation or dilution of substances. This influence cannot be simulated appropriately in conventional tissue culture conditions.

In many cases, the characterization of surfaces coated with calcium phosphates is not comparable. In many publications the figures show different roughness, structure of the surface (e.g., some polished smooth surfaces, surfaces resembling hobnails, displaying clefts at grain boundaries, openings to microporous structures below the main surface), needle-like crystals, plate-like crystals, and amorphous areas at which shear forces can hardly resist. This variety in surface structure is enlarged by variations in chemical composition and solubility of components that are partially related to the variations in crystallinity.

Apparently, the technique of coating influences the various mentioned parameters. It is not the task of this chapter to deal with coating techniques in detail (for this see Chapters 3, 4 and 6); it should be mentioned, however, that in the cited publications (Tables 4.1, 4.2) there are biomimetic calcium phosphate deposition (e.g. using simulated body fluid), wet chemical techniques with precipitation from supersaturated solution, magnetron co-sputtering, and subsequent heat treatment to increase crystallinity, pulsed laser deposition, electrostatic spray deposition, radiofrequency magnetron sputter coating, and additional heat treatment or surface modification by grinding or polishing. Therefore, it is not astonishing that the results of most of the publications cannot be compared. Nevertheless, some papers are mentioned.

The mouse preosteoblast MC3T3-E1cells were cultured on poorly crystalline calcium phosphate apatite (PCA) and compared to the behavior on tissue culture polystyrene or uncoated glass coverslips for up to 6 days. MC3T3-E1 cells on PCA displayed reduced proliferation, delayed cell cycle progression, underdeveloped stress fiber and tubulin expression, reduced focal adhesion, and decreased activation of tyrosine receptor (RTK)-Ras–extracellular signal-regulated kinase (ERK). Therefore, it was assumed that weak adhesion and reduced signaling was responsible for the reduced proliferation of MC3T3-E1 cells on PCA [44].

Human osteoblast-like cells from hip bone were cultured on: (1) pure titanium; (2) 0.8% silicon containing hydroxyapatite (Si-HA) as deposited by Magnetron co-sputtering; (3) 0.8% Si-HA heat treated at 700°C for 3 hours, thickness of the coating 600 nm. Time for culture was up to 56 days. The heat-treated Si-HA stimulated cell growth, deposition of ECM, attachment of cells to the substratum as shown by vinculin attachment points, and development of cytoskeleton shown by actin and deposition of calcium phosphate in the ECM [45].

Table 4.2 Selected *in vivo* studies on calcium phosphate coatings

In vivo animal species implantation site	Materials	Results	Reference
New Zealand white rabbits, femoral condyles—9 days	Implants of Ti6Al4V with two or three layers of beads coated with either inorganic or organic route carbonated HA thin films (1 μm). Uncoated implants for control	Both HA coatings enhanced early bone ingrowth and fixation versus uncoated implants	Gan et al. Biomaterials, 25, 2004, 5313–5321
New Zealand white rabbits, tibia—2 weeks	Porous Ti6Al4V, thin calcium phosphate sol-gel coating (1 μm) versus uncoated surfaces, morphometry	Coated implants display faster bone ingrowth and more bone, more complete fill of the pores	Nguyen et al. Biomaterials, 25, 2004, 865–876
New Zealand white rabbits, back—1, 4, 8, 12 weeks	0.1, 1.0, 4.0 μm CaP on TiO_2 discs, RF magnetron-sputtered Heat treatment at present and up to 4 weeks	After 1 week, 0.1 and 1.0 μm CaP disappeared. Amorphous CaP (4 μm) replaced by O_3-apatite	Wolke et al. Biomaterials, 24, 2003, 2623–2629
Texcel X continental sheep, femoral condyle—6 and 12 weeks	Pure HA Si-HA 0.8 and 1.5 wt% Si Granules and powders, no coating	SEM, high-resolution TEM HA voids after 12 weeks 1.5 wt% Si-HA > 0.8 wt% Si-HA > HA dissolution, Si increases bioactivity of HA	Porer et al. Biomaterials 24, 2003, 4609–4620
Sprague-Dawley rats, medullary cavity of the femur—7, 28, 56 days	Titanium Kirschner wire, diameter 1.4 mm, sandblasted and electrochemically coated with HA, thickness of the coating 2 μm	Coated material shear strength 27 MPa, uncoated 8 MPa. Histomorphometry HAp-coated bone implant contact 68%, uncoated 26%	Schmidmaier et al. J. Biomed. Mater. Res B (Appl. Biomater.) 63, 2002, 168–172
Beagle dogs HA coated dental implants in the mandible—3 and 15 weeks	Dental implants, plasma spraying, controls calcitite coating with 10% soluble phases versus heat-treated 95% crystalline HA coating	Less direct bone apposition at surfaces with high crystalline coating and less pullout forces for high crystalline coatings. Macrophages with HA particles at fibrous interfaces	Burgess et al. Clin. Oral Implant. Res. 10, 1999, 257–266

(continued)

Table 4.2 (continued)

In vivo animal species implantation site	Materials	Results	Reference
Male Japanese white rabbit tibia—4, 8, 16 weeks	Ceria stabilized tetragonal zirconia alumina, four surface preparations: (a) Uncoated polished (b) Uncoated microporous (c) Submicron HA-coated microporous with SBF (d) 4 μm HA-coated microporous with SBF	Best results in detachment test > 25 N failure load for (d) and (c) Bone-bonding ability for (d) and (c)	Takemoto et al. J. Biomed. Mater. Res. A 78, 2006, 693–701

Human primary osteoblasts, donated by patients, were expanded and cultured on three substrates and tissue culture polystyrene. Pulsed laser deposition of octacalcium phosphate (OCP) or Mn doped (0.55%), carbonate (5%), or HA (Mn-CHA) was done. The thickness of the coatings was about 800 nm for Mn-CHA and 1 μm for OCP. The surfaces were slightly different in surface roughness and morphology. Proliferation of osteoblasts was best on Mn-CHA and OCP, as was the development of alkaline phosphatase and collagen type I up to 21 days. Transforming growth factor-β1 (TGFß1) level was highest for Mn-CHA and a little less for OCP after 14 and 21 days of culture. The presence of TGFß1 indicated stimulation of growth and differentiation of osteoblasts [46].

Human fetal osteoblast-like cell line (hFOB 1.19) and murine fibroblast cell line L929 were cultured on Si wafers or titanium (Ti, polished or etched) that had been coated with OCP by pulsed UV laser deposition. No differences were found for adhesion of hFOB between control tissue culture polystyrene (TCPS), Ti, and OCP but lower hFOB on OCP compared with TCPS; there were no differences with uncoated Ti. DNA replication and caspase-1 activity of hFOB were not affected by the materials. It was concluded that after 3 days L929 fibroblasts and hFOB adhere with normal morphology, proliferate, and remain viable on OCP coatings [47].

In an additional study, poorly crystalline calcium phosphate apatite crystals (PCA) were formed at low temperature by precipitation on TCPS, giving some granular structure and a rather smooth surface. For up to 25 days, primary rat calvaria osteoblasts and MC3T3-E1 osteoblasts were cultured on the PCA thin film on TCPS or on the culture dish material (control). After 1 hour there were more cells attached to the PCA surfaces compared to TCPS. However, after 3 and 6 days there was statistically no difference between PCA and TCPS.

Both cell types expressed alkaline phosphatase. Calcification nodules developed with calvarial and MC3T3-E1 cells. There were more nodules at the surface of PCA with osteocalcin than on TCPS. MC3T3-E1 cells expressed osteoblast marker genes such as alkaline phosphatase, osteocalcin, ostconectin, and osteopontin [48].

These *in vitro* studies and others mentioned in Table 4.1 [49] were mainly performed using osteoblast-like cells or cells with some ability to express features of osteoblasts. The rationale for this procedure is to some extent unclear as the first cells that control a foreign surface are not osteoblasts but macrophages. Therefore, it would be much more realistic if the primary reactions of macrophages were studied. There are two arguments in this context: (1) According to the rule elaborated in 1969 by Frost [34], the sequence of events in bone remodeling comprises (a) activation, (b) resorption, and (3) formation—the so-called ARF rule. (2) In Fig. 4.7a,b, the early phase of a cellular reaction to an implant can be seen: the appearance of macrophages. In the presented case, macrophages are on the surface of bone bonding glass ceramic (Ceravital). The question arises as to why these macrophages appear after 3 days postoperatively and disappear and leave room for ostcoblasts after less than 7 days? Do they move away, or do they disappear owing to apoptosis? Do they leave remnants of cell membrane, receptors of cell organelles at the surface, to condition the ground for osteoblasts or fibroblasts? There is impressive documentation of osteoclast activity at the surface of implants at an early stage after implantation and even later, as well as *in vitro* coupling of resorption and formation [25, 35].

Thin CaP coatings on metals, alloys, and polymers (e.g., TCPS, glass) show better osteoblast growth (i.e., more viable cells) than uncoated substrates (Table 4.1). There is, however, one exception: When the coating displays poorly crystalline calcium phosphate, cell proliferation is reduced, the cell cycle phase is delayed, and cell attachment and signal transduction are impaired [44]. Other coatings with less amorphous phases display positive results (i.e., increased cell proliferation and differentiation). One important parameter might be a sufficiently stable ground for cells. It seems that osteoblasts need some firm ground on which to attach and to express stress fibers of actin. Up to now it has been unclear whether the amorphous calcium phosphate areas attract more and more active macrophages or resorbing multinuclear cells (osteoclasts or mineraloclasts).

Some *in vitro* studies (Table 4.1) [49, 50] with thin CaP coatings controlled the expression of proteins or substances that are known to be features of the osteoblast lineage, such as alkaline phosphatase, osteocalcin, osteonectin, bone sialoprotein, osteopontin, collagen I. These markers and mineralizing nodules are basic for an acceptable coating intended for clinical studies or application in human patients. The question arises, however, whether this expression of osteoblast markers predicts early bone bonding and the load-bearing ability of the coated material in a specific implantation site. The current conclusion is that this question cannot be answered on the basis of *in vitro* tests with osteoblasts. It would be necessary to investigate more, prognostically relevant cell lines that contribute to tissue formation at the interface of coated implants. It should be determined which genes are activated in what cells when substances are released from coatings. When a bone fracture or a surgical bone trauma is healing, the release of material from the coating layer should interfere positively, not negatively, with differentiation of the cells. A positive step in this direction was published [51]. The release of ions from the coating acted beneficially for the adhesion and development of osteoblasts [51]. It was found that the release of Mg and carbonated HA coated on Ti6Al4V up-regulated key intracellular signaling proteins (Shc, Ras/Mapkinase pathway, c-fos) in human bone-derived cells (HBDCs) and that attachment and differentiation of HBDC was stimulated. Results from those investigations can improve the guidelines for manufacture of second-generation biomaterials in this field.

There are other thin CaP coatings that were doped with molecules other than just calcium and phosphate (e.g., silicon, Mn-doped carbonate apatite, octacalcium phosphate, structured apatite with small or large plate-like apatite). Interestingly there are also reports on inhibitory effects of released material from coatings (Table 4.1).

4.4 In Vivo Evaluation of Thin CaP Coatings

It was shown in numerous experiments by Kokubo [42] and his group as well as by other, much earlier investigators (Hench, Jarcho, de Groot) [6, 52, 53] that surfaces covered with precipitates of HA by exposure to simulated body fluid or other coating techniques as well as solids containing apatite favor the development of bone when implanted in tissue, especially in a bony implantation site. The question arises about the principle of this process, induced and enhanced by the deposition of HA on implant surfaces. Porter et al. [54] demonstrated, in addition to what was known and derived from Hench's experiments, that silicon-doped HA particles in the condyles of sheep favor the deposition of apatite (i.e., mineralization of ECM). Degradation of the Si- substituted or Si-doped HA at the surface produced imperfections in the material's structure; and after dissolution of the silicon to the surroundings, the fine structure of the voids enhanced the deposition of HA and of bone. There are other examples in which the leaching of substances from the implanted material inhibited the mineralization of the prebone to mineralized bone [38]. The responsible chemical species for this inhibition of mineralization were oxides of Al, Ta, Ti, Sb, and Zr. Examples are depicted in Fig. 4.7c,d. The molecular mechanism of this inhibition of mineralization has not yet been completely elucidated.

Insofar as there are similarities in the acceptance of implant surfaces regarding *in vitro* and *in vivo* studies, some basic information on animal experiments is presented in Table 4.2 [54–63]. The spectrum of animals used in pertinent experiments is rather small. There were mainly rats, rabbits, dogs, goats, and sheep. The authors of the experiments usually investigated one animal species to judge the material's chemistry and physics when they want to apply it as a therapeutic tool in human patients.

Whereas in earlier experiments the implantation time was considered to be as long as months and preferentially years, more recent experiments considered mainly short-term tests. An example was already mentioned in Table 4.2: Gan and Pilliar [55] used porous Ti6Al4V conical cylinders or cylinders with two to three layers of metal beads displaying interconnecting pores that were left uncoated (for a control) or with an inorganic or organic route CaP coating for only 9 days in distal epiphyses of rabbits. The average thickness of the coating was 1 μm [55]. These implants were loaded in pullout tests to determine the interfacial bonding strength. There was no significant difference between inorganic and organic route CaP coatings, although statistically there was a significant difference between coated versus uncoated specimens. It must be assumed that after 9 days the mineralization of new bone cannot be as dense as possible and that therefore the maximum possible mechanical fixation of the coated porous implants was not yet reached. The organic and inorganic route CaP coatings proved strong enough to withstand mostly the loads and especially the shear forces of the pullout tests. There was only separation between coating layer and metallic substrate at the outermost regions of the sintered particles. Good attachment of the CaP coating could be expected from the evaluation of the interface strength measurements [56–58]. The authors did not report on osteoclastic resorption of the coating. Moreover, they considered the long-term stability of the calcium phosphate coating as a minor problem because the implant stability was maintained by bone ingrowth into the porous layer. The primary purpose of the coating was to provide an early boost in the initial healing response (i.e., to promote osteoconductivity).

Another study [59] with 0.1, 1.0, and 4.0 μm thick radiofrequency (RF) magnetron-sputtered CaP coatings on roughened titanium implants described the disappearance of the CaP thin coatings depending on the thickness—the 0.1 and 1.0 μm thick coatings having been dissolved after 1 week and the presence of other phases after a short 30 seconds, with heat treatment of 425° to 475°C with crystalline and amorphous phases and OCP. The 4 μm thick coatings showed apatite and amorphous phases after heat treatment. The latter coatings were still found partially after 8 and 12 weeks. The surroundings of the implanted disks in the back of rabbits displayed an inflammatory response after 1 week, with a decline in the number of inflammatory cells and development of a fibrous capsule after 8 and 12 weeks [59]. How the coating was lost was not mentioned, and especially there is no information on the question of chemical dissolution of the CaP coating or the interference with resorbing cells (i.e., osteoclasts or mineraloclasts). The mechanism of mineral absorption or resorption connected with the activity of cells was described for hot isostatic pressed HA that was implanted into the femur of rabbits [60].

The incorporation of silicate into HA has been shown [54] to increase significantly the rate of bone apposition to HA bioceramic implants. This was proven in an experiment in which 0.8 or 1.5 wt% Si-HA particles were implanted into the femoral condyles of 2- to 3-year-old Texcel X Continental sheep and explanted after 6 and 12 weeks. Controls did not contain Si in the HA. TEM revealed focal dissolution of the material in the order of 1.5 wt% SiHA > 0.8 wt% Si-HA > pure HA , suggesting that silicate ions increase the solubility of the HA. This increased solubility and the corresponding defects increase the apposition of bone to these bioceramics. It seems that this principle has not yet been introduced to new thin CaP coatings.

Pure titanium rods were coated 2 μm thick with HA in an electrochemical process [61]. They were implanted in the femur medullary cavity of Sprague-Dawley rats and biomechanically tested versus uncoated titanium wire [61]. The coated rods revealed a more than threefold increase in shear strength. This corresponded in some respect to the 2.6-fold increase of bone–implant contact. The follow-up intervals of the experiment were only 7, 28, and 56 days after implantation. Therefore, the long-term results of the thin coating, thickness 2 μm, are still awaited, considering this experiment.

There are arguments in favor of thin CaP coatings based on an experiment in which pulsed laser deposition (PLD) of HA was compared with plasma spraying (PS) [62]. The titanium rods were grit-blasted or additionally HA coated using PLD or PS. The rods were implanted in the tibias of rabbits and harvested

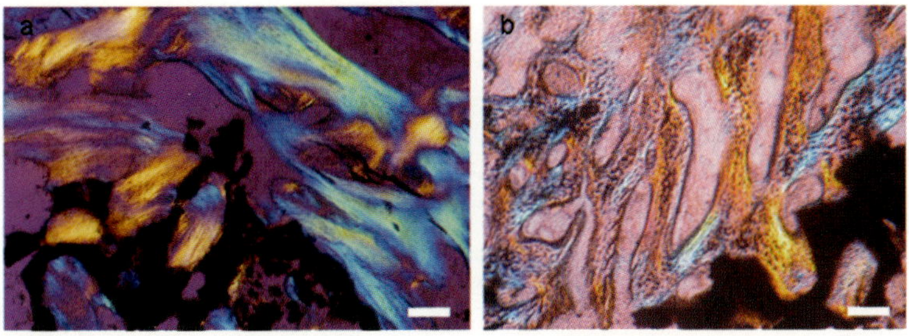

Chapter 2, Fig. 5 Polarized light micrographs of human biopsy harvested (**a**) 4 months and (**b**) 1 year after spinal arthrodesis using macro/micro porous biphasic calcium phosphate (MBCP) ceramic. Lamellar bone with osteocytes and Haversian systems have formed in contact with the residual MBCP (*black areas*). *Bar* = 500 μm

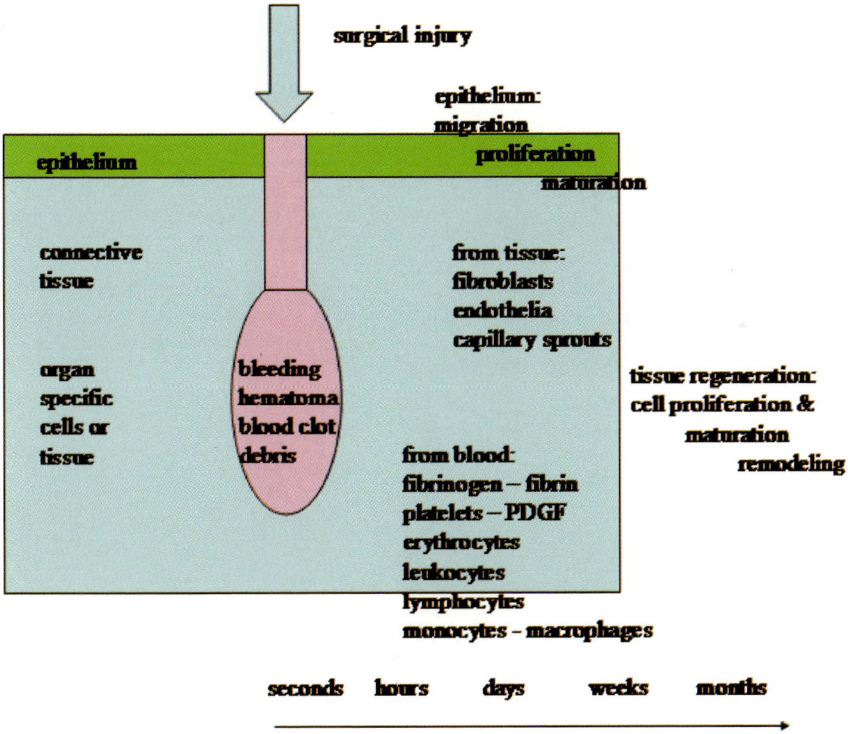

Chapter 4, Fig. 1 Main events after surgical injury and wound healing as a function of time. *PDGF*, platelet-derived growth factor

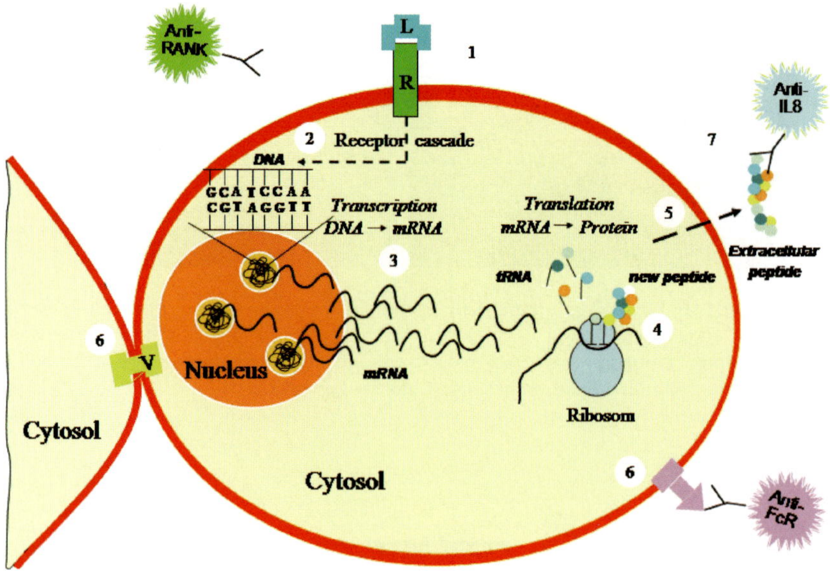

Chapter 4, Fig. 2 (*1*) Cell with transmembrane receptor (e.g., RANK). (*2*) Receptor cascade for intracellular signal transduction with molecules such as TRAF6, c-Src, NF-κB, ERK, and MAPK traveling into the nucleus. (*3*) Molecules such as FOS, JUN, TRAP, and NFATs activate DNA transcription to mRNA. (*4*) Thereafter, mRNA leaves the nucleus through pores and goes into the cytosol, where it is taken up at ribosomes where the mRNA template is translated to proteins or polypeptides. Transfer RNA (tRNA) picks up amino acids, which are composed as determined by the mRNA template. (*5*) The new proteins or peptides are controlled by chaperones and are bonded by ubiquitin and destroyed in proteasomes (not shown), used intracellularly, or secreted. Alternatively, they can be used to build receptors (*6*) (e.g., FcR) or extracellular peptides and proteins (*7*). Molecules such as vinculin (*V*) and integrins attach the cell membrane to other cells

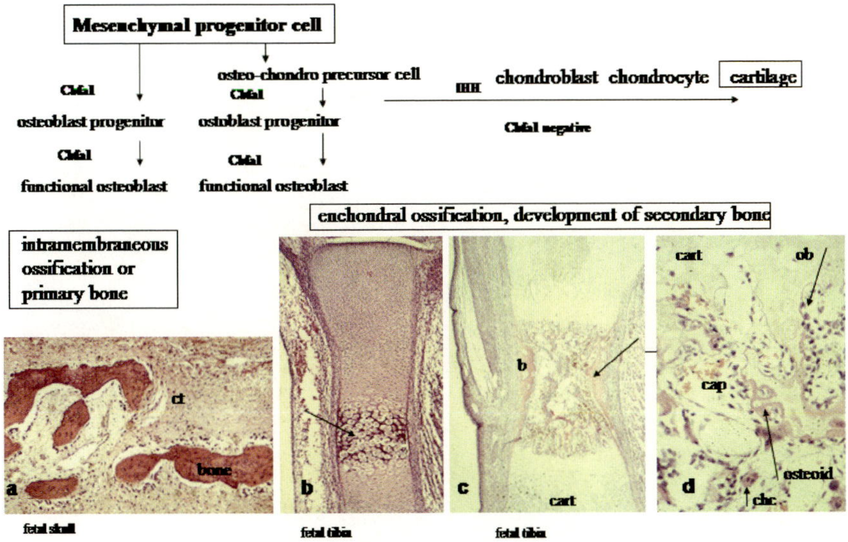

Chapter 4, Fig. 4 Development of intramembranous ossification, enchondral ossification, and cartilage. **a** Trabecular bone in connective tissue (*ct*) of the fetal skull. **b–d** Enchondral ossification of the fetal tibia. **b** In the middle of the tibia there is mineralized cartilage and bone (*b*) development. Later stages are seen in **c** and **d** with mineralized cartilage (*cart*), chondroclasts (*chc*), capillaries (*cap*), and osteoid covered by osteoblasts (*ob*). The various stages of bone and connective tissue differentiation can be observed during healing of fractured or surgically injured bone. Sections of tissue were formaldehyde-fixed, decalcified by EDTA, and stained with hemalaumn and eosin

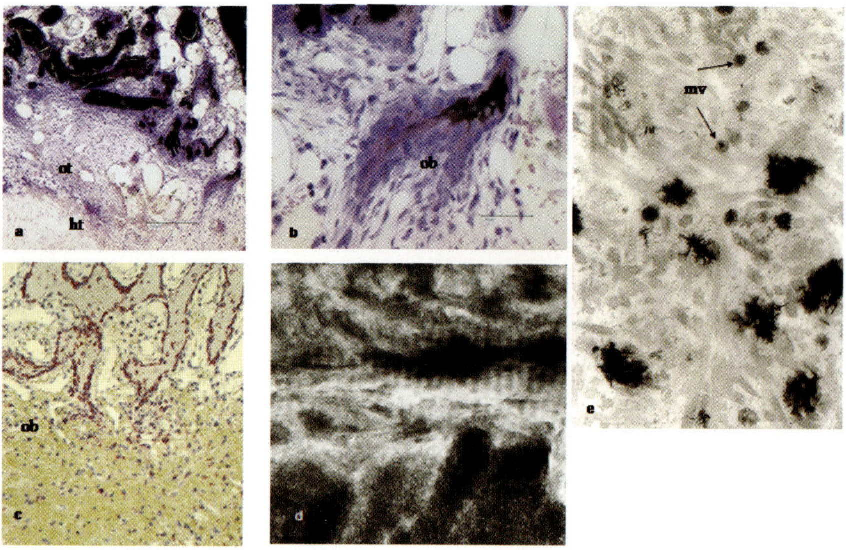

Chapter 4, Fig. 5 Early stage of bone healing. **a** Seven days after operation, the edge of a drill hole, diameter 4 mm, is seen sagittally in the distal femur epiphysis of a Chinchilla rabbit with bone trabeculae; there are fragments of lamellar bone and new primary bone with the beginning of mineralization (*black areas*). Adjacent to the left lower corner is organization tissue (*ot*) with new capillaries in young fibrous tissue with macrophages degrading erythrocytes from the hematoma (*ht*). **b** At the same time, osteoblasts (*ob*) and some fibroblasts proliferate and mineralize the extracellular matrix (*ECM*) (*black areas*). **c** They express collagen Iα1 transcripts stained red (*dark areas*) by in situ hybridization and cover new bone trabeculae. These osteoblasts are derived from undifferentiated cells that are able to mineralize their ECM with the help of matrix vesicles (*mv*) shown in **e**. **d** Mineralized bone matrix is in continuity with compacted nanometer-sized apatite (organoapatite on the bottom) demonstrating bone bonding to artificial apatite, seen by TEM. Collagen spacing is 65 nm. **a, b** von Kossa & Paragon stain. **c** In situ hybridization with cDNA probe to detect collagen I α1. **d, e** TEM

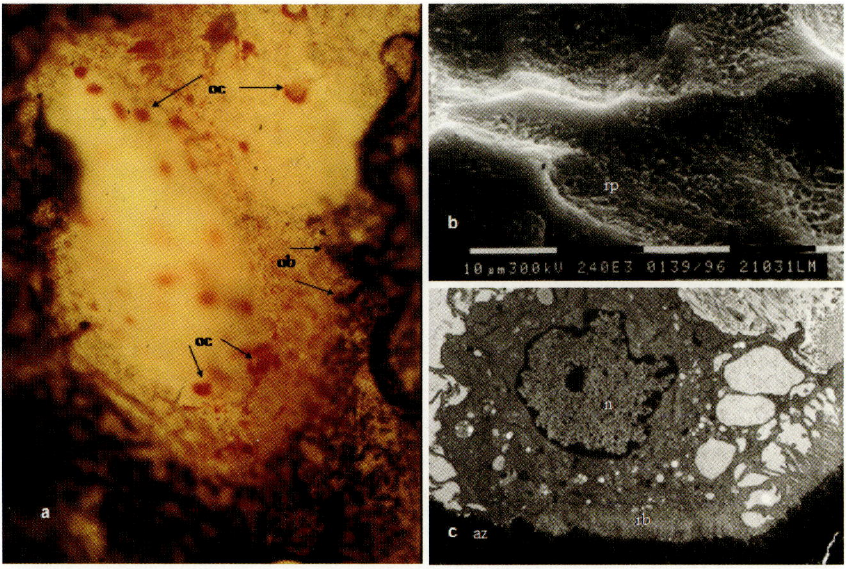

Chapter 4, Fig. 6 **a** Internal surface of a Chinchilla rabbit humerus midshaft with a large resorption zone in the center and top of the bright area in which dot-like TRAP-positive cells, osteoclasts (*oc*), display projections contacting each other. In the right and left periphery and at the bottom, the black dotted area with osteoblasts (*ob*) positive for collagen Iα1 transcripts that were visualized using a radioactive method that shows black silver particles. Only a few areas are in focus owing to the curved surface of the diaphysis. The diameter of osteoclasts ranges up to 60 μm. **b** SEM view of the surface of the resorption zone with remnants of fibers interrupted by collagenase digestion in resorption pits (*rp*), indicating the surface morphology to which osteoblasts usually stick when they begin to attach for deposition of ECM of (lamellar) bone. **c** TEM view of a section through an osteoclast on top of organoapatite. At the periphery of the mineralized material is a zone of attachment (*az*) to the right lamellar structure of the ruffled border (*rb*), where the low pH of secreted protons dissolve mineral. At the center is one nucleus (*n*) and vacuoles

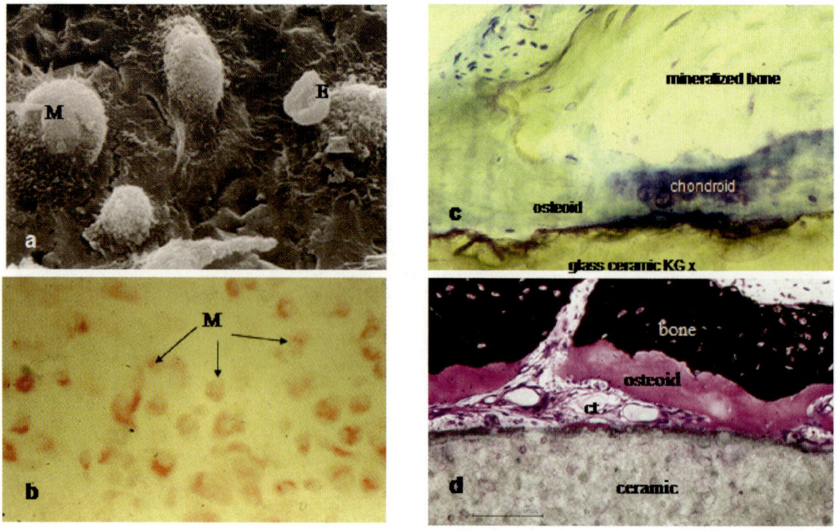

Chapter 4, Fig. 7 Macrophages (*M*) at the surface of bone bonding glass ceramic KG Cera [38] 3 days after implantation into the femur of a Sprague-Dawley rat. **a** SEM shows the diameter of the erythrocyte (*E*) to be 7 μm. **b** Macrophages stained for acid phosphatase with red signal (*dark*). Macrophage diameters are 10–20 μm. **c** Inhibition of mineralization at the interface of glass ceramic KGx 245 days after implantation in the diaphysis of the rat femur. KGx contains (in wt%) SiO_2 34, $Ca(PO_3)_2$ 12, Na_2O 3.5, CaO 23, Al_2O_3 15, Ta_2O_5 12.5 [38]. Sawn section. Giemsa stain. **d** Inhibition of mineralization with a broad zone of osteoid and connective tissue (*ct*) at the surface and surrounding calcium zirconium phosphate [$CaTi_xZr_{4-x}(PO_4)_6$ with x = 0–4] 84 days after implantation into the distal Chinchilla femur epiphysis. Sawn section. Von Kossa & Paragon stain. *Bar* = 100 μm

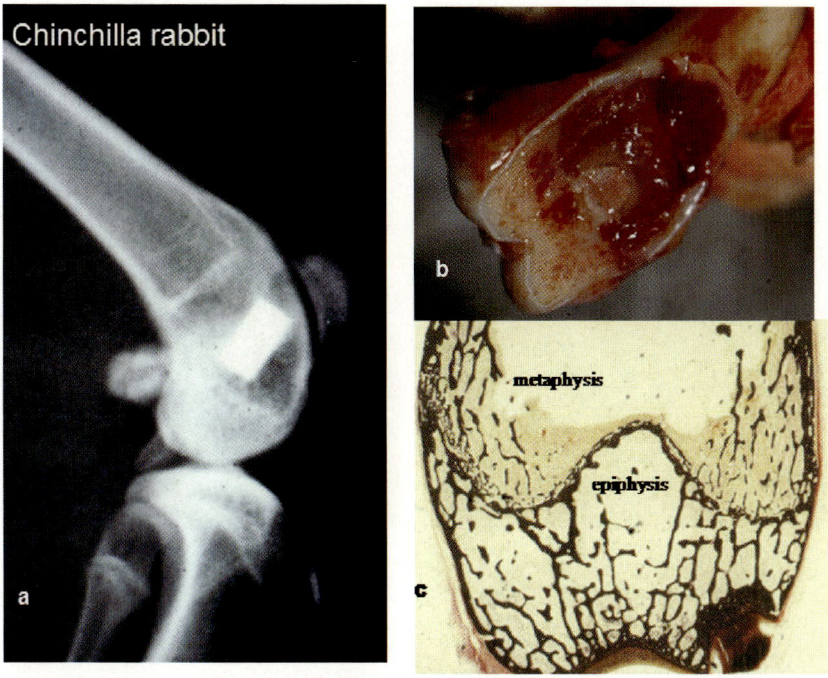

Chapter 4, Fig. 9 **a** Implantation site in the distal femur epiphysis of a Chinchilla rabbit below the patella sliding plane with an implant in a radiographic view. **b** Freshly cut surface in the frontal direction through the implantation site with an implant in situ. There is trabecular bone below the joint cartilage with fat and hematopoietic tissue in red in the metaphysis of the femur. **c** Undecalcified, formaldehyde-fixed, methylmethacrylate-embedded, sawn section of the distal femur of a Chinchilla rabbit stained with von Kossa & Fuchsin to demonstrate the mineralized trabecular bone structure and bone marrow as well as cartilage and ligament

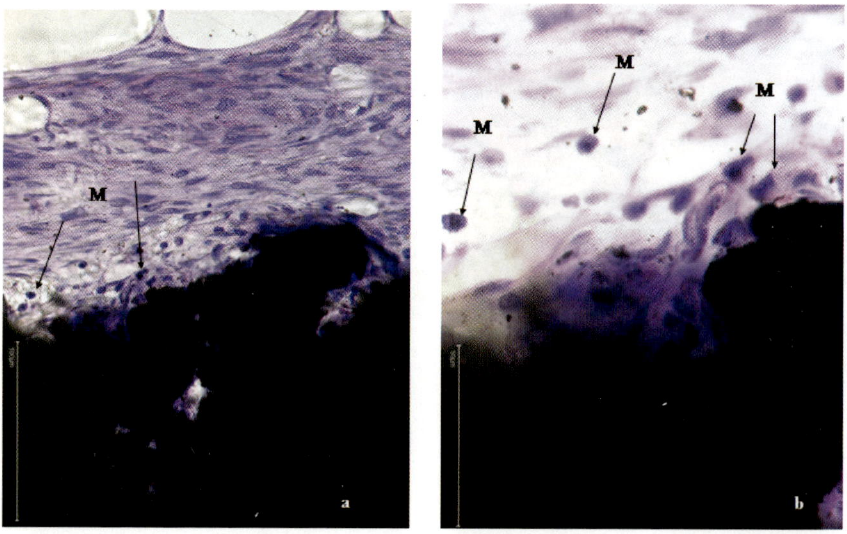

Chapter 4, Fig. 10 **a** Plasmapore® and organoapatite-coated implant 7 days after insertion into the distal femur epiphysis of a Chinchilla rabbit with young fibrous tissue and a few mononuclear cells and macrophages (M). Sawn section. Von Kossa & Paragon stain. *Bar* = 100 µm. **b** Macrophages at the nanometer-thin organoapatite coating on top of the Plasmapore® titanium coating 7 days after implantation. Sawn section. Von Kossa & Paragon stain. *Bar* = 50 µm

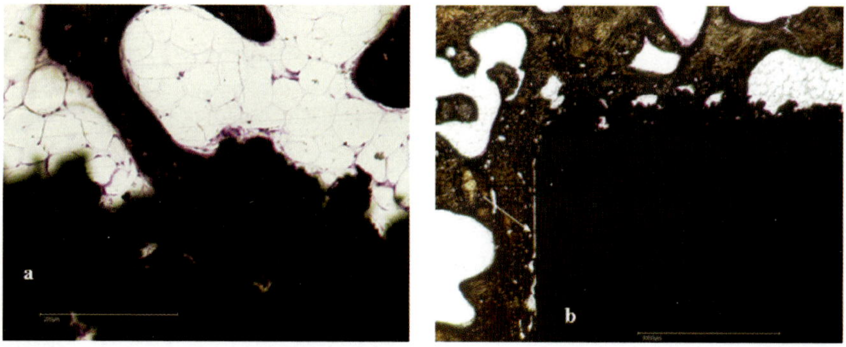

Chapter 4, Fig. 11 **a** Attachment of one bone trabecule to the organoapatite and Plasmapore®-coated periphery of the implant cylinder 84 days after implantation. In the surrounding area is a thin fibrous layer with only a few macrophages and fibroblasts and bone marrow. Sawn section. Von Kossa & Paragon stain. Bar = 200 µm. **b** Trabecular bone attaches to the Plasmapore® and organoapatite-coated periphery of the implant cylinder but not at the flat, uncoated dorsal part of the cylinder (arrow) 84 days after implantation in the distal femur epiphysis. Sawn section. Von Kossa & Paragon stain. *Bar* = 1000 µm

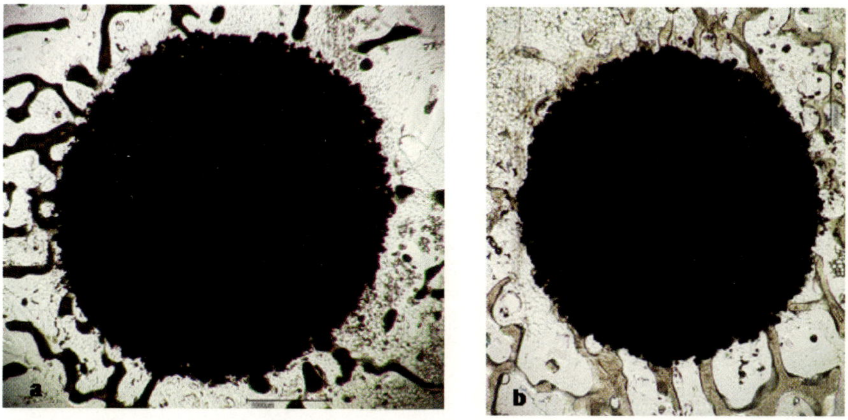

Chapter 4, Fig. 12 a,b Plasmapore® and organoapatite-coated Ti cylinder attached to trabecular bone in the distal femur epiphysis 84 days after implantation in a Chinchilla rabbit. Only a few bone trabecules are seen at the interface, with mostly soft tissue. The density of trabecular bone is largely normal, as depicted in Figure 9c. Sawn sections. **a** Von Kossa & Paragon stain. **b** Giemsa stain. *Bars* = 1000 μm

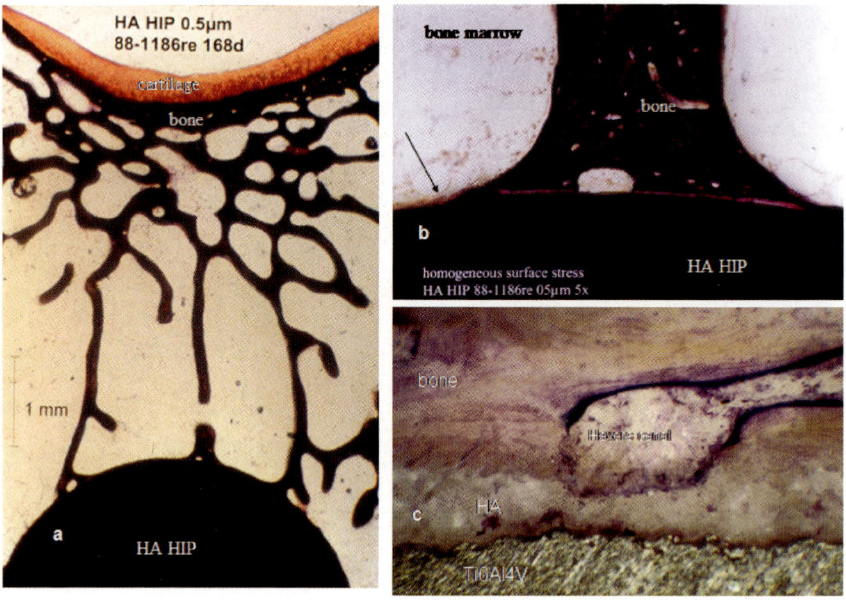

Chapter 4, Fig. 13 a Trabecular bone bonding to the surface of a hot isostatic pressed hydroxyapatite cylinder (diameter 4 mm, surface roughness Rt 0.5 µm) 168 days after implantation into the distal femur epiphysis of a Chinchilla rabbit. **b** The middle trabecule in **a** displays foot-like enlargement near the implant and adjustment of the implant cylinder surface to a surface contour (*arrow*), indicating a homogeneous surface stress state. This contour must have been made by mineraloclast(s). Note the soft tissue void in the trabecule near the implant surface near the middle of the strout according to the neutral axis of the load. **c** Bone bonded to a thick HA-coated Ti6Al4V stem of a femur component belonging to a total hip replacement system of a 64-year-old man 6 months after implantation. In the middle, a Havers canal has expanded into the HA coating owing to resorption of the HA. Cellular details cannot be discriminated any more due to progressed autolysis (postmortem specimen). Undecalcified sawn sections, von Kossa & Fuchsin stain

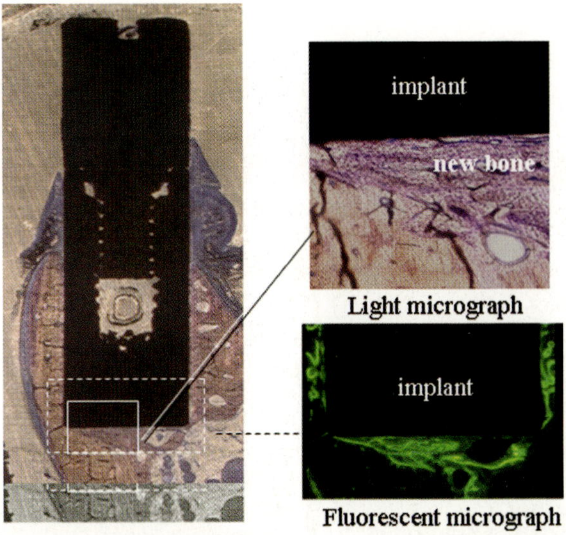

Chapter 6, Fig. 13 Light and fluorescence micrographs of the bisphosphonate-coated Ti implant–bone interface 12 weeks after implantation in a beagle dog

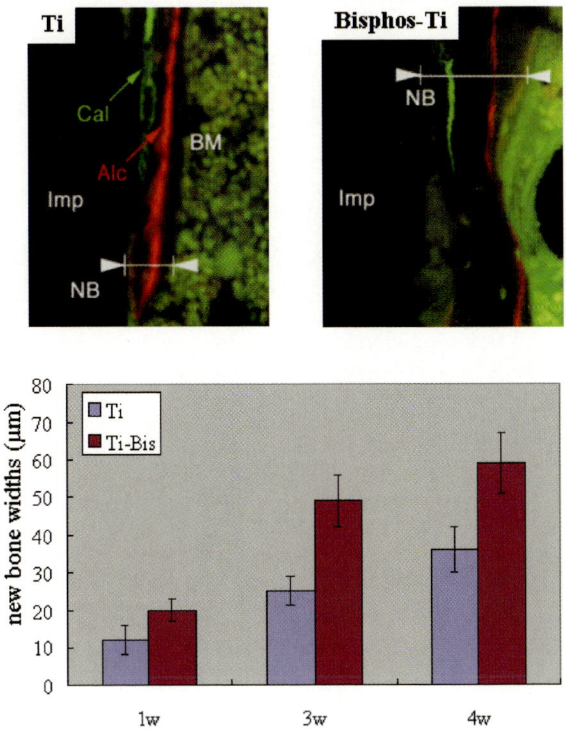

Chapter 6, Fig. 14 *Top* Confocal laser scanning microscopy. *Cal*, calcein (1 week); *Alc*, alizarin complexone (3 weeks); *BM*, xxxxxx; *Imp*, xxxxxxx; *NB*, xxxxxx. *Bottom* New bone width of Ti and bisphosphonate-immobilized implants in Wistar rats

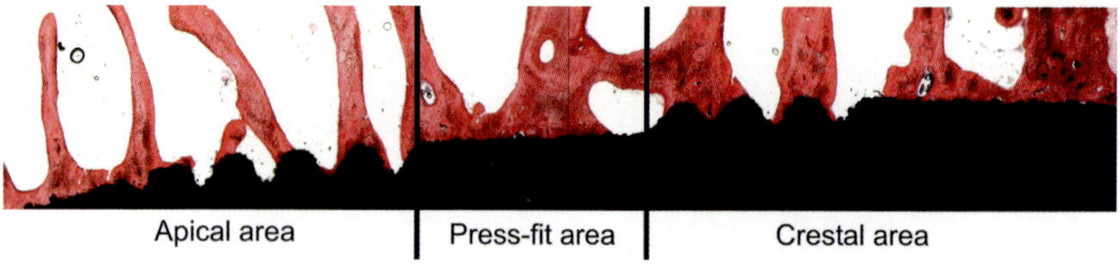

Chapter 10, Fig. 11 Light micrograph of one side of an implant with CHA coating. Bone contact is visible along the surface of the entire implant. From [70], with permission from Blackwell

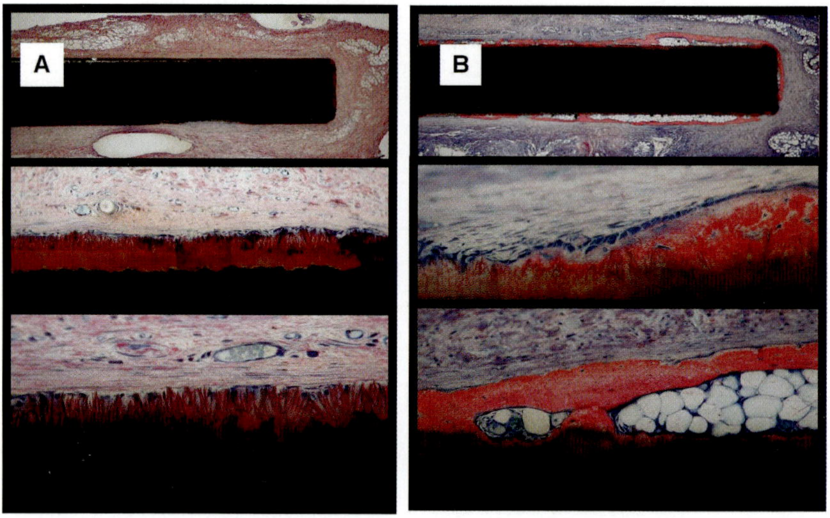

Chapter 11, Fig. 4 **A** Light microscopy images (low-, intermediate-, and high-magnification views) of a titanium alloy disk bearing an OCP coating 5 weeks after implantation at a subcutaneous site in a rat. No bone tissue has been deposited (80 μm thick section stained with McNeal's tetrachrome, basic fuchsine, and toluidine blue O). **B** Light micrographs (low-, intermediate- and high-magnification views) of a titanium alloy disk bearing octaCaP coating into which bone morphogenetic protein2 (BMP-2) had been incorporated, at 5 weeks after subcutaneous implantation in a rat. Bone tissue has been deposited both directly on the coated disk and at some distance therefrom, within the connective tissue capsule (80 μm thick section stained with McNeal's tetrachrome, basic fuchsine, and toluidine blue O)

24 weeks after implantation with the surrounding bone. HA-PLD showed the highest percentage of bone contact and bone linear density and the lowest lacunae contact and lacunae linear density. This result speaks for the usage of the HA-PLD technique for thin CaP coatings.

It can be expected that with more time the coating is better absorbed and that a more or less uncoated metallic implant subsists. The advantage of thin coating would be early bone apposition or bonding to the metal surface. At a later stage, when the coating has been absorbed, the positive effect would be minimal if not zero.

Although the following investigation [63] did not use a thin coating (the coating was 50–75 μm), it is mentioned here because it describes the influence of crystallinity and solubility on bone bonding and soft tissue at the interface. The different crystallinity (75% vs. 95%) of plasma-sprayed HA coatings at the surface of dental implant cylinders (4 mm diameter, 10 mm length) was investigated in the mandible of beagle dogs after 3 and 15 weeks [63]. The crystallinity of the plasma-sprayed coating on titanium alloy was increased by a hydrothermal treatment of 75% to 95%. Statistically, there was no difference between the two coatings regarding the pullout force at failure after 3 and 15 weeks after implantation. The extent of bone apposition was also statistically not different between the two coatings, being approximately 40% after 3 weeks and 90% after 15 weeks. Histology showed in both types of coatings either bone apposition with bonding or soft tissue with some macrophages. Phagocytosed HA particles could be identified in some macrophages. This was interpreted as proof of *in vivo* degradation of the coating. This fact implies that after a prolonged time the coating should have disappeared irrespective of the thickness.

In another comparative study, rectangular Ti6Al4V implants with square cross sections and an oblique diameter of 4.6 mm were also inserted in the mandible of beagle dogs. They were either (1) polished or (2) coated with collagen; (3) coated with mineralized collagen; (4) coated with collagen and HA; or (5) coated with HA using a special procedure in which there was a change between electrochemical deposition of HA and the growing of an anodic oxide layer [64]. The thickness of the coatings was < 5 μm. After 1 and 3 months, the implants were retrieved and analyzed mainly using morphometric methods. The best result concerning the development of bone in the cortical and cancellous bone areas was obtained with the pure HA coating (type 5), and the least result was observed with pure Ti6Al4V. Bone began to develop at the corners of the rectangular implants in the round bore hole; then the planes between the corners were covered by bone; and finally the rest of the hole filled up with bone and Havers' systems. This pattern of bone development demonstrates the influence of the implantation bed for the outcome of bone healing. In other words, the bridging of the gap between the bore hole and the implant surface takes time; and the smaller the gap, the shorter is the time for bone growth to achieve fixation of the implant. There is another important result of this experiment. It can be postulated that the introduction of collagen (type 2), mineralized collagen (type 3), and collagen and HA (type 4) inhibited bone development. Apparently, the tissue reaction did not profit from the collagen that was introduced into the coating of the implant. This should be a warning for all those investigators who intend to increase bone healing by adding substances perhaps at the wrong time, at the wrong place, or with the wrong concentration.

The next experiment deals with the surface preparation and coating of ceria stabilized tetragonal zirconia alumina ceramics (Ce-TZP) [65]. The surface of the 15 × 10 × 2 mm plates was (1) uncoated and polished; (2) acid-treated and heated to corrode the Ce-TZP particles to create a microporous surface structure; (3) coated with submicron thick HA; (4) coated with 4 μm thick HA using a biomimetic procedure with simulated body fluid (SBF). There were clear morphological differences in the structure of the four dissimilarly prepared surfaces. The plates were implanted in the proximal tibia of rabbits and examined after 4, 8, and 16 weeks postoperatively. The detachment test provided best results for surfaces of groups (3) and (4)—i.e., failure loads around 25 N. Back-scattered SEM showed bone bonding to the implant surfaces. At 16 weeks, remains of the coating could not be detected by high resolution back-scattered SEM in group (4). The intended function of the thin coating was to provide early fixation and bonding of mineralized tissue to the surface of the implant.

Plasmapore®-coated Ti6Al4V cylinders were additionally coated by organoapatite using a wet chemical technique to cover the pore surfaces. The procedures for organoapatite coating of the cylinders were described in detail by Hwang et al. [66]. The objectives of the study were to find out whether thin coating with organoapatite improves bone development at porous Ti6Al4V cylinders. Controls were implant cylinders without organoapatite coating. Following DIN 47868, the maximum surface roughness $R_T$was 109 μm (SD 8.1 μm), and the thickness of the porous structure was 75 μm. The thickness of the organoapatite coating was in the order of 250 Å [66]. The surface structure of the coated implant cylinder is depicted in Fig. 4.8. The cylinders

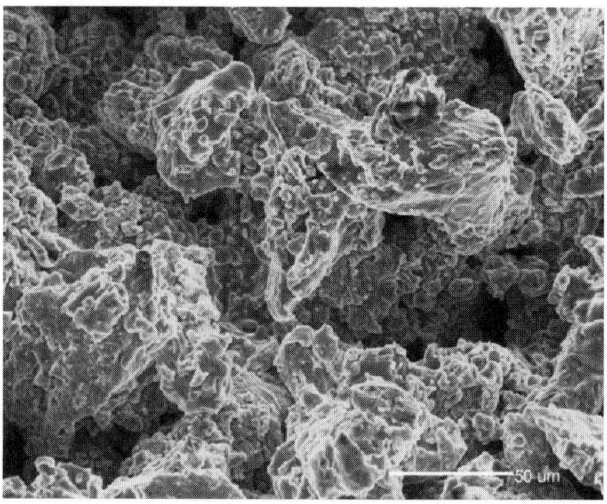

Fig. 4.8 Plasmapore®-coated and additionally organoapatite-coated titanium cylinder. SEM after sterilization and before implantation. Roughness according to DIN 4768 Rt 109 μm (SD 8.1 μm)

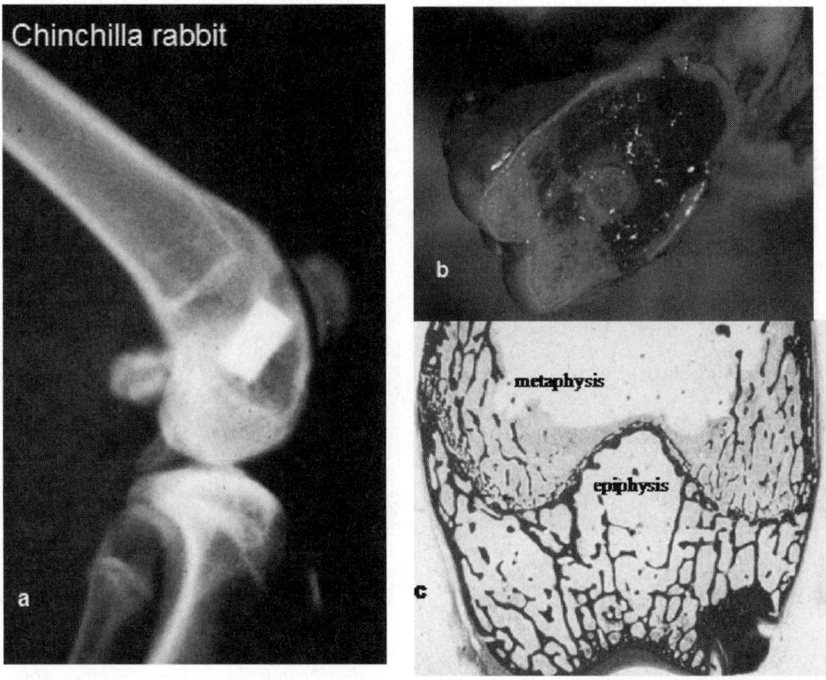

Fig. 4.9 **a** Implantation site in the distal femur epiphysis of a Chinchilla rabbit below the patella sliding plane with an implant in a radiographic view. **b** Freshly cut surface in the frontal direction through the implantation site with an implant in situ. There is trabecular bone below the joint cartilage with fat and hematopoietic tissue in red in the metaphysis of the femur. **c** Undecalcified, formaldehyde-fixed, methylmethacrylate-embedded, sawn section of the distal femur of a Chinchilla rabbit stained with von Kossa & Fuchsin to demonstrate the mineralized trabecular bone structure and bone marrow as well as cartilage and ligament (*See* Color Insert)

(length 8 mm, diameter 4 mm) with organoapatite coated or uncoated surfaces were implanted into the distal femur epiphysis of Chinchilla rabbits for 7, 28, and 84 days. Figure 4.9a,b shows the implantation site in the distal femur epiphysis of Chinchilla rabbits. Bone trabecules in the area were oriented as in Fig. 4.9c. The histology of undecalcified sawn sections, prepared as in [2], reveals fibrous tissue with some macrophages near the surface of the implants 7 days after implantation (Fig. 4.10). However, after 28 and 84 days, trabecular bone had developed up to the porous, organoapatite coated or uncoated circumference of the cylinders (Figs. 4.11, 4.12). Interestingly, the flat nonporous uncoated dorsal plane of the cylinders was covered with a plate of bone (Fig. 4.11b) and not with trabecular bone as at the circumference of the cylinder (Figs. 4.11a,b, 12). Morphometry of the tissues at the implant interface (e.g., bone, osteoid, chondroid) and soft tissue allow more detailed interpretation of the findings. Most important is the increased percentage of bone at the circumference of organoapatite-coated implants versus uncoated implants after

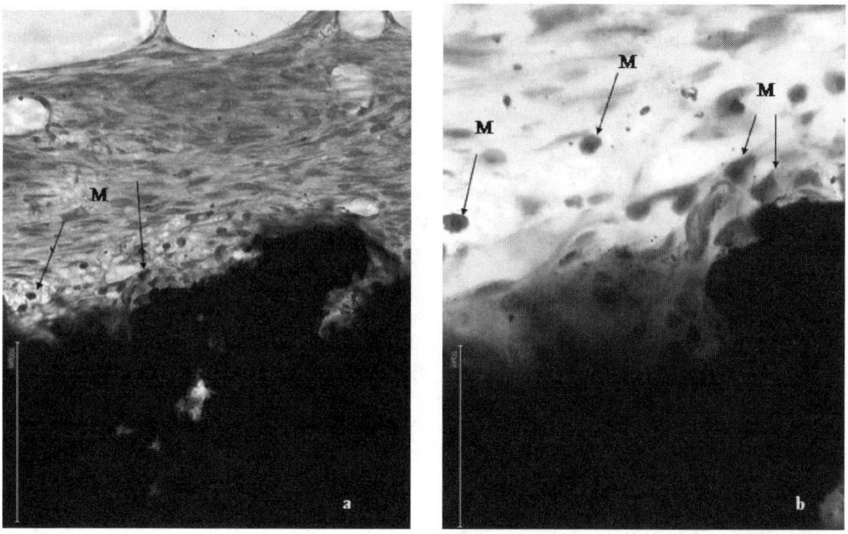

Fig. 4.10 **a** Plasmapore® and organoapatite-coated implant 7 days after insertion into the distal femur epiphysis of a Chinchilla rabbit with young fibrous tissue and a few mononuclear cells and macrophages (M). Sawn section. Von Kossa & Paragon stain. *Bar* = 100 μm. **b** Macrophages at the nanometer-thin organoapatite coating on top of the Plasmapore® titanium coating 7 days after implantation. Sawn section. Von Kossa & Paragon stain. *Bar* = 50 μm (*See* Color Insert)

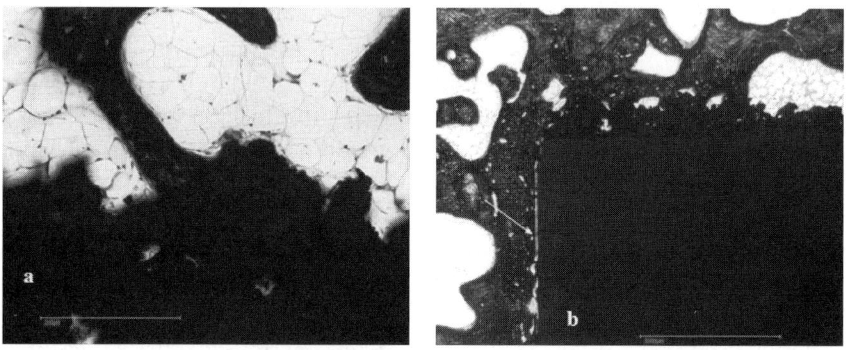

Fig. 4.11 **a** Attachment of one bone trabecule to the organoapatite and Plasmapore®-coated periphery of the implant cylinder 84 days after implantation. In the surrounding area is a thin fibrous layer with only a few macrophages and fibroblasts and bone marrow. Sawn section. Von Kossa & Paragon stain. Bar = 200 μm. **b** Trabecular bone attaches to the Plasmapore® and organoapatite-coated periphery of the implant cylinder but not at the flat, uncoated dorsal part of the cylinder (arrow) 84 days after implantation in the distal femur epiphysis. Sawn section. Von Kossa & Paragon stain. *Bar* = 1000 μm (*See* Color Insert)

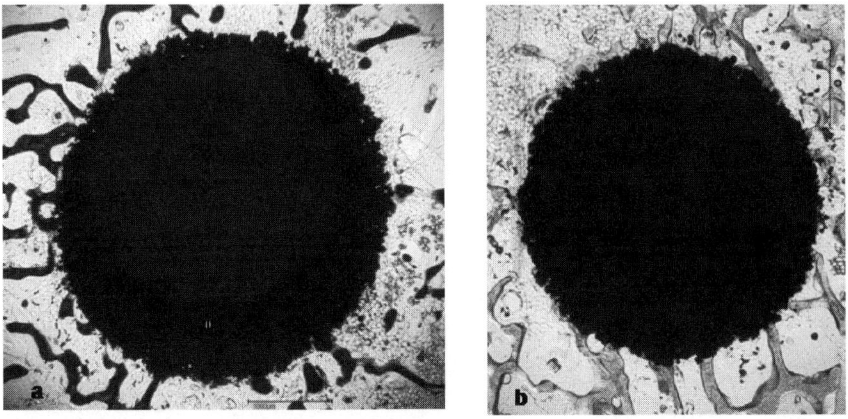

Fig. 4.12 a,b Plasmapore® and organoapatite-coated Ti cylinder attached to trabecular bone in the distal femur epiphysis 84 days after implantation in a Chinchilla rabbit. Only a few bone trabecules are seen at the interface, with mostly soft tissue. The density of trabecular bone is largely normal, as depicted in Figure 4.9c. Sawn sections. **a** Von Kossa & Paragon stain. **b** Giemsa stain. *Bars* = 1000 μm (*See* Color Insert)

Table 4.3 Percentage of bone at the interface of organoapatite coated and uncoated cylinders

Cylinder	No. of animals[a]	7 Days	28 Days	84 Days
Organoapatite coated	6	0	56.4 ± 7.4	48.6 ± 16.8
Uncoated	4	0	33.6 ± 1.5*	42.9 ± 4.8

Results are the mean ± SEM
[a]Four sections per animal.
*$P < 0.05$, *t*-test

28 days (Table 4.3). After 84 days there is no difference between bone attached to coated or uncoated cylinders. We assume that this outcome can be connected with the degradation and absorption of the coating. The result demonstrates a short-term benefit for bone attachment to an implant surface covered by a thin organoapatite coating. Comparable results were described for thick coatings with OCP and biphasic calcium phosphate 12 weeks after implantation into the femurs of goats [67].

4.5 Considerations for Predicting Clinical Performance of CaP Coatings

This section presents some principles of regulations concerning the testing institution and the validity of the test methods. Retrieval studies of successful and failed implants should be mandatory.

An important outcome of these observations and considerations is that bone trabecules fixed to the porous metallic structure of the implant provide a sufficient biomechanical support. In other words, it is not necessary that the entire surface of an implant be covered by bone to provide sufficient biomechanical support. The attachment of bone to implant surfaces follows the abovementioned principles of bone apposition to osteoclast lacunae. Whether the implant surface is made of pure metal, metal alloy, or ceramics, appropriate surface morphology with some roughness is necessary. There is no implant surface with the chemistry and morphology of bone resorption pits, including remnants of collagen fibers, surrounding ECM, and crystal structure, as shown in Fig. 4.6b. We stress the importance of following physiological structures when implant materials are to be attached to physiological ECM and cells. Therefore, all implant surfaces represent artificial structures with artificial chemistry to which macrophages, osteoclasts, and then osteoblasts have to fulfill their determined function. Included are the biomechanical requirements for physiological skeletal function of implants.

The cited *in vitro* studies provide limited information and predictions for the *in vivo* performance of implants, including surface modification by thin CaP coatings. The main argument for this statement is that the surfaces were tested using only osteoblasts. This is in contrast to the physiological mechanisms. We did not find studies in the recent literature in which the foundation of osteoclasts and their subsequent attachment, proliferation, and maturation of osteoblasts was investigated. There is another point to devalue *in vitro* studies versus *in vivo* studies: Whereas *in vivo* transport of interstitial fluid and the cooperation of various cell types in the interface can be studied, the *in vitro* studies deliver only observations and arguments that are connected to some established cell lines—primary cells of osteoblast type. These cells have not been investigated with their physiological neighbors and predecessors (i.e., macrophages, osteoclasts, mineraloclasts). Additionally, lymphocytic cells are absent in the chain of studied events. They should preferentially be investigated in an intact body (i.e., *in vivo*). Thus, there are strong arguments in favor of *in vivo* studies.

Nevertheless, *in vivo* studies with animals are providing limited arguments in favor or against certain types of surface morphology or surface chemistry of implants. There are those who argue against animal experiments with the statement that the results are not directly interpretable in favor of or against human application of implants. It is not acceptable to favor and perform investigations with human patients owing to ethical reasons. However, it should be encouraged that recipients of implants allow postmortem examination for the benefit of future implant-receiving patients. This would in some way honor the positive effects connected with implantation of various kinds of implants.

Examples of possible information by retrieval studies are presented in Figs. 4.13 and 4.14. The degradation of HA coating on the surface of a Ti6Al4V femoral stem can be seen in the area of a Havers canal, where the absorption zone is located (Fig. 4.13c). In Figure 4.14a,b, the HA-coated shaft of a total hip replacement demonstrates extended resorption or absorption

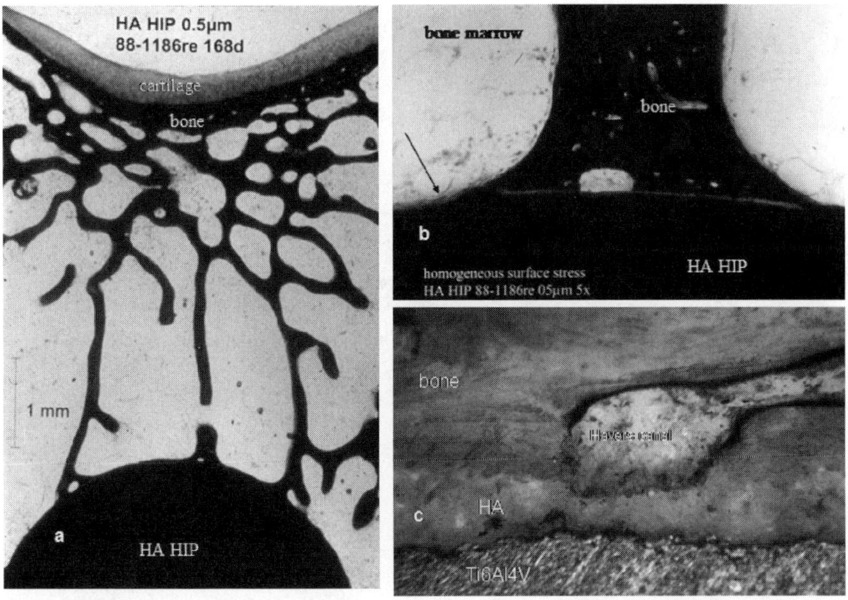

Fig. 4.13 **a** Trabecular bone bonding to the surface of a hot isostatic pressed hydroxyapatite cylinder (diameter 4 mm, surface roughness Rt 0.5 µm) 168 days after implantation into the distal femur epiphysis of a Chinchilla rabbit. **b** The middle trabecule in **a** displays foot-like enlargement near the implant and adjustment of the implant cylinder surface to a surface contour (*arrow*), indicating a homogeneous surface stress state. This contour must have been made by mineraloclast(s). Note the soft tissue void in the trabecule near the implant surface near the middle of the strout according to the neutral axis of the load. **c** Bone bonded to a thick HA-coated Ti6Al4V stem of a femur component belonging to a total hip replacement system of a 64-year-old man 6 months after implantation. In the middle, a Havers canal has expanded into the HA coating owing to resorption of the HA. Cellular details cannot be discriminated any more due to progressed autolysis (postmortem specimen). Undecalcified sawn sections, von Kossa & Fuchsin stain (*See* Color Insert)

areas. The morphology of the defects in the thick HA coating indicates a favorable result considering the activity of mineraloclasts or osteoclasts. It could also be shown in an experiment that the interstitial fluid leaches implant surfaces where particles of the coating are released. These particles are engulfed by macrophages (Fig. 14c) and degraded if possible. The macrophages are activated and stimulated to produce chemical species that are able to influence other cells (e.g., cytokines). The signals of macrophages with particles is known to be inhibitory for the growth or maintenance of bone whether dense and cortical or in a trabecular area. The signal molecules that are produced by macrophages (e.g., proinflammatory cytokines) are known to stimulate and maintain inflammation and reduce the mass of adjacent bone.

The prediction of such an event is not yet possible with an acceptable degree of reliability. Nevertheless, it should be possible to get some information based

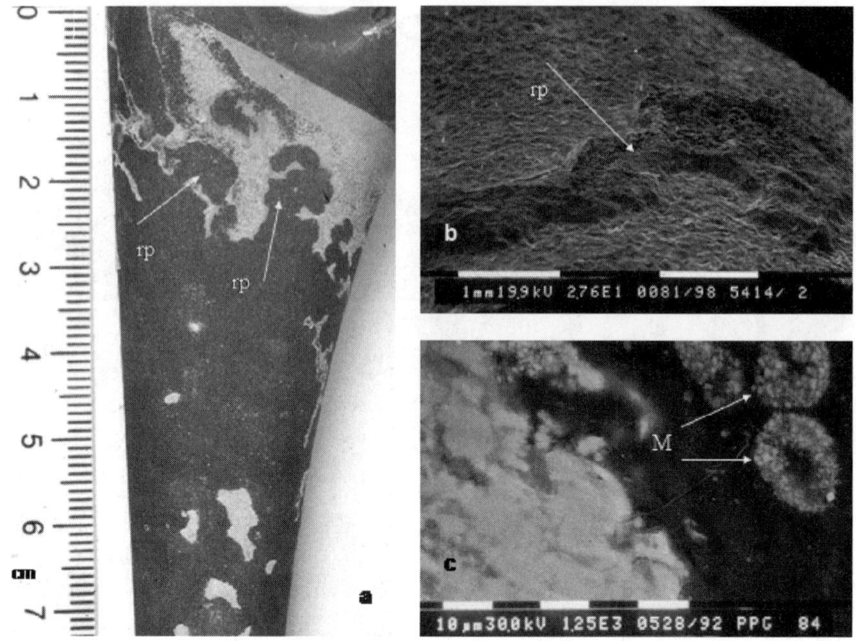

Fig. 4.14 **a** Explanted loose femoral component of a total hip replacement some months after implantation in a patient. Only a few areas have remaining thick hydroxyapatite coating. The pattern of the defects indicates resorption pits (*rp*) by osteoclasts or mineraloclasts. **b** Enlarged view of the defects and remnants of the HA coating as well as the roughness of the metallic stem in a retrieved specimen after operation for replacement of the implant. No further information was available. **c** Details of the dissolution of an HA implant in a Chinchilla rabbit femur 84 days after implantation, with street-like diminished density of the ceramic on the left, release of particles, and particles engulfed in macrophages (M). **a** Macrophotograph. **b** SEM. **c** Back-scattered mode of SEM, demonstrating the density of structures

on the changes in cell reactions, especially regarding macrophages, osteoblasts, and osteoclasts, and the activation or inhibition of the pertinent genes. At present, we are at the point of data acquisition in this field. It can be expected that in the near future techniques will be developed to investigate changes in the activity of cell receptors in order to determine the intracellular zones for signal transduction, activation of genes, and secretion of proteins and peptides. The extracellular products should provide a new and even more reliable prediction for further behavior of cells exposed to released substances from implant surfaces such as those with thin CaP coatings. In any case, the material released from thin CaP coatings doped with additional material (e.g., Si, Mg, Mn) should not have negative effects on cell proliferation, differentiation, or the interaction of cells and that of cells with the ECM.

Acknowledgments Plasmapore®-coated Ti6Al4V cylinders were supplied by Aesculap AG, Tuttlingen, Germany. The organoapatite coating of these cylinders was provided by J.J.

Hwang and S.I. Stupp, Northwestern University, Evanston, IL, USA. The experimentation with coated and uncoated cylinders was performed by L. Pröbster, (Tübingen) and Konstanze I. Grun (Berlin).

References

1. Rubin's Pathology, 4th edition. E. Rubin, Editor-in-Chief. Lippincott Williams & Wilkins, Philadelphia, 2005. ISBN 0-7817-4733-3.
2. Handbook of Biomaterials Evaluation, 2nd edition. Andreas von Recum, editor. Taylor & Francis, Philadelphia, 1999. ISBN 1-56032-479-1.
3. Biomaterials Science, 2nd edition. Buddy D. Ratner, Allan S. Hoffman, Frederick J. Schoen, Jack E. Lemons, editors. Elsevier Academic Press, Amsterdam, 2004. ISBN 0-12-582463-7.
4. Bone Engineering. Editor John E. Davies. em squared incorporated, Toronto, 2000. ISBN 0-9686980-0-X.
5. L.L. Hench, J.M. Polak. Science 295 (2002) 1016.
6. L.L Hench, R.J. Splinter, W.C. Allen, T.K. Greenlee. J. Biomed. Mater. Res. Symp. 2 (1971) 117.
7. H. Brömer, E.Pfeil, H.Käs. German Patent No. 2,326,100, 22.9.1975.
8. T. Nakamura, T. Yamamuro, S. Higashi, T. Kokubo, S. Itoo. J. Biomed. Mater. Res.19 (1985) 685.
9. J.C. Myers, S. Spiegelman, D.L. Kacian. Proc. Natl. Acad. Sci. U S A 74 (1977) 2840.
10. M.S. Krug, S.L. Berger. Meth. Enzymol. 152 (1987) 316.
11. J. Sambrook, E.F. Fritsch, T. Maniatis. Molecular Cloning, 2nd Edition, Cold Spring Harbor, NY, 1989.
12. G.L. Bubbone. Clin. Chem. 31 (1985) 164.
13. R.W. Davis. Rapid DNA purifications for enzymatic and hybridization analysis. Methods of Enzymology 65 (1980) 404.
14. S.P. Fodor, J.L. Read, M. Pirrung, L. Stryer, A.T. Lu, D. Solas. Science 251 (1991) 767.
15. R. Guimil, M. Beier, M. Scheffler, H. Rebscher, J. Funk, A. Wixmerten, M. Baum, C. Hermann, H. Tahedl, E. Moschel, F. Obermeier, I. Sommer, D. Buchner, R. Viehweger, J. Burgmaier, C.F. Stahler, M. Muller, P.F. Stahler. Nucleosides Nucleotides Nucleic Acids. 22 (2003) 1721.
16. H. Matsumura, S. Reich, A. Ito, H. Saitoh, S. Kamoun, P. Winter, G. Kahl, M. Reuter, D. H. Kruger, R. Terauchi. Proc Natl Asssoc Sci U S A 100 (2003) 15718.
17. M. Baum, S. Bielau, N. Rittner, K. Schmid, K. Eggelbusch, M. Dahms, A. Schlauersbach, H. Tahedl, M. Beier, R. Guimil, M. Scheffler, C. Hermann, J.M. Funk, A. Wixmerten, H. Rebscher, M. Honig, C. Andreae, D. Buchner, E. Moschel, A. Glathe, E. Jager, M. Thom, A. Greil, F. Bestvater, F. Obermeier, J. Burgmaier, K. Thome, S. Weichert, S. Hein, T. Binnewies, V. Foitzik, M. Muller, C.F. Stahler, P.F. Stahler. Nucleic Acids Research, 31 (2003) 23 e1515.
18. V. Velculescu, L. Zhang, B. Vogelstein, K. W. Kinzler. Science 270 (1995) 484.
19. P. Angenendt, L. Nyarsik, W. Szaflarski, J. Glökler, K.H. Nierhaus, H. Lehrach, D.J. Cahill, A. Lueking. Analytical Chemistry 76 (2004) 1844.
20. S. Horn, A. Lueking, D. Murphy, A. Staudt, C. Gutjahr, K. Schulte, A. König, M. Landsberger, H. Lehrach, S.B. Felix, D.J. Cahill. Proteomics 6 (20064) 605.
21. K. Kato, M. Toda, H. Iwata. Biomaterials 28 (2007) 1289.
22. P. Pavlickova, A. Knappik, D. Kambhampati, F.Ortigao, H. Hug. Biotechniques. 34 (2003) 124.
23. P. Ducy, T. Schinke, G. Karsenty. Science 289 (2002) 1501.
24. B.G. Keselowsky, D.M. Collard, A.J. Garcia. Proc Natl Assoc Sci U S A 102 (2005) 5953.
25. Boyde, S.J. Jones. Microscopy Research and Technique 33 (1996) 92.

26. J.D. De Bruijn, C.A Van Blitterswijk, J.E. Davies. J. Biomed. Mater. Res. 29 (1995) 89.
27. J.A. Hunt, P.J. Laughlin, B.F. Flanagan. Biomaterials 18 (1997) 1449.
28. K. Anselme. Biomaterials 21 (2000) 667.
29. H. Kojima, T. Uemura. J. Biol. Chem. 280 (2005) 2944.
30. M. Hughes-Fulford. Science STKE 2004, re12 (2004).
31. G. Karsenty. Genes Dev. 13 (1999) 3037.
32. A.H. Reddi. Cytokine and Growth Factor Reviews 8 (1997) 11.
33. D. Amir, C. Müller-Mai, H. Wendland, U. Gross, J. Sela. Biomaterials 10 (1989) 585.
34. H.M. Frost. Calc. Tissue Res. 3 (1969) 211.
35. S.J. Jones, C. Gray, A. Boyde. Anat. Embryol. 190 (1994) 339.
36. N.S. Cunningham, N.A. Jenkins, D.J. Gilbert, N.G. Copeland, A.H. Reddi, Se-Jin Lee, Growth Factors 12 (1995) 99.
37. A.H. Reddi, J. Orthop. Sci. 2 (1997) 55.
38. U. Gross, V. Strunz. J. Biomed. Mater. Res.19 (1985) 251.
39. R. G. T. Geesink, K. De Groot And C. P.A.T Klein. Clin. Ortho. Rel. Res. 225 (1987) 147.
40. J. E. Davies, N. Baldan. J. Biomed. Mater. Res. 36 (1997) 429.
41. J. Zhang, X. Zhang, C. Müller-Mai, U.M. Gross. J. Mater.Sci: Mater. Med. 5 (1994) 243.
42. T. Kokubo, H. Takadama, Biomaterials 27 (2006) 2907.
43. Y. Yamada, A. Fujimoto, A. Ito, R. Yoshimi, M. Ueda, Biomaterials 27 (2006) 3766.
44. Y.-J. Lee, J. S. Ko, H-M. Kim. Biomaterials 27 (2006) 3738.
45. E.S. Thian, J. Huang, S.M. Best, Z.H. Barber, W. Bonfield. Biomaterials 26 (2005) 2947.
46. Bigi, B. Bracci, F. Cuisinier, R. Elkaim, M. Fini, I. Mayer, I.N. Mihailescu, G. Socol, L. Sturba, P. Torricelli. Biomaterials 26 (2005) 2381
47. G. Socol, P. Torricelli, B. Bracci, M. Iliescu, F. Miroiu, A. Bigi, J. Werckmann, I.N. Mihailescu. Biomaterials 25 (2004) 2539.
48. J.-Y. Hong, Y.J. Kim, H.-W. Lee, W.-K. Lee, J.S. Ko, H.-M. Kim. Biomaterials 24 (2003) 2977.
49. Y.-F. Chou, W. Huang, J.C.Y. Dunn, T.A. Miller, B.M. Wu. Biomaterials, 26 (2005) 285.
50. M.C. Siebers, X.F. Walboomers, S.C.G. Leeuwengurgh, J.G.C. Wolke, J.A. Jansen. Biomaterials 25 (2004) 2019.
51. H. Zreiqat, S.M. Valenzuela, B. Ben Nissan, R. Roest, C. Knabe, R.J. Radlanski, H. Renz, P. J. Evans. Biomaterials 26 (2005) 7579.
52. K.A. Thomas, J.F. Kay, S.D. Cook, M. Jarcho. J. Biomed. Mater. Res. 21 (1987) 1395.
53. C.P. Klein, A.A. Driessen, K. De Groot, A. Van Den Hooff. J. Biomed. Mater. Res. 17 (1983) 769.
54. A.E. Porter, N. Patel, J.N. Skepper, S.M. Best, W. Bonfield. Biomaterials 24 (2003) 4609.
55. Lu Gan, R. Pilliar. Biomaterials 25 (2004) 5303.
56. Lu Gan, J. Wang, A. Tache, N. Valiquette, D. Deporter, R. Pilliar. Biomaterials 25 (2004) 5313.
57. Lu Gan, J. Wang, R. M. Pilliar, Biomaterials 26 (2005) 189.
58. H.Q. Nguyen, D.A. Deporter, R.M. Pilliar, N. Valiquette, R. Yakubovich. Biomaterials 25 (2004) 865.
59. J.G.C. Wolke, J.P.C.M. Van Der Waerden, H.G. Schaeken, J.A. Jansen. Biomaterials 24 (2003) 2623.
60. C.M. Müller-Mai, C. Voigt, U. Gross. Scanning Microscopy 4 (1990) 613.
61. G. Schmidmaier, B. Wildemann, P. Schwabe, R. Stange, J. Hoffmann, N.P. Südkamp, N.P. Haas, M. Raschke. J. Biomed. Mater. Res B 63 (2002) 1689.
62. C. Peraire, J.L. Arias, D. Bernal, J. Pou, B. Leon, A. Arano, W., Roth, J. Biomed. Mater. Res. A 77 (2006) 370.
63. A.V. Burgess, B.J. Story, W.R. Wagner, P. Trisi, M.A.Pikos, S.A. Guttenberg. Clin. Oral Impl. Res. 10 (1999) 257.

64. H. Schliephake, D. Scharnweber, M. Dard, S. Robetaler, A. Sewing, C. Hüttmann. J. Biomed. Mater. Res. 64 A (2003) 225.
65. M. Takemoto, S. Fujibayashi, M. Neo, J.Suzuki, T. Kokubo, T., Nakamura, J. Biomed. Mater. Res. A 78 (2006) 693.
66. J.J. Hwang, K. Jaeger, J. Hancock, S.I. Stupp. J. Biomed. Mater. Res. 47 (1999) 504.
67. P. Habibovic, J. Li, C. M. Van Der Valk, G. Meijer, P. Layrolle, C. Van Blitterswijk, K. De Groot. Biomaterials 26 (2005) 23.

Chapter 5
Pulsed Laser Deposition of Thin Calcium Phosphate Coatings

Betty León

Abstract This chapter reviews the work performed by the international research community on the production of thin calcium phosphate (CaP) coatings by pulsed laser deposition (PLD). Studies on the mechanisms of the technique shed light on the scientific bases for optimization of the coatings beyond empirical work. The relations between the physicochemical coating properties and the various processing parameters are presented. PLD can produce extremely thin, dense, well adhering CaP coatings with extraordinary controlled chemistry and crystallinity. No postdeposition thermal annealing is needed. Different CaP phases and morphologies can be deposited, so the degree of resorption may be adapted to a specific medical application. Coatings with graded composition or graded crystallinity can readily be produced, not only on metal substrates but also on polymers. *In vitro* and *in vivo* testing with various cells and animal models have verified similar or better osseointegration of the PLD coatings compared to the commercially available plasma-sprayed coatings, with improved adhesion properties and without risk of delamination or detachment of the coating. The technique is mature enough for an industrial scale-up and the start of clinical tests with real dental or orthopedic implants.

5.1 Introduction

Shortly after the invention of the first high-power ruby laser during the early 1960s, it became clear that this new intense radiation could be used to vaporize and deposit thin films [1]. However, the major breakthrough for the wider application of this technique did not arrive until the late 1980s, when it was triggered by the successful growth of high T_c superconducting films in 1987 [2]. These new applications were propelled by the development of lasers with shorter pulses and therefore with very high peak power density.

B. León (✉)
Departmento de Física Aplicada, E.T.S.I. Industriales, University of Vigo, Lagoas-Marcosende s/n, 36200 Vigo, Spain
e-mail: bleon@uvigo.es

B. León, J.A. Jansen (eds.), *Thin Calcium Phosphate Coatings for Medical Implants*, DOI 10.1007/978-0-387-77718-4_5,

Pulsed laser deposition (PLD) is also called laser ablation, stressing the significance of the fast vaporization phenomenon that takes place in the target material that leads to deposition and growth of the film on the substrate. The basic idea of PLD and its experimental implementation is rather simple. A high-power laser provides the energy source to melt and vaporize materials from a target. Owing to the high power density of a focalized pulsed laser, the ablated material forms a plasma plume consisting of a collection of highly excited molecules, atoms, ions, and electrons, which expand in a vacuum or a gas environment, transporting the material that condenses on a substrate. Pulsed lasers with high repetition rates allow growth of a thin film of the desired material.

Bulk bioactive calcium phosphate ceramics (CPCs) show excellent biocompatibility and are therefore useful materials in the field of orthopedic surgical applications. Among them, hydroxyapatite (HA) —$Ca_{10}(PO_4)_6(OH)_2$)— is widely used because its chemical and crystallographic structure is similar to the apatite of living bone. Despite the ability of solid sintered HA to guide bone formation along its surface and to achieve bone fixation by tight bonds, this material is brittle and thus susceptible to fatigue failure [3]. Therefore, the main clinical application of CPCs as bulk material is limited to bone fillers for bone defects or bone cavities [4]. Its use in load-bearing applications is limited to serve as coating on metal devices, where the substrate provides the necessary mechanical properties [5]. The metal substrates usually utilized are pure titanium, titanium alloys, and cobalt-chromium alloy [6]. HA-coated titanium implants are known to be able to form a chemical fixation to the bone with a strength comparable to that of the cortical bone itself.

Most commercially available HA coatings are produced by the plasma-spray technique (PS), but this method does not allow controlling crystallinity, phase composition, or morphology; and the final coating can have properties diverging from the starting HA. HA-polystyrene (PS)-coated prostheses in hip arthroplasties allow early fixation of the femoral stem. They also enhance the stability of the acetabular component, reducing the period of rehabilitation and improving functional activities. However, after almost a decade and a half of HA-PS application in preclinical and clinical fields, several coating-related factors have been associated with the failure of the implants. First, poor coating-to-substrate adherence may produce delamination of the coating from the microstructured metal base after implantation due to low resistance to high shear and tensile forces. Second, the physicochemical instability of the HA-PS coating is liable for its degradation, and HA particles may be released into the immediate environment, causing an inflammatory and osteolysis process in surrounding tissues [7] and accelerating polyethylene wearing processes of the acetabular component [8]. Third, microbiologically, the presence of a HA-coated implant surface, rich in calcium, may increase the risk of bacterial infection. Although it remains unclear if the HA coating itself is the primary cause of implant failure [9], the eventual negative aspects mentioned above may compromise the longevity of this type of plasma-sprayed coating.

Several approaches have been followed to overcome plasma-sprayed coating instability:

- The use of more stable apatites such as high crystalline fluoroapatite, which shows greater physicochemical stability under physiological conditions [10]
- Post-plasma-spraying treatments to reduce its amorphous fast resorbable parts [11]
- Plasma-sprayed composite coatings (adding titanium or bioactive glass particles to the HA) to improve the coating stability [12], the metal-coating bonding strength [13], or the biological properties [14]

There are alternative application techniques, which allow reduction of the final thickness of the coating, such as electrophoretic deposition ([15] and Chapter 9 in this book) ion beam deposition ([16] and Chapter 6 in this book), radio-frequency magnetron sputtering ([17] and Chapter 7 in this book), hot isostatic pressing [18], biomimetic methods ([19] and Chapter 11 in this book), and pulsed laser deposition [20].

Uniform coating with the desired thickness, composition, and crystallinity can be obtained by applying PLD, the achievements of which is reviewed in this chapter.

Compared to the commercially available plasma sprayed coatings, PLD coatings offer many general advantages:

- They can be much thinner but still cover the titanium substrate densely to prevent ion release into the body from the implant. The reduction in thickness lowers the risk of delamination.
- Their composition is homogeneous, and it can be well controlled. In addition, films can have gradient composition, thereby being able to tailor their bioactivity or resorption to match the dynamics of bone growth.
- PLD films do not require preceding grit-blasting preparation of the substrate for efficient adherence.
- Their morphology, however, follows that of the substrate, thus conserving a previous texturing or structuring production step if it should be appropriate.

The first reports on PLD of calcium phosphate (CaP) thin films date back to 1992, when Cotell [20] and Torrisi [21] published their pioneering work, using an excimer laser and a ruby laser, respectively. Since then, many other groups [22–33] have conducted extensive and intensive research for studying the influences of the processing parameters on the quality of the thin CaP films for medical applications. Properties such as the chemical composition, morphology, structure, and the interface to the titanium substrate have been studied, this last one being a key factor in the adhesion and mechanical properties of the coating. *In vitro* and *in vivo* testing has demonstrated that this technique can produce well adhered coatings that improve the osseointegration capability of implants in contact with bone.

5.2 Description of the Technique

Figure 5.1 depicts a typical experimental system for PLD. A pulsed laser beam is focused through a transparent window at a 45° angle of incidence onto the target, situated inside a high vacuum chamber. A low base pressure inside the vessel ($< 10^{-3}$ Pa) ensures control of the processing atmosphere. Therefore, turbomolecular pumps and pressure measuring equipment (Pirani and Penning gauges) are currently used. Gas inlets, valves, and Baratron devices provide control over the processing pressure. Vacuum, oxygen, inert gas, water vapor, or mixtures of the last two have been investigated as processing environment at pressures ranging up to some tens of Pascals [34]. The rotation of the target prevents crater formation, fast erosion of the target surface, and deviations of the plasma plume. The substrates are positioned at a certain distance parallel to the target on a heated substrate holder. Temperatures can range from room temperature to around 800°C. Because high fluences are needed for laser ablation, most of the work accomplished to date has been centered on excimer and Nd:YAG lasers. Only Torrisi's group [21, 35, 36] utilized the ruby laser, and Antonov [37] has rarely applied TEA-CO_2 lasers.

5.2.1 Mechanism of PLD

As simple as the experimental setup for PLD coatings is, as complex are the physical mechanisms involved in the various stages of the process. First, the

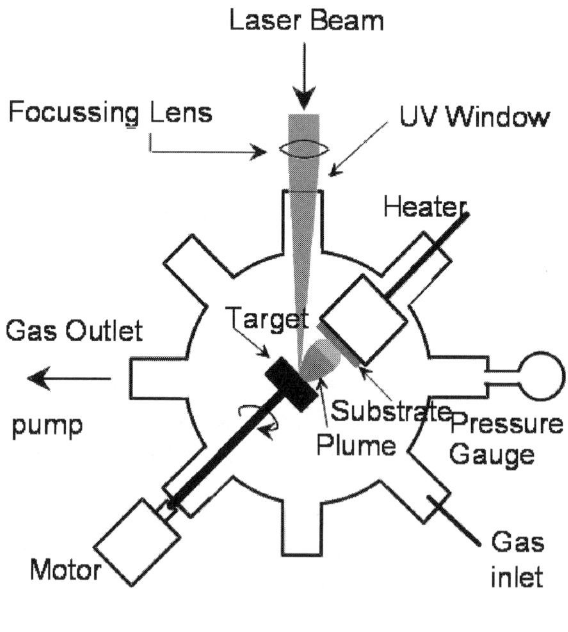

Fig. 5.1 Typical experimental system for pulsed laser deposition. From [72], with permission from Elsevier

photons from the laser pulses must be absorbed by the target material, leading to thermal, electronic, exfoliational, and hydrodynamic sputtering of material off the surface [38]. By cumulative laser irradiation, the target surface may suffer morphological and chemical modifications that affect the previously mentioned sputtering effects. Periodic surface structuring of the surface, cone formation, surface segregation, laser fluence dilution, and plume deflection may take place. In the time scale of the few tens of nanoseconds' duration of the laser pulses, an ablation plume is generated, consisting of a high pressure (~10–500 atm) bubble of hot plasma (T = 5000 K) formed less than 50 μm away from the target surface [39]. The expansion of this bubble has been fluid dynamically modeled, involving linear pressure gradients; however, interbeam collisions result in hydrodynamic effects, such as Knudsen-layer formation, redeposition of material on the target, and shock fronts. The expansion produces a supersonic beam similar to that generated from a pulsed nozzle jet, except for the plasma effects. Different species may have differing angular distributions, which can lead to stoichiometry variations in the deposited films. Moreover, particulates (also called droplets) are generated in some cases. Their sizes, chemistry, and microstructure depend on the processing conditions and material type. Theoretically, it has been suggested that the properties of PLD films are derived from the fact that the vapor has a high degree of supersaturation (10^5 J/mol), a high degree of ionization (~50%), and high mean kinetic energy (~1000 eV) [40]. However, under experimental growth conditions in the presence of ambient gases, a large number of gas phase collisions take place on the way from the target to the substrate that reduce both the ion fraction and the kinetic energy. The nucleation and growth of the film on the substrate also involve many processes such as atomic deposition, reevaporation, cluster nucleation and growth, species diffusion within the surface, and cluster dissociation. Each of these processes may involve a different free energy change. Apart from the density and energy of the condensing particles, their ionization degree and type, and the physicochemical properties of the substrate, the main processing parameter governing the film growth mode is the substrate temperature.

5.2.1.1 Interaction Between the Laser and the Calcium Phosphate Target

The interaction between the laser photons and the target depends primarily on the absorption coefficient of the target material for the laser wavelength. The higher the absorption is for the used wavelength, the more efficiently the energy of the laser pulses is coupled to the target surface. Extensive work performed on high T_c superconductors documented that shorter wavelengths lead to higher absorptivities and therefore to shorter penetration depths of the laser light. This general experience has been observed for calcium phosphates too. Guillot-Noël et al. [29] measured the absorptivity of various CaP powders that were pressed and sintered. They demonstrated that the higher the optical absorption coefficient, the lower was the droplet density on the surface of the deposited films.

Low absorptivity produces greater penetration depths, larger volume heating with a thicker layer of melted material, and the occurrence of a subsurface superheating effect once the evaporation begins, which leads to particle or droplet ejection. Higher optical absorption coefficients enable to restrict the heating to the outermost surface region. This results in increased heating efficiency, with more laser energy available for ablation and less for inefficient deep target heating. Thus, the evaporation process begins also at earlier times. The absorption edge of the CaP is around 200 nm [41], so several authors [32, 42] have studied the wavelength dependence of the density and size of droplets on the surface of the PLD CaP coatings. The coatings obtained with the KrF laser wavelength ($\lambda = 248$ nm) have a granular surface with the presence of droplets on their surface, whereas the coatings deposited with the ArF laser wavelength ($\lambda = 193$ nm) [43] have a smooth surface morphology, free of droplets with fine polygonal crystallites of 100 to 500 nm and columnar structure (Fig. 5.2).

At even greater wavelengths, when using the third-harmonic generation (THG) wavelength of the Nd:YAG laser ($\lambda = 355$ nm), the deposited coatings show a granular, not columnar, morphology, incorporating droplets of rather irregular shape and a wide range of sizes (30 nm to 4 mm) [44]. Moreover, the coatings produced with the THG of the Nd:YAG laser are rougher than those grown with the fourth harmonic (FHG, $\lambda = 266$ nm)-generated radiation [42].

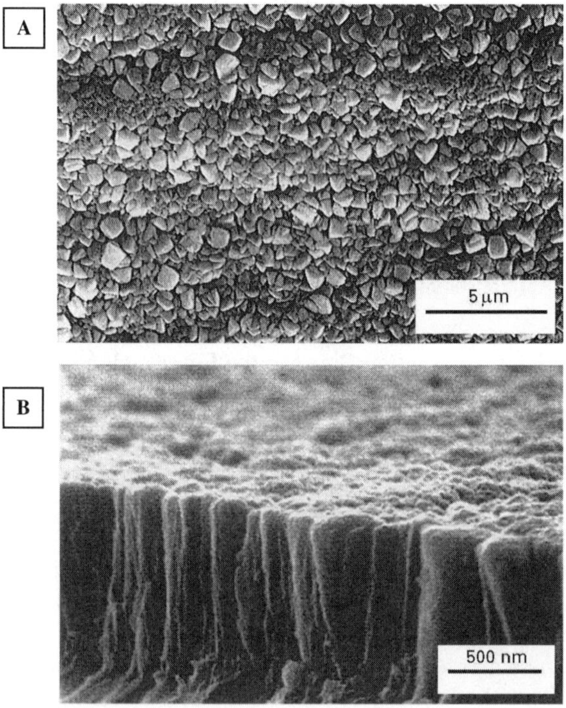

Fig. 5.2 Argon fluor excimer (ArF) laser deposited hydroxyapatite (HA) coating at high magnification, revealing that (**A**) it is formed by a network of polygonal-shaped HA crystallites and (**B**) it has columnar structure. From [43], with kind permission of Springer Science and Business Media

In fact, for the ArF laser [45] the absorption coefficient for sintered targets was calculated to be in the order of 10^5 cm^{-1}. This value is two orders of magnitude higher than that measured for the ruby laser ($\lambda = 694$ nm) [36], one order of magnitude above the measured at $\lambda = 500$ nm [46], and the same order of magnitude as the tricalcium phosphate targets doped with Mn used by Guillot-Noël et al. [29] to increase their absorption. Correspondingly, the target ablation threshold (Φ_o) was 0.09 J/cm^2 with the ArF laser, which is lower than the threshold with the KrF laser (Φ_o = 0.6 J/cm^2 [47]) and far below the onset of ablation for the ruby laser (Φ_o = 4.5 J/cm^2 [21]). Therefore, the efficiency of the ArF laser in ablating HA targets is much higher owing to its shorter wavelength even if the pulse energies available from commercial equipment are lower than the energies delivered by the other laser types.

The target density greatly influences the film morphology. The application of pressures up to 400 MPa [48] during preparation of the pellets without sintering leads to HA target densities of 1.7 g/cm^3 (54% of the theoretical HA density). However, uniaxial pressing at 81 MPa and sinterization at 1260°C for 4 hours with heating and cooling rates of 2.5°C min^{-1} yield densities of at least 3.0 g/cm^3 (95% of the theoretical HA density, $\rho_{HA} = 3.156$ g/cm^3 [49]). These high-density targets were utilized by García-Sanz et al. [43] with the ArF laser to produce the droplet free films shown in Fig. 5.2. Nevertheless, when using the KrF laser, the presence of droplets could not be avoided; although by using target sintering temperatures of 500° to 1100°C [50] films with varying grain sizes were obtained. Therefore, droplet-free, smooth coatings with the smallest grain sizes (100–500 nm) can be obtained with a combination of low-wavelength (ArF laser) and high-temperature sintered pellets.

More recently, some authors have attempted to improve even more the bioactivity and stability of the CaP thin coatings by varying the composition of the PLD targets. Ferro et al. [51] have added 10% fluorapatite to HA before sintering to improve the *in vivo* stability of PLD coatings; but the use of a rather long wavelength (532 nm), high laser fluence, room temperature growth, and vacuum environment has yielded no crystalline but greatly disordered amorphous coatings. Ferraz et al. [52] mixed into the HA target 1.5 wt% of CaO-P_2O_5 glass without sintering, with the aim of increasing the bioactivity of HA-PLD coatings produced with the ArF laser. In an immersion experiment in simulated body fluid (SBF), the films produced from the glass–HA targets induced earlier formation of natural apatite and better defined crystallinity than the films produced from the pure HA targets. By adding silicon (Si) powder to HA when producing the target, Si-substituted HA coatings have been deposited on titanium (Ti) substrates with the same laser [53]. The Si atoms are efficiently transferred to the coatings, and its incorporation in the coating was linear to its presence in the targets, so fine control of Si content was achieved. The Si atoms are present in the form of ortho-silicate groups (SiO_4^{4-}), which prefer to substitute CO_3^{2-} groups instead of PO_4^{3-} groups. The silicon substitution does not provoke the formation of new secondary crystalline phases, causing only a decrease in the crystallinity degree of the coatings.

György et al. [54] successfully produced Mn^{2+}-doped carbonated apatite films with the aim of improving cell adhesion. Mn^{2+} ions activate a family of receptors that mediate cellular interactions with extracellular matrix (ECM) and cell surface ligands. The KrF laser was used under dynamic oxygen pressure of 10 Pa at 400°C.

Furthermore, Suda et al. [55] compared films prepared from HA and HA(10%) + TiO_2 targets on titanium dioxide thin films, which were aimed at producing films with both bioactivity and photocatalytic properties for decomposing organic materials and bacteria. They used the SHG-mod a Nd:YAG laser (λ = 532 nm) and have annealed the films at 900°C to obtain high crystallinity.

These approaches of target composition modifications can open new optimization alternatives and improve performance for coatings produced by this technique in the future.

5.2.1.2 Dynamics of the Ablation Materials (Laser Plume)

When a pulsed laser beam impinges on a material surface at low laser energy density, small quantities of neutral and ionized species are photodesorbed from the surface. To obtain reasonable film growth, deposition rates in the order of 1 Å/pulse are needed, which implies that sufficient material should be removed from the target. Therefore, the threshold fluence in laser ablation is defined as the energy density at which measurable material removal takes place. If the laser energy increases beyond this threshold, significant material is ablated and a light-emitting plasma plume is generated. The exponential increase in the vapor pressure with temperature predicted by the Clausius-Clapeyron equation determines the evaporation threshold. At these laser fluences, the rapid heating rates overcome the radiation and thermal diffusion losses, and evaporation proceeds nonlinearly. For a KrF laser with a photon energy of 5 eV, a plasma plume temperature of T = 5.000 K can be attained, which is well above the boiling point of most materials.

In situ plasma diagnostic techniques have determined the nature, density, and kinetic energy of the species existing in the plasma generated by the laser ablation of HA targets. Guillot-Noël et al. [29] studied the ablation plume formed with the third and fourth harmonics of a Nd:YAG laser with in situ time- and space-resolved optical emission spectroscopy. Serra et al. [56–59] used fast intensified CCD imaging and optical emission spectroscopy with bandpass filters to study the dynamics of the generated plume. They studied KrF, ArF, and the THG of Nd:YAG laser ablation of HA targets as a function of the processing parameters. Three emitting populations were identified when ablation was performed in vacuum. The fastest distribution (velocity $\sim 10^4$ m/s), a plume-like shaped component, is an atomic population, dominated by emissions of neutral CaI, OI and PI, and ionic CaII species, with some contaminants (MgI, SiI, SiII, NaI). The other two near-isotropically expanding glow regions can be ascribed to molecular radicals (the faster one: velocity $\sim 10^3$ m/s) and to hot particulates ejected from the target (the slower one: velocity ~10^2 m/s). The molecular radicals correspond to a calcium oxide (Ca_xO_y) of unknown stoichiometry. With the KrF laser and for laser fluences in the range 2.1 to 4.8 J/cm^2, the emission of light species, atoms and molecules, is more significant for higher target densities. On the other hand, for lower target densities, the amount of hot particulates released from the target is greater, thus corroborating the advantage of the target sintering approach to obtain smoother thin HA coatings. With regard to the dependence of laser energy density, the emission is dominated by neutral calcium (Ca I) at all laser fluences [56]. The increase of fluence results in an increase in the ionic calcium contribution (Ca II) and makes apparent the presence of neutral phosphorus (P I) and oxygen (O I) as emissive species in the plasma. The molecular contribution of calcium oxides (Ca_xO_y) to the emission decreases with laser fluence. Summarizing, the effect of a background water atmosphere changes not only the shape and dynamics of the HA laser ablation plume but also the composition of its emissive species.

A parallel analysis [59], under identical conditions but with an ArF laser, revealed again the presence of the first two plasma clouds, and the absence of the third glow region, consisting of hot particles. This fact substantiated once more the advantages of using the short wavelength ArF laser to prevent or even eliminate the droplet presence in the PLD HA films.

With the THG of Nd:YAG lasers the detected plume species are similar to the excimer case except for oxygen, whose importance as an emissive species is stronger [60]. In water vapor atmospheres, there is again confinement of the ablated species in a shock front.

Based on the cited studies about the species present in the plume and their velocities, Arias el al. [61] studied the relation between transport of the ArF laser-ablated material through the water vapor atmosphere and the film properties. By placing a silicon wafer substrate at various distances from the target, inside and outside the visible plume, the thickness distribution of deposited material and its composition (Ca/P ratio and CO_3^{2-} content) were studied. This study is important for a potential scaling up of the laboratory research system to a commercial PLD coater.

The thickness homogeneity was better than 20% at ± 10 mm from the plume center for substrates situated 48 mm from the target. For dental and orthopedic applications, the more suitable target–substrate distances would be those greater than the stationary plume length because they produce more homogeneous HA coatings regarding the thickness. Shorter distances originate undesired phases and surface damage.

Before discussing the influence of the gas atmosphere composition on the obtained CaP coatings, it should be pointed out that the laser capacity to evaporate the target material is greatly influenced by the gas environment; this implies that at the target surface the ablation rate also depends on the gas type and pressure [62]. The ablation rate decreases linearly with pressure for all ambient gases (O_2, Ar, and H_2O vapor) but with different slope depending on the atmosphere.

In a water atmosphere, the situation is more complex than in the case of other gases owing to the formation of different CaP phases after the melting and the resolidification cycle that takes place at the surface of the target following impingement of each laser pulse. Based on the phase diagrams of the system CaO-P_2O_5 in the presence and absence of H_2O, after the first pulse in a H_2O atmosphere the resolidified target surface, initially a nonstoichiometric HA (Ca/P = 1.7), becomes a combination of a more stoichiometric HA and calcium oxide. On the other hand, in the absence of H_2O the resolidified material is a combination of tricalcium phosphate (TCP) and tetracalcium phosphate (TTCP), which has the same melting point as HA (1680°C) and is lower than that of calcium oxide (2300°C). This fact may indicate that after the first laser pulse the activation energy ΔE of desorption of the target particles from the surface becomes higher in a H_2O atmosphere than in other environments and can explain, in addition, the presence of other CaP phases in the coatings under certain processing conditions, as described in the next section.

Summarizing, from the point of view of target interaction with the laser photons and material transport through an atmosphere, the most efficient way to obtain PLD coatings is to use an ArF excimer laser to ablate sintered targets with a density as high as possible in a water vapor atmosphere. Less work has been performed in the field of tuning the target composition to eventually optimize the film bioactivity even further.

5.3 Physicochemical Properties of PLD Coatings: Nucleation and Growth on the Substrate

When analyzing the physicochemical properties of CaP PLD of thin coatings in view of their application for medical devices, one concludes that the relevant properties of these films are the chemical composition (CaP phases), their morphology (roughness, grain sizes), their structure (crystallinity), and their mechanical behavior. These properties control their *in vitro* and *in vivo* performance, as described in Chapters 2 and 5.

Probably one of the main advantages of PLD over other thin film deposition techniques is its ability to attain directly pure, crystalline HA coatings with no further thermal annealing step aiming at the necessary hydration of the coating, leading to its crystallization. Notwithstanding, process parameters should be well controlled.

The main processing parameters that influence the phase composition and structure of PLD CaP coatings are the substrate temperature and the gas environment. However, their impact differs depending on the laser wavelength, the range of laser fluences, the pulse repetition frequency, and the target utilized. Therefore, it is extremely difficult to compare the work reported in many published articles because in most cases several of these parameters differ, making direct comparison impossible. Here, we summarize the main results contained in the complete list of papers published in this field at the end of the present chapter (Table 5.5), trying to establish general trends when possible.

In 1993, Cotell [34] summarized the processing window (temperatures and gas environment) leading to the diverse CaP phases for ablating pressed and low temperature sintered (550°C) HA targets with a KrF laser. For substrate temperatures $T_{sub} > 700°C$, in O_2 and inert gas/water vapor environment, β-TCP and TTCP were obtained, whereas for O_2 and temperatures of 400° to 700°C α-TCP was the favored phase. Crystalline HA was achieved within this same temperature range but in an inert gas/water vapor atmosphere. For either any gas and temperatures below 400°C or nonreactive gas and $T_{sub} > 400°C$, amorphous layers were formed. For the same temperature, O_2 ambient favors α-TCP and Ar/water environment promotes crystalline HA.

Since the HA structure needs OH ions to stabilize its crystalline structure, most of the work performed thereafter used a water vapor atmosphere only, demonstrating that PLD does not require a postdeposition annealing step to rehydrate the HA molecule as sputter and plasma deposition techniques reportedly require (see Chapter 7). The gases in the deposition chamber have three main functions [23]: They (1) reduce the kinetic energy of the species so that good crystalline quality of the films can be obtained; (2) control film stoichiometry by promoting a hydration reaction between the film species and water or its decomposition products; and (3) prevent reevaporation of the volatile phosphorus from the coating by maintaining the gas at over-pressure.

5.3.1 Pressure Dependence

When considering the pressure dependence of coatings deposited in pure water vapor ambient ($T_{sub} = 575°C$, nonsintered targets) with the KrF excimer wavelength [32] and high laser energy density (3.5 J/cm^2), if the pressure was below 50 Pa, TTCP (Ca/P = 2) was formed in addition to HA. For pressures above this value, α-TCP (Ca/P = 1.5) was promoted instead of TTCP. This evolution was consistent with the hypothesis that the Ca/P ratio diminishes for increasing water pressure [23] because more phosphorus can be retained in the coating. However, with lower laser wavelength (ArF laser) and the same conditions, no crystalline phases different from those of HA were found. Preferential orientation in the (100) direction, crystallite size and hydroxylation have a maximum at around 50 Pa [32]. Even at a much lower temperature ($T_{sub} = 455°C$) and laser fluence (0.8 J/cm^2) the only crystalline phase detected was HA for pressures between 30 and 80 Pa [31] using sintered targets made of carbonated HA (Ca/P = 1.7). Above and below this water vapor pressure range, coatings became amorphous, as shown in Fig. 5.3, where the x-ray diffraction (XRD) patterns of the coatings produced by ArF PLD at different water pressures are depicted. A detailed infrared-spectroscopic analysis, combined with unit-cell calculations based on the XRD spectra [49] allows us to conclude that almost all the OH incorporated in the apatitic

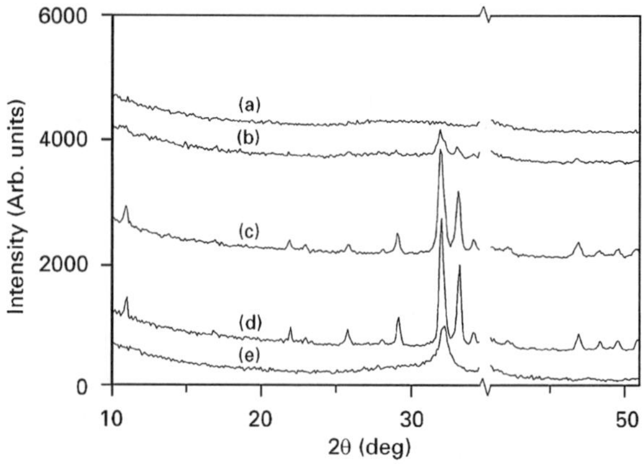

Fig. 5.3 X-ray diffraction (XRD) patterns of coatings produced by ArF pulsed laser deposition (PLD) at 455°C and different water vapor pressures: (*a*) 80; (*b*) 60; (*c*) 45; (*d*) 30; (*e*) 15 Pa. Laser fluence: 0.8 J/cm^2. From [31] with kind permission of Springer Science and Business Media

phase comes from the water vapor atmosphere, not from the target hydroxyl. Therefore, a minimum water vapor pressure is needed to obtain a crystalline coating, but this minimum pressure depends on the substrate temperature. At 455°C, it is ~30 Pa, whereas at 575°C it is < 15 Pa. The composition of the coatings at pressures of 15 to 80 Pa follows the general formula

$$Ca_{10-x-y+u}(PO_4)_{6-x-y}(HPO_4)_x(CO_3)_y(OH)_{2-x-y+2u}$$

where carbonate (CO_3^{2-}) and orthophosphate (HPO_4^{2-}) ions may substitute the PO_4^{3-} or the OH^- ions in the apatite lattice. At high pressures the crystallinity is lost, provoked by a decrease in hydroxyl ions due to the incorporation of orthophosphate, which competes with carbonate in phosphate substitution. At the same time, coatings become Ca-deficient.

At too low pressure, however, high carbonate incorporation is responsible for the amorphization of the coating (Fig. 5.4). The carbonate substitution for phosphate increases the Ca/P ratio and deforms the HA unit cell. Figure 5.5 [31] shows the carbonate content of coatings versus the unit-cell parameter for carbonated apatites (CHAs) produced by PLD at 455°C, in comparison to CHA powders produced by high temperature synthesis [63] and by precipitation in aqueous solution [64]. As depicted, despite being a vacuum method at relative high temperatures, PLD yields coatings that are more similar to those obtained by the wet method than those obtained by high temperature sintering. At high pressure, the orthophosphate substitution for phosphate is predominant, and the coatings become Ca-deficient (Fig. 5.6).

5.3.2 Temperature Dependence

The temperature of the substrate primarily modulates the crystallinity of the coatings. Below 400°C no crystalline coating can be deposited (Fig. 5.7) at 45 Pa

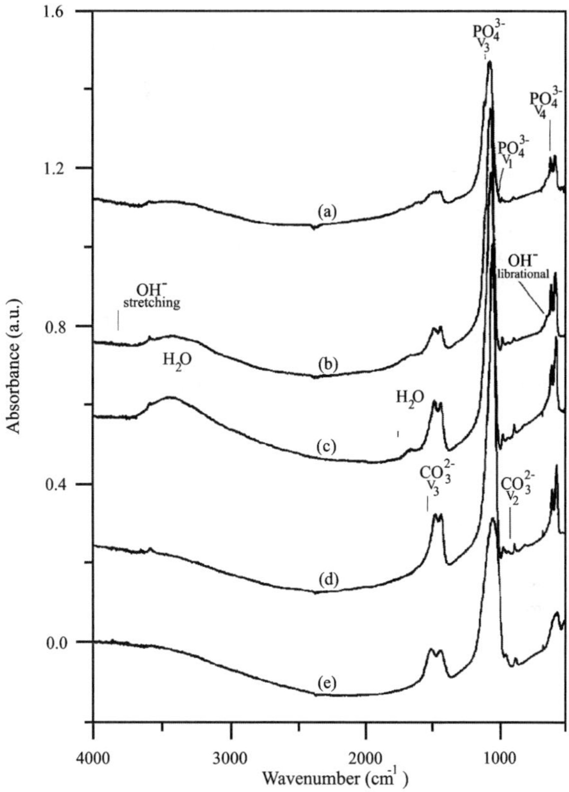

Fig. 5.4 Fourier transform infrared spectra of coatings produced by ArF PLD at 485°C and various water vapor pressures. (*a*) 80; (*b*) 60; (*c*) 45; (*d*) 30; (*e*) 15 Pa. Laser fluence 0.8 J/cm^2. From [49], with permission from Elsevier

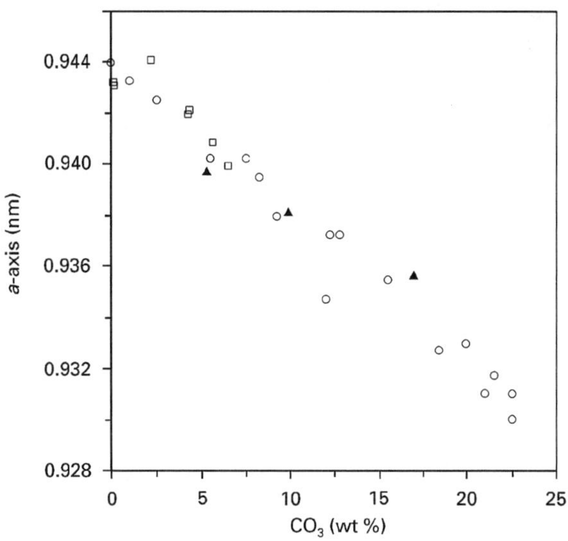

Fig. 5.5 Unit-cell parameter *a* versus CO_3 content for various HA production methods. *Circles*, data from [64]; *squares*, data from [63]; *triangles*, coatings produced by ArF pulsed laser deposition. From [31] with kind permission of Springer Science and Business Media

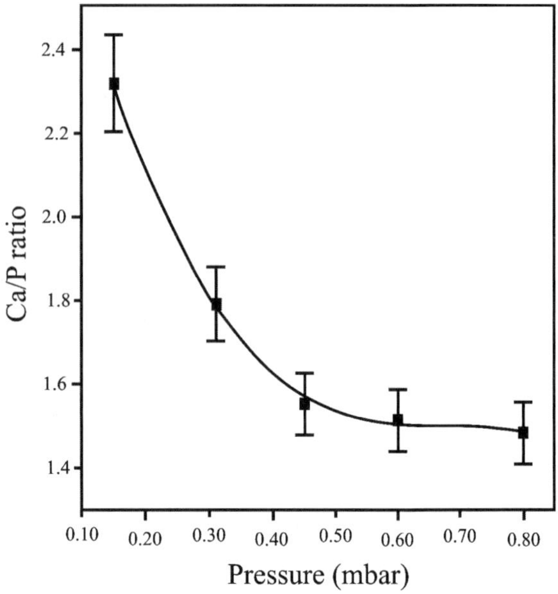

Fig. 5.6 Calcium phosphate (Ca/P) ratio of pulsed ArF laser-deposited coatings as a function of the pure water pressure; $\lambda = 193$ nm, 20 Hz, $\tau = 20$ ns, $\phi = 0.82$ J/cm^2, d = 4.5 cm, T_{sub} = 485°C, ρ_{target} = 3.0 g/cm^3, $(Ca/P)_{target}$ = 1.72. From [49], with permission from Elsevier

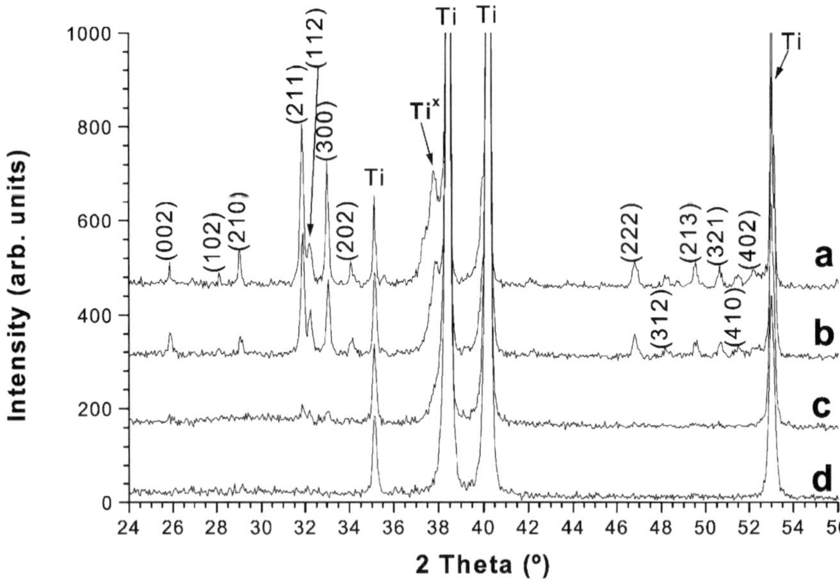

Fig. 5.7 XRD patterns of ArF laser coatings produced at 45 Pa and various substrate temperatures. (*a*) 460°C; (*b*) 400°C; (*c*) 350°C; (*d*) 300°C. Laser fluence 1.2 J/cm^2. From [73], reprinted with permission of Elsevier

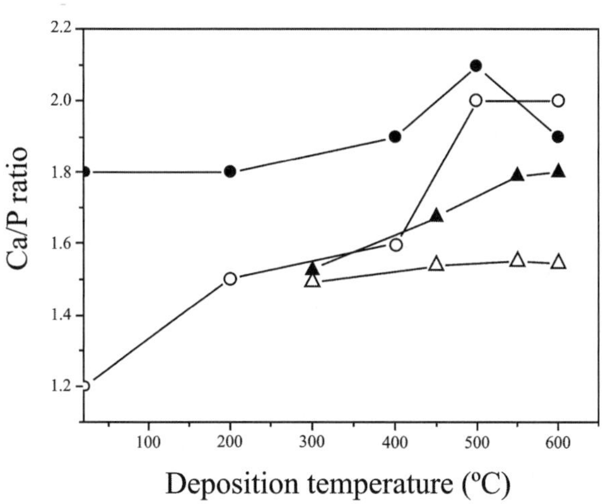

Fig. 5.8 Ca/P ratio of PLD coatings versus the substrate temperature. *Triangles*, ArF laser [72], with processing parameters the same as in Fig. 5.6. However, water pressures were 45 Pa (*open triangles*) and 30 Pa (*filled triangles*). *Circles*, Nd:YAG (THG) laser [124]: $\lambda = 355$ nm, 10 Hz, $\tau = 10$ ns, $\Phi = 3.1$ J/cm^2, d = 4 cm, $\rho_{target} = 1.5$ g/cm^3, $(Ca/P)_{target} = 1.7$. Water pressures were 10 Pa (*filled circles*) and 45 Pa (*open circles*)

water pressure and 1.2 J/cm^2 laser energy density of ArF laser. The Ca/P ratio of the coatings from ArF laser PLD tends to be lower (1.5) than the original target ratio (1.7), and it increases with temperature owing to greater incorporation of carbonate ions substituting phosphate into the HA structure, as shown in Fig. 5.8, for 30 Pa water pressure. However, at 45 Pa pressure, this dependence is negligible.

When the THG radiation of a Nd:YAG laser is used [44], again a water-containing atmosphere together with a minimum temperature of 400°C is needed to deposit crystalline CaP phases (in this case a mixture of HA, α-TCP, and β-TCP phases). These coatings have a higher relative content of α-TCP than those obtained with KrF laser (Fig. 5.8), probably owing to the higher deposition rate obtained with Nd:YAG, as faster deposition with the 248 nm excimer wavelength also favors the formation of α-TCP.

Comparison of films produced with the FHG wavelength of the Nd:YAG laser ($\lambda = 266$ nm) and those obtained with the THG [65] resulted in a higher Ca/P ratio in the films obtained with the 266 nm wavelength (1.82) than with 355 nm radiation (1.77). The original Ca/P ratio of the targets was much lower (1.65). Because the FHG wavelength of the Nd:YAG laser is close to that of the KrF excimer laser, it is not surprising that Blind et al. [48] found optimized parameters similar to those of Fernández-Pradas et al. for the KrF laser [32], as has been noted.

5.3.3 Fluence Dependence

Figure 5.9 shows the laser fluence dependence of the Ca/P ratio of coatings deposited with the ArF laser at T_{sub} = 490°C, 45 Pa water pressure, and a target–substrate distance of 4.8 cm [66]. Although the targets have a Ca/P ratio of 1.7 with 4.4 wt% of carbonate, the coatings have a higher ratio for energy densities below 1.2 J/cm^2, tending toward the original target composition for more intense laser fluence. This behavior finds its explanation in the incongruent melting of HA. HA is a material that cannot be in equilibrium with its own melt. It suffers several transformations before becoming liquid. When its temperature is raised: (1) It loses the carbonate as CO_2 gas, decomposing into CaO and stoichiometric HA. (2) The stoichiometric HA and the CaO react to form TTCP, which coexists with part of the HA. (3) The stoichiometric HA decomposes into TCP and TTCP. (4) TCP melts, whereas TTCP keeps its solid state. (5) TTCP melts. This process is not reversible, as the degasified CO_2 lost in the first step cannot be reincorporated. Thus, the resolidified material is not the starting one but a mixture of CaO and nonstoichiometric HA with a higher melting point; the melting point of CaO is higher (2300°C) than that of HA (1680°C).

For low energy densities, if the ablation depth is not equal to or higher than the molten depth in each pulse, the remaining upper layer of the target is Ca enriched, as is the coating produced after the first ablation pulse. However, for higher laser fluences, the pulse energy is enough to ablate the higher temperature melting CaO on the surface together with deeper parts of the target, and the coating composition equals that of the original target. Jelínek et al. [25] also observed greater Ca enrichment for lower energy densities in KrF laser experiments than for more intense fluence. Despite using such elevated energy

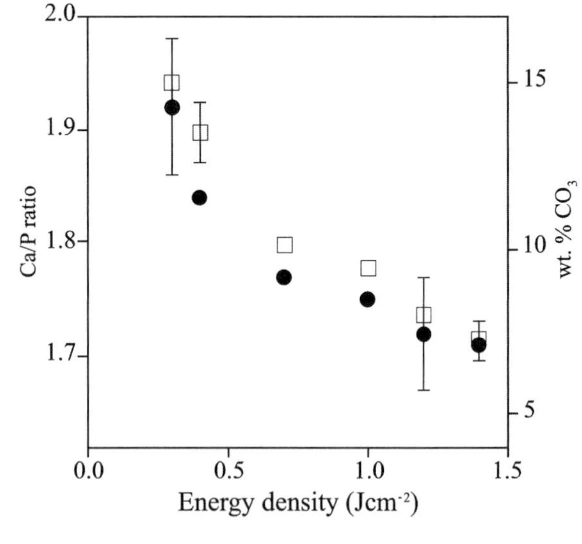

Fig. 5.9 Ca/P ratio and carbonate content of ArF laser deposited coatings as a function of the energy density [66], processing parameters are the same as in Fig. 5.6. Water pressure was 45 Pa; d = 4.8 cm, T_{sub} = 490°C. Reprinted with permission from Elsevier

densities (3 and 13 J/cm^2), they did not achieve congruent deposition at 500°C, 20 Pa water vapor pressure, and a target–substrate distance of 7.5 cm. On the other hand, Antonov et al. [67] needed 9 J/cm^2 to achieve congruent KrF-PLD of HA coatings grown at room temperature and 2 Pa residual air pressure (i.e., no water atmosphere), substantiating the effect of the gas environment on the laser ablation process of the target.

Having in mind the possible industrial application of PLD, the stability of the deposition rate as a function of time is an important issue that deserves attention. In the case of the KrF laser, Fernández-Pradas et al. [68] determined that there is a certain fluence between 1.3 and 2.2 J/cm^2, below which the deposition rate diminishes with the number of pulses; above it, the opposite behavior is observed. They related these findings primarily to the effective area increase of the ablated crater in the target surface as a function of the ablation time. However, in this study the surface composition change described described by Arias et al. [66] with regard to the fluence dependence has not been considered. At low fluence, the target surface is enriched in CaO due to the heating and melting cycles, and therefore its surface melting point is increased. Thus, the deposition rate should also drop with increasing number of pulses at low laser energy density. The longer wavelength of the KrF laser compared to the ArF laser implies a larger penetration depth due to its lower absorption coefficient. Therefore, it is not surprising that the fluence at which the pulse number dependence of the deposition rate changes for 248 nm lies between 1.3 and 2.2 J/cm^2, somewhat higher than the energy density at which congruent composition coatings can be obtained with the ArF laser (1.2 J/cm^2).

5.3.4 Pulse Repetition Rate Dependence

If we aim at potentially scaling up the PLD technique, it would be straightforward to think that the deposition rate can be readily augmented by increasing the pulse repetition rate. It has been demonstrated that the slowest particulate compounds of the plume travel at around 100 m/s, and the fastest one travels two orders of magnitude faster [69]. This means that the time needed by all species to arrive at the substrate placed at a 5 cm distance would be at most 0.5 ms. Accordingly, one could grow HA at a 2000 Hz pulse repetition rate based only on the time needed to transport material from the target to the substrate. Actually, there are other growth-limiting factors.

As can be seen in Fig. 5.10, the deposition rate per pulse augments with increasing repetition rate until about 1 Å/pulse at 80 Hz and T_{sub} = 460°C and 45 Pa. For higher frequencies, the deposition rate shows a steep rise, but the coating becomes amorphous. When the time interval between pulses increases for lower frequencies, the Ca/P ratio and the carbonate incorporation drop slightly and the crystallinity of the coatings is enhanced. Some kind of unknown desorption mechanism may take place both at this temperature and at

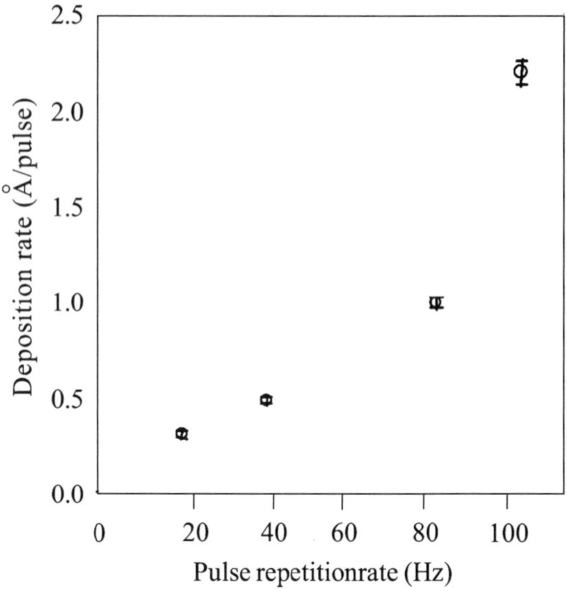

Fig. 5.10 Deposition rate per pulse for the coatings produced with the ArF laser at various pulse repetition rates. From [71], reprinted with permission from Elsevier

frequencies between 20 and 80 Hz, resulting in an almost linear dependence of the deposition rate per pulse on the pulse frequency, with only slight differences in Ca/P relation and carbonate incorporation. On the other hand, there seems to be a maximum deposition rate at which crystalline HA coatings may be grown, when considering film growth originated by the neutral and ionized species formed in the plasma plume. The droplet growth through the ablated particulates is not included in this consideration. This maximum deposition rate depends on the diffusion length of arriving surface species or ad-atoms at the growing surface for them to enable the building of a polycrystalline structure. The diffusion length depends on the surface temperature. At a given substrate temperature there is a limitation to the number of arriving species that can be accommodated in the crystalline structure. In the case of HA, Fernández-Pradas [70] found a maximum value of 0.9 Å/pulse for the KrF laser at 575°C, whereas Arias et al. [71] obtained 1 Å/pulse for the ArF laser at 460°C—values that are in good agreement. It is likely that by raising the temperature for the ArF laser a higher value may be obtained, but then the titanium–HA interface is usually damaged, thus compromising the mechanical properties of the coating.

5.3.5 Preferential Orientation

PLD HA films can have preferential orientations with regard to the usual powder standard XRD pattern. Strongly preferential (002) orientations were reported by Cotell [34] in samples deposited at 500°C in He/H_2O and Kr/H_2O, being stronger in the last gas mixture, in which the films showed fewer particulates. Hence, she concluded that the (002) orientation resulted from the columnar part of the film, whereas the other peaks in the XRD pattern stem from the random orientation of the incorporated droplets.

However, most studies [23, 25, 32, 72] have obtained preferential growth in other crystallographic directions. With the KrF laser, Jelínek et al. [25] found the preferential orientation to change from (300) to (002) and (112) according to the deposition conditions. With a laser fluence of 3.5 J/cm^2 at 575°C and a very short target–substrate distance (2 cm), it was found that the coatings have the highest degree of hydroxylation at a water vapor pressure of 50 Pa. They also have the best crystalline properties, corresponding to films of pure HA for the ArF laser beam and of almost pure HA for the KrF beam, both oriented preferentially in the (100) direction. For much lower or higher pressures in the ArF laser experiment, the orientation was closer to the random standard distribution of orientations. At roughly the same temperature, pressure, and fluence range, Singh et al. [23] obtained the same results on silicon substrates.

The substrate temperature also influences the crystal orientations. Mayor et al. [72] observed that when they reduced the temperature from 525°C to 485°C, the XRD pattern of the ArF laser deposited films resembled more the standard random distribution of orientations. Therefore, one can conclude that at lower temperature ($\leq$ 485°C), the preferential orientation is lost. It is not clear what causes the growth of the crystallites to be not randomly distributed but with (100) planes parallel to the substrate surface. Cotell suggested that some degree of epitaxy may take place. Jiménez et al [73] found the (002) preferential orientation at 300°C with the ArF laser when crystal seeds were formed first at high ionization current (see modification of PLD techniques) and the rest of the coating at lower ionization current. Under electrical discharges, a higher concentration of OH^- and H^+ is generated at the substrate surface. Simultaneously, the film is bombarded with electrons, and it tends to grow in the orientation that needs the lowest energy to nucleate, which in the case of HA is the (002) direction [74].

5.3.6 Influence of the Substrate Material

Albeit most of the work performed on PLD of CaP coatings has used pure titanium (primarily in dental implants) or titanium alloy (Ti-6Al-4V) (in orthopedic devices), for certain characterization techniques, such as transmission electron microscopy (TEM), silicon wafers were the adequate reference substrate for studying the coatings. Notwithstanding, a warning is required in this context because the preferential orientation often observed in PLD of HA—with (100) planes parallel to the substrate surface [23]—depends considerably on the rugosity and the chemistry of the silicon surface ([75, unpublished results]. Preferential orientation was much more pronounced in Si (100) substrates than in Si (111) when the native oxide was etched in HF acid (HF) for 10 minutes for both substrates. Similarly, HF-etched Si (100) for 30 minutes (rugosity 0.30 nm) and methanol-washed Si (100) (maintaining the amorphous native silicon oxide) displayed no preferential orientation compared to Si (100), whereby the native oxide was etched away for just 10 minutes. These last two treatments leave a surface with a rugosity of 0.15 nm. Furthermore, it was calculated that the distance between the silicon atoms in the (100) plane (0.38 nm) geometrically matches the distance between the OH^- ions in the <100> direction of the HA crystal (0.34 nm, according to Legeros and Legeros [76]). Hence, hydroxyl ions could link to the silicon atoms of the Si (100) planes, and from then on the (100) HA planes would build up parallel to the substrate surface, resulting in this preferred orientation growth. Consequently, the larger roughness of a metallic substrate would not permit preferential orientation for temperatures below 485°C. Thus, it is clear that one cannot automatically transpose the results obtained on one substrate to those obtained on any other, especially from Si to titanium or its alloys.

5.3.7 Interface Between HA and Titanium

Because crystalline HA coatings are obtained for temperatures above 400°C and under a hydrating reactive atmosphere, the titanium surface oxidizes during the deposition time. Titanium oxides are known to be brittle; therefore, to improve coating adhesion on titanium implants, the nature and properties of the interface between the CaP thin coating and the titanium alloy are of paramount importance.

Fernández-Pradas et al. [77] conducted an elegant study of the interface of KrF-laser-deposited coating and the Ti-6Al-4 V substrate by correlating the information provided by secondary-ion mass spectrometry (SIMS), scanning electron microscopy (SEM), Raman spectrometry, grazing incidence XRD, and x-ray photoelectron spectroscopy (XPS). The coating was deposited with a laser fluence of 2.2 J/cm^2, a target–substrate distance of 4 cm, a pure water vapor atmosphere at 45 Pa, and a substrate temperature of 575°C, conditions corresponding to the best KrF laser-produced coatings. The results obtained with the various characterization techniques at this rather high temperature show that the interface between the CaP coating and the titanium alloy is a complex system where diffusion and oxidation processes occur. Although the original coating thickness was 0.9 μm, the interface had a thickness of about 1.5 μm. The bulk coating consisted of HA and α-TCP, and the interface constituted a graded layer of mixed CaP and amorphous titanium oxide.

There was a zone of 0.35 μm with interdiffusion of substrate elements into the coating and coating components into the substrate oxide layer, probably promoted by the high deposition temperature. No XRD reflections corresponding to any titanium oxide were detected. Crystalline Ti_2O_3 seemed not to be present, although its amorphous phase was detected by Raman spectrometry. Titanium alloy reflections were broad, probably indicating oxygen incorporation into the titanium alloy lattice. Neither titanium phosphates nor calcium titanates were observed. Because the oxygen content of the oxide layer diminishes with depth until it is only incorporated in solid solution in the titanium alloy, oxygen diffusion into the substrate has been demonstrated. For the titanium substrate, the HA coating acts more as a diffusion barrier for oxygen incoming from the gas than as an oxygen source during deposition.

In fact, using the ArF laser at even higher temperatures (650°C), Jiménez et al. [78] found that an extremely thin (25 nm thick) buffer layer of HA, grown at the lower temperature of 460°C, can protect the interface efficiently from the formation of TiO_2 at the higher temperature at which the rest of the coating (1 μm total thickness) is produced. The interface studies integrated the information provided by XRD, Fourier transform infrared (FTIR) spectrometry, and XPS. Under the high temperature processing conditions (60 Pa water pressure, gas flow 30 Pa L/s), the buffer layer prevented formation of rutile at the interface but provoked formation of titanium hydride ($TiH_{0.71}$) and stressed titanium there owing to diffusion of both oxygen and hydrogen into the substrate. As explained later, these phases compromise the mechanical performance of the coatings. In this study, the undesirable phases could be eliminated by doubling the water vapor flow to 60 Pa L/s. Thus, the stronger gas flow drags out the hydrogen resulting from water dissociation at the hot surface during coating deposition. At 460°C and with the ArF laser, none of these deleterious phases have been found at the interface; thus, the mechanical performance is markedly better.

5.3.8 Octacalcium Phosphate Thin Films

Octacalcium phosphate (OCP)—$Ca_8(HPO_4)_2(PO_4)_4 \cdot 5H_2O$—occurs as transient compound in the precipitation of HA and biological apatites; therefore, it plays a crucial role in the *in vivo* mineralization of bones and teeth. Its structure consists of apatitic layers similar to HA separated by interlayers containing structural water molecules. The similarity between the structures of OCP and HA is the reason OCP easily converts to HA in aqueous solution. Therefore, the use of OCP has been proposed as a coating for stimulating bone growth. However, it cannot be processed at high temperatures because it decomposes at 200°C [79, 80].

5.3.9 Deposition on Other Materials

The ArF laser has been used to fabricate HA thin films on polymer materials such as polyimide (PI), polytetrafluoroethylene (PTFE), silicone rubber (SR), and polyethyleneterephthalate (PET) [28] at a substrate temperature of 100°C in a residual oxygen atmosphere. Thereafter, samples were heat-treated in an oxygen and water vapor environment to crystallize the films at various temperatures below the melting point of the polymer substrates.

Crystalline HA films were obtained on the PI and PTFE substrates with annealing temperatures of 360°C and 320°C, respectively, but not on the other substrates, for which the melting point was < 300°C. The temperature of this treatment leading to crystalline films is rather low compared to temperatures needed in the sputtering technique. The reduction in the crystallization temperature is probably due to the presence of apatite crystal nuclei already formed in the thin film by the strong excitation effect unique to the excimer PLD technique. The KrF laser has also been used to deposit CaP coatings at room temperature and 2 Pa residual air pressure on the following polymer surfaces: Teflon (PTFE) and polyethylene (PE) [37] as well as poly-L-lactide (PLA) and poly-ϵ-caprolactone (PCL) [81]. The same group of investigators [82] has also deposited PLD coatings with the ArF laser on α-Al_2O_3, SiO2//Si (100), and $SrTiO_3$ for biomaterials and bioelectronic hybrid layered structures. They measured (for the first time) the electrical properties of 1 μm thick HA films with a Ca/P ratio of 2.03 to 2.08. The dielectric constant was 5.7 (25°C, 1 MHz), and the loss tangent was typically < 2%. The breakdown electric field was as high as 10^4 V/cm. Furthermore, by depositing onto glass substrates and further photolithographic patterning [83], they tested the specific adsorption of diverse proteins on the patterned HA coating. This technique may be useful for developing a chromatographic chip, biosensors, and scaffolds for tissue culturing. By tailoring the preferred orientation of the film, positively or negatively charged surfaces may be prepared that have a differentiated adsorption capability for biological molecules.

More recently, Antonov et al. [84] tested thinner (100 and 300 nm thick) layers than those produced by them in another study [37] as sublayers for biomimetic growth of thicker CaP layers in SBF. In their SBF immersion experiments, only the coatings grown at very high fluence (9 J/cm^2) built up large plate-like crystallites on and around the initial laser-deposited macroparticles (droplets). The coatings obtained at reduced fluence have decreased their thickness after immersion, probably owing to their smaller content of crystalline droplets and their rather amorphous structure [85].

Deposition of HA with the ArF laser has also been successful on biomorphic silicon carbide substrates [86], a new type of material for implant devices that has improved mechanical properties and has incorporated a porous network, following the natural vascular system of wood. Results are similar to those obtained on titanium substrates. Moreover, it was found that because of the forward velocity of species in the PLD plasma plume, the coating penetrates the porous surface of the biomorphic substrate to a certain extent.

5.4 Modifications of the PLD Technique

Seeking for a more efficient way to multiply the number density or the energy of highly reactive species on the growing surface, some authors have proposed modifications of the usual PLD technique by adding an energy source to the experiment, apart from the ablating laser. Nelea et al. [87] proposed an ultraviolet (UV)-assisted KrF-PLD system. A low-pressure mercury (Hg) lamp with a fused silica envelope was installed inside the PLD chamber. It allows ~85% of the emitted 184.9 nm radiation (~6% of the 25 W output) to be transmitted. The UV in situ irradiation enhances gas reactivity and increases bombardment of the surface film with excited species from the laser plasma. These effects proved beneficial for film densification and tensile bonding to the substrate but provoked decomposition of the HA into TTCP, dicalcium phosphate (DCP) (whitlockite), $Ca_2P_2O_7$, and CaO, which may seriously compromise the stability of the coating.

Instead of decomposing oxygen in situ with a UV lamp, Katto et al. [88] proposed use of a split beam of the ablating KrF laser to laser-assist the laser ablation method (LALA) to improve coating adhesion and crystallinity by in situ photonic annealing when growing at room temperature. The ablation beam had an energy density of 1.5 J/cm^2, and the annealing beam had a fluence of 0.2 J/cm^2. The Ca/P ratio of the coatings was 2.2, suggesting the presence of TTCP and/or other amorphous Ca-enriched phases, in agreement with the results obtained with the in situ UV lamp annealing [87]. The in situ irradiated and nonirradiated coatings were tested in a 1.5 $\times$ SBF immersion experiment. Nonirradiated coatings were dissolved after 1 day, whereas the laser annealed coatings remained but reduced their Ca/P ratio to 1.0 after immersion. A small peak at 31.7° in the XRD spectra of the irradiated samples suggests that a small number of microcrystals were induced by the optical annealing, serving as seeds for HA growth in SBF.

Another variation of this LALA method [89] uses the high energy output of the KrF laser to ablate the target, and a different laser, an ArF laser, as the assisting laser. In this experiment, the coating properties depended on the synchronization of the assisting pulsed irradiation and the incoming ablated particles. Only then could the assisting beam photons impart photothermal and photochemical excitation energy to these particles and thus accelerate the migration and crystallization processes. Even so, it remains to be demonstrated if such higher experimental complexity is of practical significance.

A much simpler and inexpensive PLD modification approach consists in creating an autonomous electrical discharge between the target and the substrate with a direct current (DC) power supply (0–1000 V, 800 W), resulting in ionization currents between 0 and 80 mA [73]. With this configuration, a plasma with a high ion concentration is obtained around the substrate, leading to dissociation of the water molecules ($H_2O \rightarrow H^+ + OH^-$). Two studies were performed: (1) keeping the ionization current at 40 mA and varying the substrate temperature between 300° and 460°C and (2) changing the ionization current in the range 0 to 60 mA and maintaining the substrate temperature at 300°C.

The coating structure tends to grow in the orientation, which needs the lower energy to nucleate, which in the case of HA is the (002) direction [74]. A current of 40 mA allowed reduction of the temperature to obtain crystalline coatings from 400°C without current to 350°C. At 300°C, an ionization current of 60 mA is necessary to start to see HA peaks in the XRD patterns. To elucidate how the ionization current induces the crystallinity of the coatings, a coating was produced at a substrate temperature of 300°C and an initial ionization current of 80 mA during the first 10% of the coating growth process and 40 mA during the other 90%. Its XRD pattern (Fig. 5.11) shows better crystallinity than the coatings produced at a more intense ionization current (60 mA) during 100% of the growing time. Therefore, it can be concluded that the seeds for crystallization are formed during the initial growth steps because of the additional energy provided by the ionization. Once these crystal seeds are formed, less energy is necessary to grow the crystalline coating; one-half of the seeding ionization current is sufficient. The application of low ionization currents has

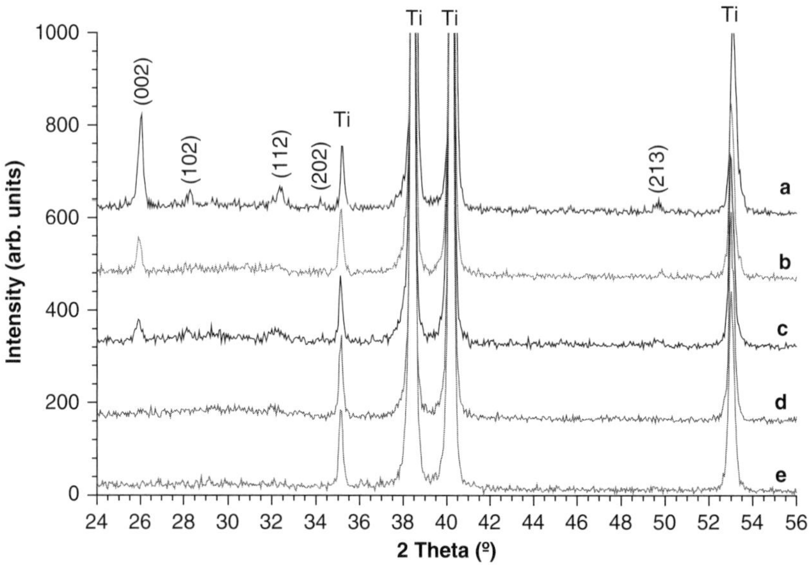

Fig. 5.11 XRD patterns of the coatings produced at a substrate temperature of 300°C and an ionization current of: (*a*) 80 mA during the first 10% of growth and 40 mA during the last 90%; (*b*) 60 mA; (*c*) 40 mA; (*d*) 20 mA; (*e*) 0 mA. From [73], with permission from Elsevier

been highly effective in reducing the minimum temperature for obtaining crystalline HA coatings down to 300°C, which can be extremely useful for coating thermal-sensitive devices, such as polymers.

Likewise, a radiofrequency (RF) plasma source was applied to assist the PLD process [90]. The deposition rate was increased, and the crystallinity of the HA films was improved owing to decreased carbonate incorporation.

5.5 Mechanical Properties of the PLD Coatings

Application of thin CaP coatings to orthopedic implants involves a series of conditions necessary for improving the performance of commercial plasma-sprayed coatings. Apart from inducing faster bone regeneration and bonding between the implant surface and the newly formed bone, thin CaP coatings should be well adherent, and they should not release particles that could damage other components of the implant device. Moreover, their elastic modulus should have an intermediate value, between that of the substrate and that of the bone, to reduce the intrinsic residual stresses in the implantation area. Several factors determine the mechanical performance of the PLD coatings.

- Their morphology, either columnar or globular
- Their structure, either crystalline or amorphous
- Their thickness
- Their interface with the substrate.

We have already described the processing conditions leading to the diverse morphologies and crystallinity of CaP coatings, and the factors affecting the interface composition and its thickness have been addressed. As for the thickness, in general it affects the mechanical performance of coatings owing to increases in stress accumulation with increasing thickness [91]. Thus, if bioactivity of a thin CaP coating is safeguarded by its composition, the coating has to be as thin as possible with regard to its mechanical properties.

5.5.1 Adhesive Bond Strength

When considering the bond strength of HA coatings, either plasma-sprayed or PLD thin coatings, as measured in a pullout experiment it should be noted that the bond strength for a typical plasma-sprayed coating in reality measures the bond strength of the adhesive resin to a grit-blasted titanium surface. This point becomes clear in Fig. 5.12, which shows an SEM cross section image of a typical commercial plasma-sprayed coating specified to be 50 μm thick. Because the adhesive resin penetrates the plasma-sprayed coating's pores and cracks, if the modus of failure is cohesive the value measures the cohesive failure of an HA-resin composite. If the failure is adhesive, the measured value is a

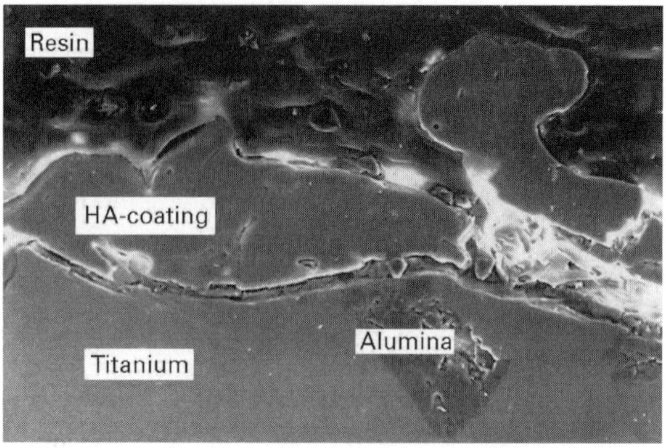

Fig. 5.12 Cross-sectional view of a polystyrene (PS)-HA coating. Note the microcracks penetrating the coating surface and even reaching the substrate. A large crack along the coating–substrate interface can be clearly appreciated, as can an embedded alumina particle from the grit-blasting roughening step. From [43], with kind permission of Springer Science and Business Media

combination of the real adhesion strength of the HA coating to the metal substrate and that of the resin to the metal surface.

Moreover, the plasma-sprayed coating needs a previous grit-blasting treatment performed with ceramic powder (usually Al_2O_3 or SiC) to add a mechanical interlocking contribution to the coating–substrate bonding mechanism. This grit-blasting treatment leads to surface contamination and to the eventual release of these highly abrasive particles. Figure 5.12 also shows an alumina particle embedded into the titanium and clearly demonstrates that parts of the plasma-sprayed coating are not bonded to the substrate because the resin is in contact with the metallic substrate.

PLD coatings are usually dense and pore-free, so the resin cannot penetrate it, as shown in Fig. 5.13. Thus, in the case of PLD coatings, the pullout test measures different strengths depending on the fracture site. If the fracture is

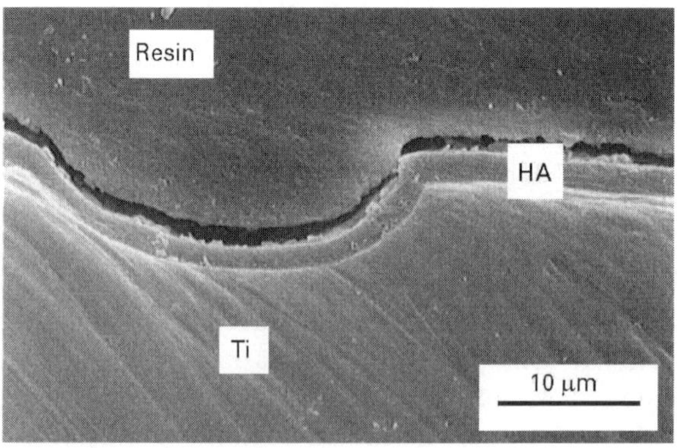

Fig. 5.13 Cross-sectional view of a PLD-HA-coated textured titanium (Ti) rod. The substrate surface texture is perfectly followed by the coating, without cracks or spallation. From [43], with kind permission of Springer Science and Business Media

Table 5.1 Tensile bond strength of pulsed laser deposited HA coatings

Laser type	Tensile bond strength [MPa]	Substrate type	$T_{substrate}$ (°C)	Reference
ArF	>58	Ti, grade 3	455	[43]
	3	Ti, grade 3	550	[95]
	30–40	Ti, grade 2	500–600	[30]
	9.8	HA/PI	room	[28]
	6	HA/PTFE	room	[125]
Nd:YAG (THG, FHG)	21.1–31.1	Ti, grade 2	0–600	[42]
Plasma sprayed	32.5	Ti, 99.3%	–	[92]

situated at the resin–coating interface, the measurement corresponds to the resin–coating bond strength. However, if the fracture takes place in the coating, the coating cohesive strength is obtained. Finally, only when the coating–substrate interface is fractured does the measurement deliver the coating–substrate bond strength. Hence, testing samples must be carefully examined after performing the pullout test for elucidating the causes for failure and for correct interpretation of the measurements.

Table 5.1 shows the tensile bond strength as reported for PLD coatings in the literature. Only four groups have described results with pullout testing: three of them on titanium or its alloys [30, 42, 43] and one on polymer substrates [28]. No pullout studies have been performed with KrF laser-produced coatings. When using the ArF laser, it becomes clear that the processing temperature plays a major role and that it should be as low as possible to mantain an interface between the coating and the substrate, which is free of brittle titanium oxide phases. The highest tensile bond strength value [43] was $\geq$ 58 MPa for crystalline HA coatings at 455°C and 1 to 2 μm thickness; and the fracture was at the adhesive resin in all cases, without spallation of the coating. This value is much better than the 30 to 40 MPa reported for 500° to 600°C [30] and 10 μm thickness, where the fracture occurred predominantly in the coating; these results indicate that with these thicker films and higher temperatures the intrinsic strength of the HA coating itself played a more critical role than that of the coating–substrate interface. Zeng et al. [42] reported values of 21 to 31 MPa with the THG- and FHG-Nd:YAG lasers. Compared to the values obtained for the plasma-sprayed (32.5 MPa [92]) and heat-treated sputtered coatings (>53 MPa [17]), the PLD coatings had improved performance, probably owing to the fact that no thermal annealing is needed to achieve sufficient crystallinity, and thus it is possible to reduce to a minimum the amount of titanium oxide at the metal– coating interface.

5.5.2 Scratch Testing

Mechanical performance of the samples has been thoroughly evaluated by scratch testing by a number of authors [20, 44, 93–95]. In general, it has been found that the lower the processing temperature is the higher is the critical load. The titanium oxide interface layer should be minimized to attain the best mechanical performance of the HA coatings [96]. However, comparison between the different results is difficult because critical loads are determined by acoustic emission and/or friction force correlation to SEM observations after the scratch experiment. Moreover, substrate roughness, spherical stylus material, and diameters are different; loading and scan velocities are not equal as well, so a direct comparison of the critical load values becomes meaningless (see section on mechanical evaluation). Notwithstanding this fact, general trends can be concluded based on each set of experiments.

When coated at 575°C [94] with the KrF laser, coatings fail under the scratch test by spallating laterally from the diamond tip, and the failure load increases as the thickness decreases. The thinner the coating, the stronger is the influence of the substrate on the scratch characteristics: The thinnest coating does not fail adhesively (but cohesively) as the thickest ones do, and it only deforms plastically because the substrate is ductile. For such a thin film, the adhesion to the substrate overcomes its own cohesive strength. However, this thinnest coating is amorphous. The influence of the interface layer on the adhesion is well documented for this same type of coatings. If deposited during an interval of only 7 minutes but held at the processing temperature for various annealing times in the water environment, the interface layer grows as described previously, and its critical load drops accordingly.

Comparable thickness dependence studies have been made with the 355 nm wavelength of the Nd:YAG laser [44]. All processing parameters were similar to those used with the KrF laser mentioned above, with the exception of the pulse duration, which in this case is much shorter (10 ns) and the larger wavelength, thus yielding a higher deposition rate (fivefold) and higher α-TCP content compared to those deposited with the KrF laser. This is probably the reason for obtaining critical loads, which are strikingly low (0.4 N for 0.4 μm thickness) compared to those obtained with the 248 nm wavelength, although the same thickness dependence trend was confirmed.

When all parameters but the temperature are kept constant, coatings produced by an ArF laser can be amorphous HA (290°C) or crystalline HA (460°C) [95]. The scratch tests for both samples indicate good coating adhesion. The amorphous coating fails cohesively, and the crystalline coating deforms plastically without detaching from the surface even at loads as high as 24.4 N, as can be seen in Fig. 5.14. Plate-like crystals of irregular shape, with sizes smaller than a few tens of nanometers, constitute this crystalline coating, with many defects at the grain boundaries. On applying load, extended grain boundary shifting takes place, and the material deforms plastically, without any spallation or detachment of the coating. The combination of shorter wavelength (193 nm) and lower temperature of deposition (460°C) has resulted in the exceptional adhesion properties of these coatings compared to those obtained under other conditions.

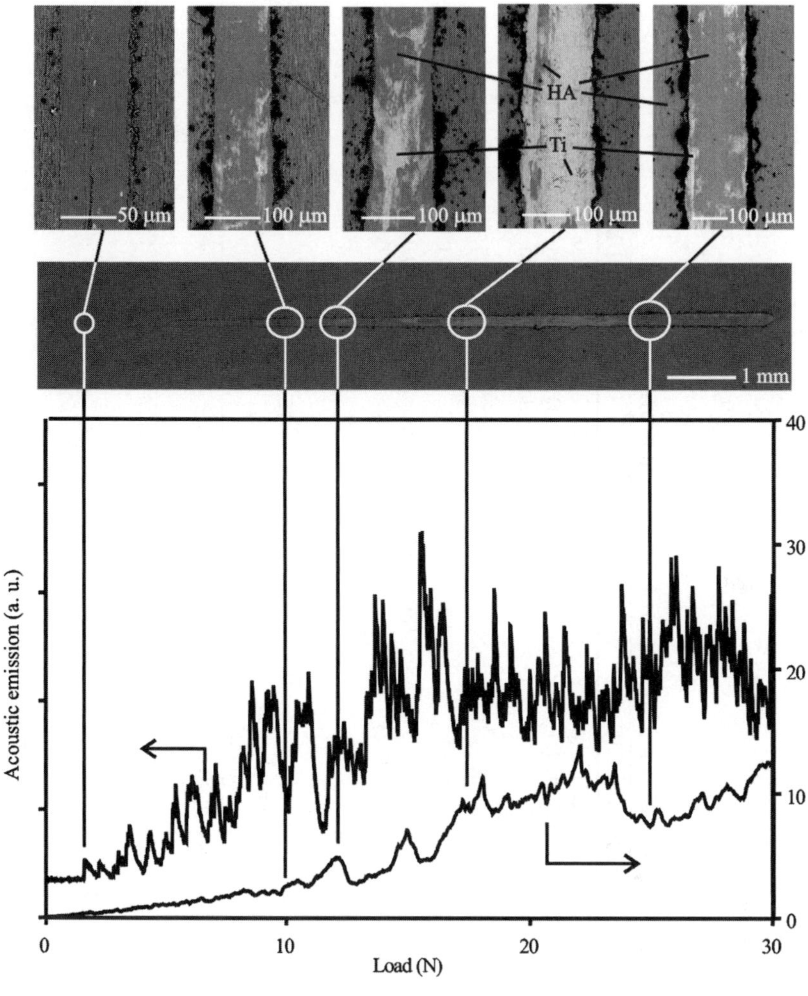

Fig. 5.14 Scratch testing of the crystalline CaP coating produced by ArF laser (T_{sub} = 460°C, 45 Pa, 1 J/cm^2) highlighting the principal events along the scratch length. From [95], with permission from Elsevier

5.5.3 Elastic Modulus and Hardness

Nanoindentation has been used to determine the elastic Young's modulus E and the hardness H of amorphous and crystalline coatings. Table 5.2 lists the results reported by various groups. When using the ArF laser [95], the obtained H and E values are in agreement with those measured in the amorphous and crystalline parts of the plasma-sprayed coatings [97]. Moreover, they demonstrate the higher ductility of these coatings compared to the titanium substrate as their H/E ratio is lower, thus explaining the material spreading on the groove

Table 5.2 Young's modulus and hardness of pulsed laser-deposited HA coatings

Laser type	$T_{substrate}$(°C)	Young's modulus E (GPa)		Hardness H (GPa)		H/E (μm)	Reference
KrF	RT + annealed 500–600	111	(PLD)	2.7	(PLD)	0.024	[87]
		170	(UV-PLD)	7	(UV-PLD)	0.041	
	RT + annealed 500–600	130	(PLD)	5	Ar^{+} implanted	0.038	[99]
	500	140	(UV-PLD)	4.5		0.032	[98]
	600	185	(UV-PLD)	7.2		0.039	
ArF	290	93	(amorphous)	1.6	(amorphous)	0.018	[95]
	460	74.4–107	(crystalline)	0.55–1.06	(crystalline)	0.006	
Cortical Bone		7–30					[126]
Ti		138.3		4.6		0.113	[95]
Plasma sprayed		73	(amorphous)				[97]
		120	(crystalline)				

Data for cortical bone and plasma sprayed coatings have been included for comparison observed during the scratch testing. The E value of the crystalline coatings lies between those of Ti and cortical bone. Hence, by varying the substrate temperature during deposition, a coating with graded Young's modulus can be easily obtained by this technique; thus, improved reduction of the intrinsic residual stresses in the implantation area can be envisaged.

Nelea et al. [87, 98] obtained higher values of E and H by in situ UV annealing for KrF laser deposition of HA coatings. Subsequent ion implantation also increases the values for the elastic modulus and hardness [99]. However, the use of higher temperatures (500°C and 600°C) may deteriorate the interface when a TiN buffer layer is not used. Despite of the improved mechanical performance obtained with these in situ or ex situ treatments, the higher complexity of the process may compromise the industrial application of these technological modifications.

Advances in the development of instrumentation for nanoindentation allow us to determine the elastic modulus and hardness as a function of the indentation depth to measure the effect of a buffer layer made of low temperature (460°C) but crystalline HA [78] deposited at the metal–coating interface of an HA film grown at much higher temperature (650°C). For layers of 1 μm thickness, the 25 nm buffer layer acts as an efficient protective diffusion barrier for oxygen, preventing growth of the titanium oxide phases at the interface. However, hydrogen from the water atmosphere decomposition can still diffuse through the coating and produce titanium hydride and stressed titanium at the interface. Depth-dependent nanoindentation has demonstrated that doubling the water flow can drag out the undesired hydrogen, and it can augment the interface E and H values to the original elastic modulus and hardness of the titanium substrate. During impact tests the fatigue resistance (cycles to failure) of the coatings produced with a buffer layer and high water flow could be raised to three to six times that of coatings produced at low water flow, indicating that the impact test can constitute a valuable tool for interface optimization.

5.6 *In Vitro* Evaluation

5.6.1 Dissolution Behavior

Depending on the chemical composition of the CaP coatings and their crystallinity, the dissolution behavior varies in diverse solutions. The type and concentration of the buffered or unbuffered solutions, their degree of saturation, and their pH value, as well as the testing time, affects their *in vitro* dissolution. Based on the solubility diagrams of the various CaP compounds [76], the dissolution of calcium phosphate ceramics (CPCs) containing CaP phases other than HA are affected by the type and amount of the non-HA phases, as the extent of dissolution decreases in the following order: TTCP >> α-TCP >> β-TCP >> HA. Thus, highly crystalline HA coatings produced with the KrF excimer laser do not dissolve in calcium-free Hank's balanced salt solution [100] when immersed for up to 120 hours at 37°C. The solution was refreshed every 12 hours. However, when deposition conditions favor the formation of multiphasic coatings, as mentioned above, the TTCP and α-TCP parts of the film dissolve completely, leading to microporosity, whereas the HA and β-TCP portions remain in the coating. Amorphous coatings show complete dissolution. Equilibrium was reached during a 24-hour immersion. Nd:YAG laser deposited coatings, composed of HA and α-TCP [101], were similarly tested, and behaved according to their composition: α-TCP dissolved rapidly depending on its amount in the coating. The 30% to 35% content of this non-HA phase dissolved completely within 24 hours.

In another calcium-free solution with a higher salt concentration, Earl's balanced salt solution (EBSS), ArF laser-deposited coatings were immersed for up to 30 day to test their stability compared to plasma-sprayed (PS) coatings (83% crystallinity) [102, 103]. Figure 5.15 shows the accumulative

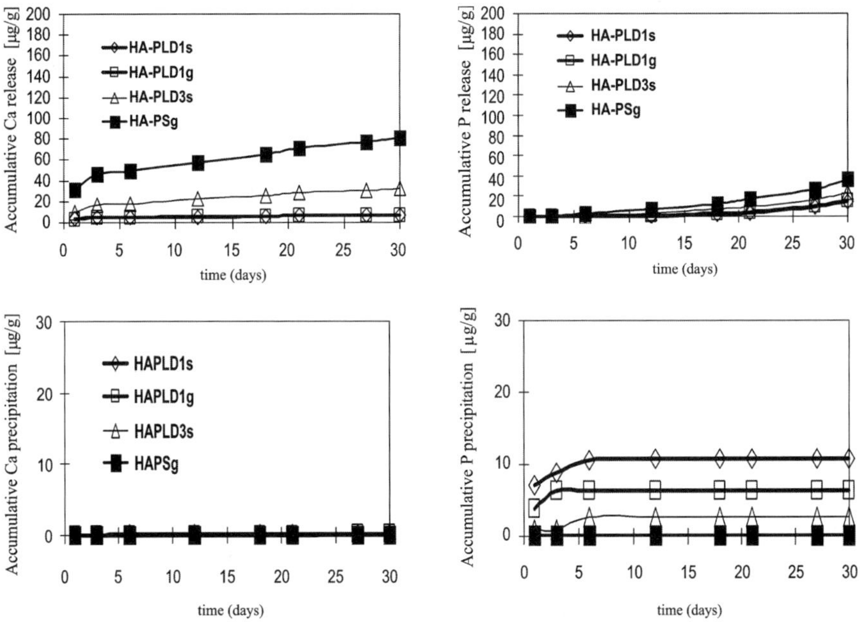

Fig. 5.15 Calcium and phosphorus release and precipitation of ArF laser-deposited carbonated HA coatings in calcium-free Earl's balanced salt solution (EBSS) compared to plasma-sprayed coatings [103]. All coatings were 2 µm thick. The initial and final Ca/P ratios are resumed in Table 5.5. For the fully crystalline PLD1 coating, the deposition conditions were 45 Pa water vapor, 460°C, and 1 J/cm^2. PLD3 coatings were a double layer (inside fully crystalline, outside amorphous, deposited at 300°C). Plasma-sprayed coatings were commercial, specified for 50 µm. Substrates are grade 3 titanium. *s*, smooth, as-machined (Ra 0.4 µm); *g*, grit blasted with 14 µm grain size alumina powder

calcium and phosphorus release and precipitation as measured by analysis of the solution composition every 3 days, when it was refreshed. The PS coatings release both Ca and P to a higher degree than any of the PLD coatings tested even up to day 30. Fully crystalline PLD coatings (PLD1), deposited on as-machined or grit-blasted titanium, showed strong release of Ca and weak precipitation of P at day 1; equilibrium was reached at day 6. However, the double layer (PLD3s), consisting of a fully crystalline inner coating with an amorphous CaP layer at the outer surface, showed similar but weaker release behavior than the PS coatings. Phosphorus precipitation from the double layer occurred later than from the crystalline films and to a lesser degree. Compared to the PS coatings, the ArF-PLD coatings are more stable in this calcium-free solution. Notwithstanding, in a complete culture medium composed of Iscove's modified Dulbecco's medium (IMDM) plus 10% fetal calf serum, the ArF laser-deposited coatings showed a dynamic equilibrium in the solution. There was Ca and P release and precipitation around the equilibrium from the early stages and continuing throughout the test (Fig. 5.16). However, in this medium the double layer showed the same behavior as the fully crystalline ones. Comparatively, for the PS coatings, Ca release was nine times greater and P release four times greater, reaching equilibrium at day 15, whereas precipitation of P and Ca did not start until days 21 and 27, respectively. Energy dispersive x-ray spectroscopy (EDX) analysis of the Ca/P ratios at the end of the tests (Table 5.3) resulted in a considerable decrease in this

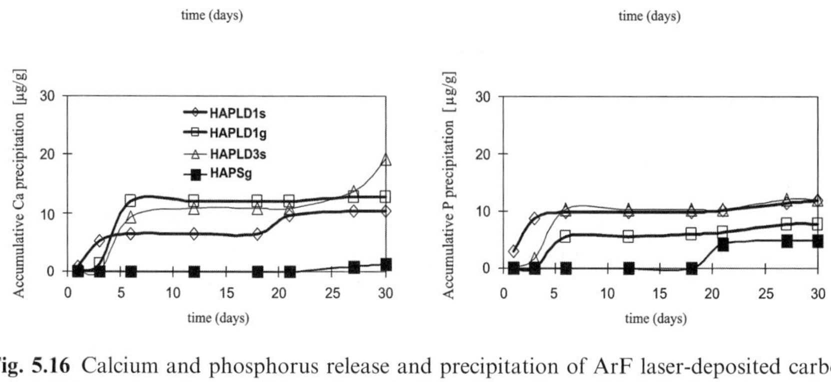

Fig. 5.16 Calcium and phosphorus release and precipitation of ArF laser-deposited carbonated HA coatings in complete culture medium [Iscove's modified Dulbecco's medium (IMDM) + 10% fetal calf serum] compared to plasma-sprayed coatings [103]. Materials were the same as in Fig. 5.15

Table 5.3 Ca/P ratios of ArF laser deposited coatings before and after immersion in Ca-Free EBSS or complete culture medium, without and with cells

		After 30 days immersion in medium		After 18 days MG63 cell culture in medium
Materials	Initial	Ca free (EBSS)	IMDM + proteins	IMDM + proteins
HA-PLD1s (smooth)	1.63	1.54	1.52	2.77
HA-PLD1g (grit blasted)	1.68	1.58	1.58	2.61
HA-PLD3s (smooth)	1.54	1.48	1.35	1.77
HA-plasma Sprayed (grit blasted)	1.55	1.46	1.41	-

Substrate was pure Ti. The smooth surfaces were as-machined. Alumina powder with 14 μm grain size was used for grit blasting. PLD1 is fully crystalline; PLD3 is double-layered (inside crystalline, outside amorphous). All PLD coatings were 2 μm thick [103]

ratio for the double layer, even stronger than for the PS coatings. This is probably the reason for the poor results of this double layer in the cell proliferation test. The dynamic equilibrium, as established early for PLD coatings, may be an explanation for their successful *in vivo* performance without strong initial dissolution and later reprecipitation steps.

Therefore, distinct types of functional coatings can be produced through pulsed laser deposition, including completely resorbable coatings consisting of amorphous CaP, intermediate resorbable ones, and dense crystalline HA thin coatings that can constitute an enduring base layer in contact with metal substrates. Moreover, by changing a single processing parameter, it is possible to obtain graded composition layers that adapt their resorbability to bone growth dynamics.

5.6.2 Cell Activity

5.6.2.1 PLD Coatings on Titanium Substrates

Parker et al. [104] cultured fibroblasts on KrF laser coatings deposited at room temperature and 2 Pa residual air pressure. Fibroblasts showed increased activity on surfaces deposited at higher laser fluences, wherein these coatings have different macroparticle sizes and distribution than those deposited at lower fluences. Ball et al. [85] presented a thorough study with human osteoblasts in this same type of material before and after annealing at 575°C and 10^{-2} Pa in a reducing hydrogen gas. Coatings deposited onto thin titanium films using 6 and 9 Jcm^{-2} were initially amorphous but became crystalline after annealing. Osteoblasts cultured on the crystalline surface were more active than those cultured on the amorphous ones as measured using alamar blue dye reduction, and they produced more alkaline phosphatase. They also had a more organized actin cytoskeleton and more focal contacts with the surface, as assessed by vinculin staining. Unannealed samples had similar behavior in all parameters, confirming that, being amorphous, the cell response was comparably low, independent of the fluence with which they were produced. Thus, a clear correlation between human osteoblast response and crystallinity may be concluded.

In an experiment with rat bone marrow cells (RBMs) three types of CaP coatings obtained by KrF-PLD were tested in an osteogenic primary cell culture to document the mode of bone tissue interface elaboration [105]. The coatings were constituted by highly crystalline HA, α-TCP + β-TCP, or amorphous calcium phosphate (ACP). Cells were cultured for 2 weeks with three medium changes per week. A morphologically distinct layer was found as the immediate interface created with each of the three types of coating exposed to the differentiating osteogenic cells (Fig. 5.17). This cement-like layer, similar to that found in bone remodeling events *in vivo* [106], was carbonated and of apatitic nature, as the apatitic crystals found in the globules synthesized by differentiating osteogenic cells [107]. The absence of this layer in the biological medium without cells supports the hypothesis that this interface layer was cellularly mediated and not the product of physicochemical events. The ability for CaP materials to form this bone bonding-promoting interlayer is normally related to the coating solubility. Notwithstanding, an extensive mature and adherent bone matrix was produced on the surface of these low solubility, highly dense, crystalline HA coatings. In contrast, on the amorphous coating this bone matrix was quite immature, probably because of the loss of the coating and consequent influence of the substrate.

In this study, the bone remodeling process was also studied in an osteoclast-enriched RBM cell culture. Although osteoclasts were not able to resorb the crystalline HA coatings, discontinuous island-like lacunae were observed on the α-TCP + β-TCP coatings. For RBM cells, the highly dense, crystalline coating did not dissolve and was osteoconductive and bone bonding. This indicates that

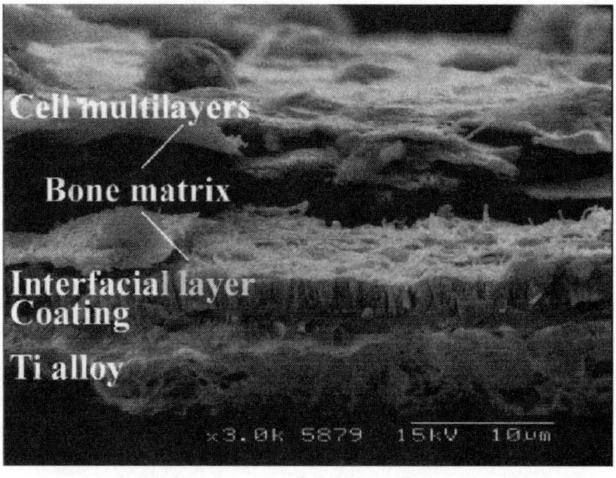

Fig. 5.17 Cross-sectional view of the bone matrix created in KrF-PLD fully crystalline HA coatings. It shows the cell multilayers, interfacial layer, coating and Ti alloy substrate. From [105], with permission from Wiley Interscience

bone growth may take place on this kind of thin coating even without previous osteoclastic resorption.

In fact, in a cellular proliferation test using MG-63 osteoblast-like cells cultivated in the same complete culture medium as was used in the release tests shown in Fig. 5.16, three types of ArF PLD coatings were tested on titanium surfaces, both as-machined (smooth: s-code) and grit-blasted (g-code). The proliferation was measured by the MTT colorimetric method at 1, 3, 6, 12, 15, and 18 days. Phenotype expression, alkaline phosphatase (ALP), total protein content, and osteocalcin content were evaluated. The coating types tested were highly crystalline HA deposited at 460°C (PLD1) and the same double layer of the cell-free test referred to above (PLD3: inside crystalline, outside amorphous). Surprisingly, this double-layer coating did not enhance either the cellular proliferation or the differentiation of MG-63 cells compared to the highly crystalline coatings [103], as shown in Fig. 5.18. No difference was observed between this coating and as-received titanium. However, the fully crystalline coating showed the highest proliferation at intermediate times, even better than that on the negative control (tissue culture polystyrene). Table 5.3 also shows the Ca/P ratio of the coating surfaces at the end of the test, after the detachment of the cell multilayer formed after 18 days in culture. Comparison of these values with those obtained in the cell-free medium allow us to conclude that the higher cell proliferation and differentiation promoted by the crystalline (PLD1) coatings has transformed the surface underneath the cells into a highly calcium-enriched layer, maybe coinciding with the interlayer observed by Cléries et al. [105] in Fig. 5.17. It is known that the degree of crystallinity of the CaP influences osteoblastic differentiation. HA with low crystallinity [108, 109] had exhibited a higher level of mineralization, greater Ca

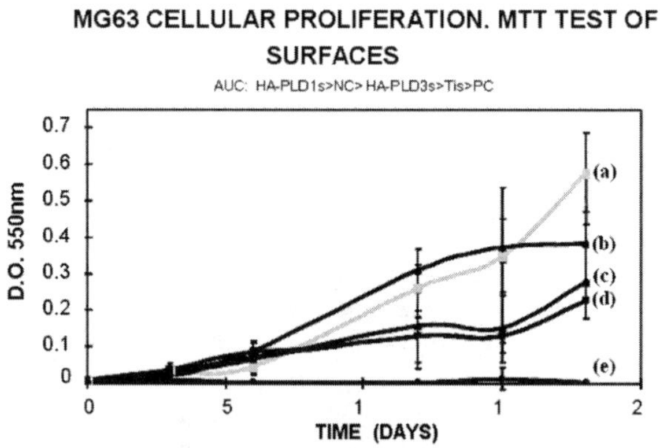

Fig. 5.18 Cellular proliferation (MTT test) of ArF laser deposited coatings on as-machined titanium [103]. (*a*) Negative control (tissue culture polystyrene); (*b*) highly crystalline HA (PLD1s); (*c*) double-layer HA (PLD3s); (*d*) bare Ti; (*e*) positive control (phenol solution 0.64 mg/ml). Materials were the same as in Fig. 5.15. *AUC*, area under the curve; *PC*, positive control; *MTT*, 3-(4,5-dimethylthiazole-2-yl)-2,5-diphenyl tetrazolium bromide

release, and enhanced ALP values than HA with high crystallinity. However, in this experiment, the double layer, being amorphous at the outside, did not favor cell activity. This was also clear from the evolution of the Ca/P ratio. The double layer did not augment the intracellular protein content of cells as did the crystalline coating. This demonstrates once more that in thin CaP coatings the bioactivity stimulation is triggered by other pathways. Osteocalcin expression was higher for the highly crystalline coatings on grit-blasted titanium (PLD1g) than on the same coating on as-machined titanium. This is probably due to a combination of the surface area effect, together with the osteoconductivity promoted by the PLD HA coatings. Extracellular matrix was formed on all crystalline PLD coated surfaces, independently of their roughness.

Fibroblasts LEP, isolated from human embryonic lungs, and macrophages from mouse peritoneum were cultured to test KrF excimer laser-deposited coatings [110]. Material toxicity, toxicity of percolates, and cell activity were evaluated. A test of mononuclear cell proliferation activity was implemented, whereby the ratio between proliferation activity of stimulated and nonstimulated mononuclear cells in the presence of sample percolates was defined as a stimulating index (SI). Very low or zero values imply cell damage or reduction of cell adherence. Too high SI can represent escalation or even abnormal cell metabolism. With an increasing Ca/P ratio, the biological properties deteriorated. Samples with Ca/P ratios > 2, with higher content of soluble components, often had high proliferation activity as expressed by an elevated SI. The blastic transformation of macrophages and coating damage also occurred more frequently. Ca/P ratios near the theoretical value of HA (1.67) were associated with SIs mostly much higher than those for the titanium alloy control, which means that the proliferation activity was increased without harming cell function.

Seydlova et al. [111] evaluated titanium alloy coated with zirconia and HA, both produced by PLD. A KrF laser was used for the zirconia buffer layer, whereas an ArF laser was utilized at 50 Pa water atmosphere, 6.2 J/cm^2, and 600°C substrate temperature for the HA coating. 3T3 murine line fibroblast and human dermal fibroblasts were cultivated, and adhesion, proliferation up to 96 hours, and fibronectin expression were evaluated. The initial Ca/P ratio was 2.2 to 2.4. References were tissue-grade polystyrene and Noritake ceramics. No cytotoxic effect was detected. However, no comparison was made to the bare titanium substrate or other CaP materials.

The biocompatibility of nanocrystalline OCP coatings produced by a KrF laser was tested [80] using human fetal osteoblast-like cell line hFOB 1.19 and murine fibroblast cell line L929. Cell proliferation, DNA replication, apoptosis, cell morphology, and cell adhesion were evaluated. Both fibroblasts and osteoblasts adhered, reached normal morphology, proliferated, and remained viable when cultured on OCP coatings, which supported the good cytocompatibility and absence of any toxicity of these coatings. No significant differences were found between these OCP coatings, the reference as-received titanium or polystyrene control.

Bigi et al. [112] compared the response of human osteoblasts to these OCP coatings (1 μm thick), Mn^{2+}-doped carbonated HA (0.8 μm), and as-received titanium. A KrF laser was used under the conditions already described for OCP and Mn-CHA deposition. Mn^{2+} ions should increase the ligand-binding affinity of integrins through conformational changes. The osteoblasts grown on OCP thin films displayed multiple cytoplasmatic extensions that could not be discerned in the cells grown on Mn-CHA coating. The reduced proliferation observed on Ti and on Ti-coated materials with respect to the control at 14 days was most likely due to the increased cellular differentiation (Fig. 5.19). Accordingly, the significant increase of the ALP levels during the second week of cell culture suggests that the cells were shifting to a more differentiated stage, whereas the observed reduction of the expression of this enzyme at 21 days might be due to extensive mineralization. The ALP activity of the cells cultivated on coated Ti is drastically higher than that of cells cultured on the control. This seems to be a clear indication of the ability of the coating to improve tissue integration. As ALP activity starts to decline after 14 days, a significant decrease of procollagen type 1 (CICP) is also observed. The different time evolution of the osteoblasts differentiation stages on the coated substrates with respect to control and Ti is further supported by the results obtained for the values of transforming growth factor-β1 (TGFβ1). At variance, TGFβ1 levels on OCP and Mn-CHA coatings increase progressively with time, so at 21 days the values are significantly higher than those obtained on Ti substrates. The progressive and high production of TGFβ1 indicates that bone growth, due to triggering of cell proliferation and differentiation, will continue after 3 weeks of implantation. However, in this study, the different composition and most likely the beneficial presence of Mn^{2+} and carbonate, counterbalanced the higher crystallinity of Mn-CHA with regard to OCP, so both materials improved the osteoblastic differentiation on coated Ti. These investigations appear to support the introduction of the two new CaPs and possibly their derivates to promote better osseointegration on various orthopedic and oral implants.

5.6.2.2 PLD Coatings on Polymer Substrates

A 3T3 mouse fibroblast cell line was cultured in DMEM with 10% newborn calf serum for 48 hours to determine the toxicity of KrF laser-deposited CaP coatings on Teflon and polyethylene substrates [37]. Samples were not annealed after deposition and were produced at room temperature and 2 Pa residual pressure. Extended dissolution took place within a few hours after immersion in SBF owing to the elevated content of amorphous or faster dissolving CaP phases. A morphological assessment of the biocompatibility was carried out by SEM using osteoblasts obtained from embryonic 20 day Wistar rat calvaria dissociated by collagenase/trypsin digestion.

Fibroblasts grown on HA-coated PE exhibit greater mitochondrial activity than those on the positive control, indicating that this surface is nontoxic. The

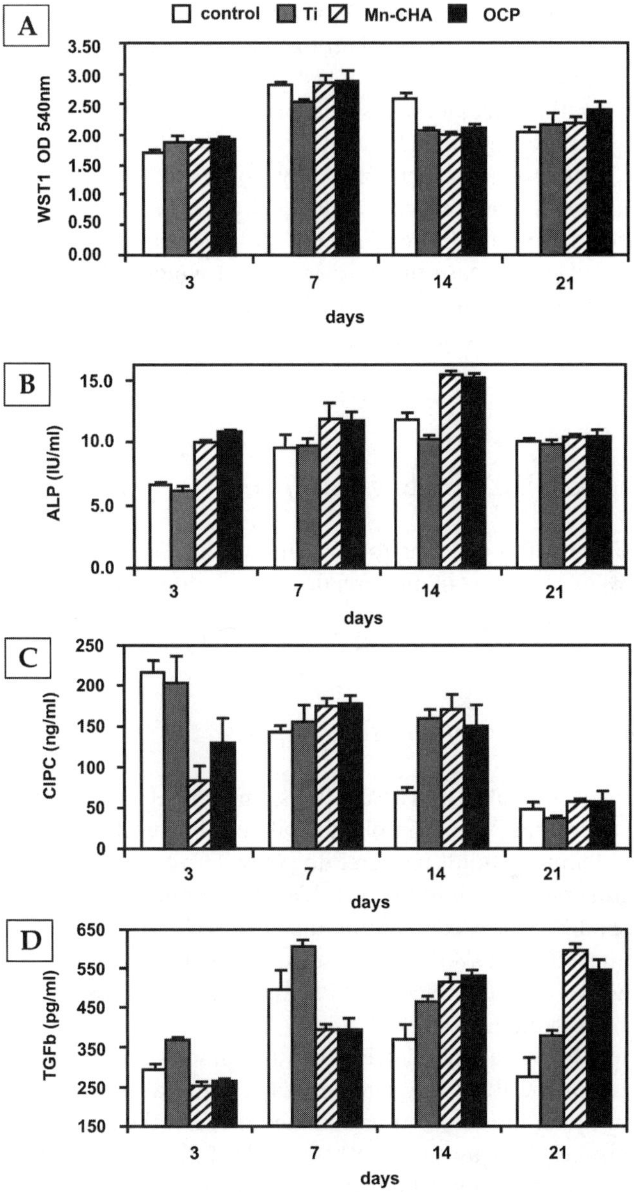

Fig. 5.19 Human osteoblast response to octacalcium phosphate (*OCP*) and M-doped carbonated HA (*Mn-CHA*) deposited by krypton fluor excimer (KrF) laser after culturing for up to 21 days. **A** Proliferation of primary osteoblasts (*WST1*). **B** Alkaline phosphatase (*ALP*) activity. **C** Collagen type I (C-terminal type I procollagen, or *CIPC*). **D** Transforming growth factor-β1 (*TGFb*) produced. Uncoated titanium was the reference. Polystyrene is the control surface. From [112], with permission from Elsevier

uncoated PE had some toxic effect. More mitochondrial activity was found on HA-coated and uncoated Teflon than on the positive control. The mean cell count of primary rat calvaria osteoblasts was significantly higher on coated Teflon than on the uncoated substrate or on the coated PE. This could be attributed to the fact that the HA coating on PE underwent extensive erosion during the culture period, such that only about 10% of the initial coating thickness remained after 6 hours of contact with SBF.

Before application of PLD coatings on polymer materials, more work has to be performed to decrease the temperature at which a bioactive protective CaP coating can be produced. It would have to be stable enough to withstand dissolution when it is in contact with body fluids as well as promote cell activity.

5.7 Efficacy of PLD Coatings *In Vivo*

The suitability of PLD coatings for implant applications has been assessed in several *in vivo* experiments in mongrel dogs [113], rats [37], minipigs [114–117], rabbits [118] and beagle dogs [119].

5.7.1 Study in Mongrel Dogs

The first *in vivo* study of PLD-HA coatings, implemented by Cotell et al. [113], consisted of cylindrical Ti rods implanted bilaterally into the cancellous bone of the proximal femur of adult mongrel dogs for 2 and 6 weeks. Four materials were tested: uncoated polished or grit-blasted titanium, plasma-sprayed (PS) HA coated, and PLD HA coated titanium. The KrF laser was used at 2 J/cm^2, Ar/water atmosphere at 78 Pa, and a substrate temperature of 610° to 630°C. PLD coatings were 0.3 μm thick, and PS coatings were 30 to 50 μm. The shear strength of bone bonding was evaluated.

The highest torsional shear strength was found for PS HA samples. The shear strength of the PLD HA samples was comparable to that of uncoated Ti-6Al-4 V samples; the values approximated those of the polished Ti and were lower than the results from the grit-blasted Ti. Large areas of the implanted PLD HA coatings delaminated under relatively low torsional stress. Failure of these samples occurred at the interface between the coating and the substrate. It did not appear from SEM examination of the implanted specimens retrieved after mechanical testing that there was bonding of bone to the intact portions of the PLD HA coating. Probably the interface layer found by Fernández-Pradas et al. [77], where titanium oxides are present, was even thicker in this experiment because of the higher temperatures used and may have been responsible for the lack of bone bonding.

5.7.2 Study in Rats

Antonov et al. [37] implanted Ti-6Al-4 V flats, coated and uncoated, into the femurs of 36 adult rats for periods of 15, 30, and 60 days. Coatings were produced with KrF and with a TEA-CO_2 laser under equal processing parameters (10 J/cm^2, room temperature, 2 Pa residual air pressure, 4 μm thick). Bone response and new bone tissue formation were analyzed by SEM and histology. Because in the preliminary test the HA coatings deposited with a CO_2 laser were one order of magnitude less stable in SBF than those deposited with the KrF laser, the as-deposited implants were annealed for 1 hour at 550°C in residual air pressure.

SEM revealed new bone formation surrounding the site of implantation of the HA-coated alloy samples only at 60 days. No significant differences in the osteogenesis process were observed between the samples coated using the two laser wavelengths. In general, osseointegration was slightly superior for the annealed than in the nonannealed samples. No inflammation was observed around the sites of implantation for any of the groups of samples; however, the uncoated samples did lead to significant fibrous tissue formation. In contrast, both the KrF laser-coated and the CO_2 laser-coated samples exhibited little fibrous tissue after 60 days and showed formation of new bone, which was in direct contact with the implant surface.

5.7.3 Studies in Minipigs

The same KrF laser wavelength was used by Dostálová et al. [115] for production of HA coatings on real dental implants machined from pure titanium (deposition parameters were 3 J/cm^2, 500°C, 1 μm thick). Mainly HA with a small additional amount of TCP was detected by XRD. Moreover, the HA films were partly amorphized. The dental implants were inserted into both halves of the lower jaws of minipigs 10 weeks after lower premolars extraction. After 16 weeks of unloaded implantation, animals were sacrificed, and samples were prepared for quantitative and qualitative evaluation.

The presence of newly formed bone around all implants was confirmed, so it could be concluded that, after 16 weeks, the implants had osseointegrated. The percentage of osseointegration for the HA-coated samples was 77.3% ± 1.3%, but there was no statistical difference between the coated and uncoated implants with regard to bone contact. These results are consistent with the values of 40% to 80% in the literature [120]. At the light microscopy level, no irritation or inflammation was visible at the coated implants, and fibrous tissue interposition was only seldom observed. The active bone formation and presence of foreign body cells could be seen in coated and uncoated reference samples. Similar results were found by the same group after 16 weeks of unloaded and 6 months of loaded osseointegration [117] in the same animal model. Samples were deposited with the same laser at 490°C. The coating material consisted of a mixture of HA, TCP, and some CaO, corresponding to the droplet containing morphology already described. TiO_2 was also detected in the XRD spectra. Under polarized and fluorescent light, no osteoclasts, macrophages, or inflammatory reaction cells, including phagocytes, were observed, and no regressive changes were apparent in any of the ground sections. In the laser-deposited samples, a layer of fibrous connective tissue occurred in about 22.5% of the implant body surface without producing a continuous layer. In the control group (bare titanium), the fibrous connective tissue between the implant and the newly formed bone occupied 34.8% (i.e., more than in the coated samples). However, these differences were not significant. The calculated area of the bone–implant interface varied from 65.2% (SE 13.5%) for titanium implants to 77.5% (SE 10.2%) for HA films. There was no significant difference (Student's t-test with probability $P = 0.05$) between the type of surface. Therefore, it is believed that the osseointegration of all HA films and the control titanium implants was similar.

5.7.4 Studies in Rabbits

A comparative study of the biological stability and osteoconductivity of HA coatings produced by ArF laser deposition and plasma spraying (PS) was conducted by Peraire et al. [118]. Deposition conditions for PLD were: 0.9 J/cm^2, 45 Pa, and 490°C. Three implant groups were used: grit-blasted titanium rods coated with PLD HA (2 μm thick), grit-blasted titanium rods coated with PS HA (50 μm thick), and uncoated grit-blasted titanium. The implantation took place in the proximal tibia of 12 mature New Zealand white rabbits for 24 weeks, at the end of which the radiographic study revealed that sham holes were completely healed. Samples were evaluated using descriptive histology and histomorphometry.

The plasma-sprayed implants showed considerable instability and reduction in thickness after 24 weeks (but with no statistical difference from the titanium group). The PLD HA group showed significant better bone apposition (Scheffé test, $P < 0.05$) than the other two groups, without signs of degradation or dissolution. The bone contact percentage for this ArF laser-deposited coatings amounted to 86% ± 4% (Fig. 5.20), a value much higher than that achieved by PLD HA coatings in other animal studies. The histology study confirmed these results: The PLD HA material surface presented good bone regeneration at both endosteal ends of the implant; the new bone was similar to the original cortical bone; and mature osteocytes were detected. Mineralized matrix in apposition to the PLD HA implant was observed in all examined areas (cortical insertion area, opposite endosteal area, bone marrow) under polarized microscopy. The central area in contact with bone marrow showed bone apposition

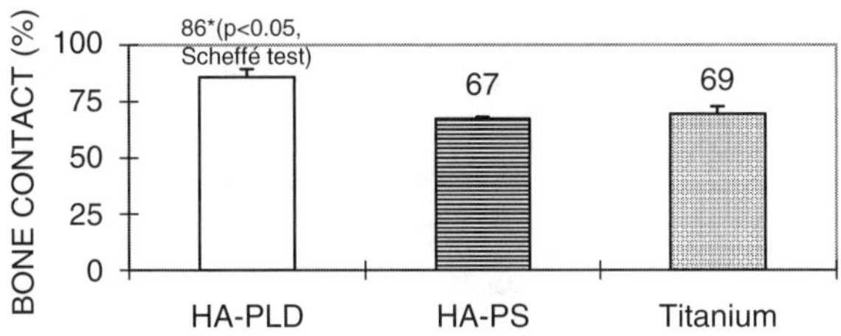

Fig. 5.20 Percentage of bone contact (numbers at the top of the bars) for ArF laser-deposited cylinders (*HA-PLD*) implanted in rabbit tibia for 24 weeks. Reference material was plasma spray-coated cylinders (*HA-PS*) and bare titanium cylinders. From [118], with permission from Wiley Interscience

areas interspersed in a thin fibrous capsule, with large trabeculae growing from the coating surface (Fig. 5.21).

In the PS HA implants, there was also good bone regeneration at the ends of the implant samples (endosteal zones), but the newly formed bone in contact with the implant surface showed a significant larger amount of remodeling lacunae. This active remodeling may be due to degradation of the coating. The PS HA coating had partially disappeared in some areas of the implants; and HA particles, coating delamination, and detachment were detected. Bone apposition areas were hardly observed at the central zone, with a slightly thicker fibrous capsule and some foci of inflammatory cells. Lymphocyte infiltration was present in three of the PS HA implants, and in two of them other inflammatory cells were also present, such as macrophages and/or neutrophils. There was no direct relation between the instability of the coating and the presence of the inflammatory infiltrate, as only one animal presented both effects at the same time.

The observations by SEM allowed us to detect the PLD HA coating on the grit-blasted titanium surface after 24 weeks of implantation (Fig. 5.22). The

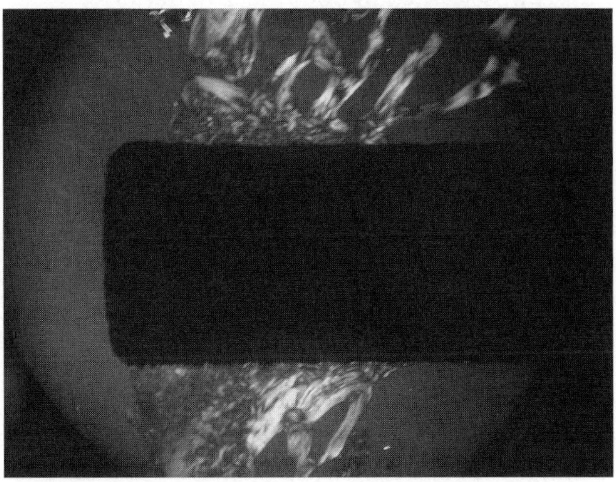

Fig. 5.21 Optical microscopy observation of the PLD-HA implants produced with the ArF laser. Trabeculae growing from the PLD coating surface in the central zone of the implant. From [118], with permission from Wiley Interscience

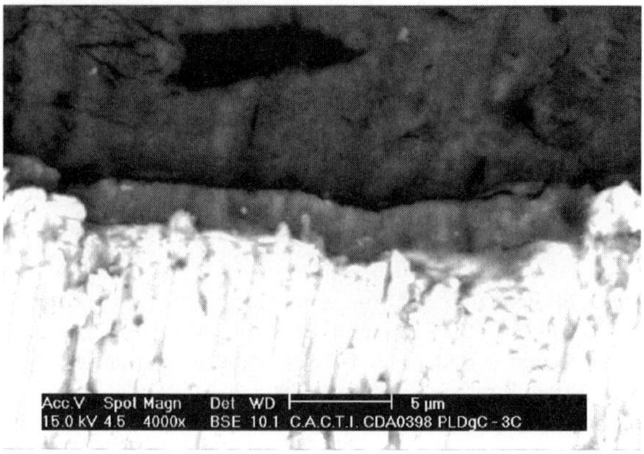

Fig. 5.22 Scanning electron microscopy cross-section micrograph of the ArF laser-deposited implant surface in contact with surrounding bone. The almost intact original 2 μm thick PLD coating could still be observed in extended areas after 24 weeks of implantation in rabbit tibia. From [118], with permission from Wiley Interscience

back-scattering image showed different contrast for bone and coating, allowing us to differentiate them. The EDX analysis indicated a higher Ca/P ratio for the coating and a more intense carbon signal for bone, mainly corresponding to the organic matrix. Remarkably, after 6 months, the almost intact 2 μm thick PLD coating could still be observed by electron microscopy in extended areas.

It should be pointed out that ArF laser coatings, as deposited under these conditions, were droplet-free, dense, and fully crystalline carbonated HA, without any other CaP present. Moreover, the Ca/P ratio was 1.77, which was closer to the theoretical value of HA than the material used in previous *in vivo* studies by other authors. In addition, the applied low temperature (490°C) maintained the interface of titanium oxides that are deleterious to the mechanical properties of the coating. Whereas other authors did not find statistical differences between coated and uncoated samples, these ArF-PLD coatings not only promoted an improved bone response with regard to titanium but also with regard to plasma-sprayed coatings. Moreover, the ArF laser-deposited coatings were shown to produce osteoconduction in zones where the bone was previously absent (i.e., in bone marrow).

5.7.5 Studies in Beagle Dogs

Although the PLD method does not need a grit-blasting step to achieve strong coating adherence to the substrate, as has been shown, the thin coating can follow any surface topography achieved through predeposition machining, cleaning, or grit-blasted roughening. Hence, PLD constitutes a suitable method to evaluate the contribution of the CaP chemistry to osseointegration, with least interference of the roughness. Therefore, Peraire et al. [119] used dog jaws to demonstrate the bone response for ArF laser-deposited coatings in an *in vivo* model similar to human oral implantation. It was considered of special interest to assess the contribution of roughness and the chemistry of the coatings to the osseointegration of the implants, not only from the histological point of view but also with regard to their mechanical bonding after implantation.

Hence, 3 months after teeth extraction, five materials were implanted in Beagle dogs: (1) smooth, as-machined, titanium plugs (Ti-s); (2) grit-blasted titanium plugs (Ti-g); (3) grit-blasted titanium plugs with HA-PS coating (HA-PS); (4) smooth, as-machined titanium plugs with HA-PLD coating (HA-PLDs); and (5) grit-blasted titanium plugs with HA-PLD coating (HA-PLDg). The PLD coating was the same 2 μm thick, dense, and fully crystalline coating as previously tested in rabbit tibia [118]. The implantation period was 12 weeks, at the end of which the radiographic study revealed that sham holes were not completely healed. This indicated that the bone had not finished its maturation process, and remodeling was still ongoing. Qualitative and quantitative analyses were performed on samples prepared for histology, whereby % bone apposition, % lacunae apposition, and % bone surface were measured. To assess bone bonding, a push-in test was used to evaluate the mean shear strength. For all the implanted materials, the central zone of the implant was surrounded by trabecular bone, whereas cortical bone was associated with the apical zone. Table 5.4 shows the results for bone apposition and mean shear strength. The mean roughness (Ra) of the surfaces was also included. No statistical differences were detected when the three coated surfaces were compared—the plasma-sprayed samples (PSg), the pulsed laser-deposited HA coatings on grit-blasted surfaces (PLDg), and those deposited on as-machined titanium (PLDs)—despite their very different roughness. However, these coated surfaces could be significantly differentiated from their corresponding uncoated counterparts. The PLDs implants improved bone apposition compared to the uncoated titanium smooth surfaces (Ti-s) (Scheffé Test) ($P < 0.05$), as the plasma-sprayed surface could be differentiated from the grit-blasted titanium surface (Ti-g). Remarkably, rough surfaces (Ti-g and PLDg) did not increase bone apposition when compared to their respectively "smooth"

Table 5.4 Bone apposition and mean shear strength of ArF laser coatings on titanium smooth and grit-blasted surfaces

		Histomorphometry		Push-in test
Group	Ra (μm)	% Bone apposition	Bone contact (μm)	Mean Shear Strength (MPa)
Ti-s	0.40	38 ± 18	2900 ± 1500	3.19 ± 0.74
PLDs	1.44	66 ± 27*	4400 ± 1800	5.14 ± 1.89
PLDg	4.25	64 ± 15	4600 ± 1100	6.76 ± 1.41
Ti-g	5.43	52 ± 14	3900 ± 1000	5.05 ± 1.08
PS	8.86	81 ± 16*	6100 ± 1100*	4.21 ± 1.32

From ref. 119, with permission

Ti-s, as-machined titanium, Ti-g, grit-blasted titanium; PLDs, pulsed laser-deposited coating on smooth Ti; PLDg, pulsed laser-deposited coating on grit-blasted Ti; PS, plasma-sprayed coating

* $P < 0.05$ Scheffé test

Table 5.5 List of articles published on pulsed laser deposition of calcium phosphate coatings

		Specificity of the particular system						Physico-chemical characterization techniques used									Testing		
		Laser type																	
				Nd:YAG															
Year	Author(s)	ArF	KrF	SHG	THG	FHG	Modifications	FTIR	Raman	XRD	SEM	EDS	TEM	AFM	RBS/SIMS	XPS/AES	Mechanical	In – vitro	In – vivo
1992	Baeri [21]						x				x				x	x			
1992	Cotell [20]		x					x		x	x				x		x		
1993	Cotell [34]		x							x	x				x		x		
1993	Torrisi. [36]						x				x				x	x			
1994	Sardin [22]	x						x		x	x				x				
1994	Singh [23]		x							x	x	x	x		x				
1994	Torrisi [35]						x	x		x	x					x			
1995	Bagratashvili [26]		x							x	x	x							
1995	Jelínek [25]		x							x	x				x		x		
1995	Serra [24]	x																	
1996	Antonov [127]		x					x				x					x	x	
1996	Cotell [113]		x								x	x				x	x		x
1996	Guillot-Noël [29]				x	x					x	x							
1996	Hontsu [28]		x							x				x			x		
1996	Parker [104]	x						x			x							x	
1996	Serra [59]	x	x																
1996	Tucker [27]		x										x		x			x	
1997	Antonov [128]		x				x							x					
1997	Arias [31]	x						x		x									
1997	García-Sanz [43]	x								x	x	x					x		
1997	Hontsu [82]	x								x		x					x		
1997	Serra [58]		x																
1997	Wang [30]	x						x	x	x	x	x		x			x		
1998	Antonov [37]		x				x				x							x	x
1998	Arias [49]	x						x				x							
1998	Cléries [100]		x						x	x	x							x	
1998	Dostálová [115]		x							x									x
1998	Fernández-Pradas [32]	x	x					x		x	x								
1998	García [129]							x		x	x								
1998	Himmlová [110]		x							x								x	
1998	Hontsu [125]	x								x	x			x				x	
1998	Mayor [72]	x						x		x	x	x							
1998	Mayor [130]	x						x											
1998	Serra [56]		x																
1998	Serra [131]		x																
1998	Serra [57]		x																
1999	Cléries [101]				x			x	x	x	x							x	
1999	Craciun [33]		x					x		x	x				x				
1999	Craciun [132]		x					x		x	x				x				

Table 5.5 (continued)

		Specificity of the particular system						Physico-chemical characterization techniques used									Testing		
		Laser type																	
				Nd:YAG															
Year	Author(s)	ArF	KrF	SHG	THG	FHG	Modifications	FTIR	Raman	XRD	SEM	EDS	TEM	AFM	RBS/SIMS	XPS/AES	Mechanical	In – vitro	In – vivo
1999	Serra [60]				x														
1999	Serra [69]		x																
2000	Arias [66]	x						x			x	x							
2000	Cléries [133]		x			x			x	x	x							x	
2000	Cléries [93]		x		x				x	x	x						x		
2000	Cléries [105]		x					x		x	x							x	
2000	Lo [134]		x					x		x	x							x	
2000	Fernández-Pradas [124]				x			x	x	x	x					x	x		
2000	Nelea [135]		x							x			x				x		
2000	Zeng [42]				x	x				x	x						x		
2000	Zeng [65]				x	x		x				x							
2000	Zeng [136]				x	x				x	x	x							
2001	Antonov [84]		x								x	x						x	
2001	Antonov [67]		x								x	x						x	
2001	Ball [85]		x							x								x	
2001	Dostálová [117]		x																
2001	Fernández-Pradas [94]		x							x	x						x		
2001	Fernández-Pradas [68]		x								x								
2002	Arias [71]	x						x		x	x	x							
2002	Arias [61]	x						x		x		x							
2002	Jelínek [116]		x																x
2002	Fernández-Pradas [44]				x					x	x					x	x		
2002	Fernández-Pradas [96]		x							x	x					x	x		
2002	Katto [88]		x				x			x	x							x	
2002	Nelea [87]		x				x				x		x				x		
2002	Nelea [137]		x				x			x							x		
2003	Antonov [81]		x								x	x						x	x
2003	Arias [95]	x						x	x	x	x	x	x	x			x		
2003	Arias,J.L. [62]	x																	
2003	Fernández-Pradas [70]		x					x	x	x	x								
2003	Katto [89]	x	x				x	x		x	x								
2003	Nelea [98]		x				x			x	x		x				x		
2004	De Aza [138]				x					x	x	x	x						
2004	Ferraz [52]	x								x	x					x		x	
2004	Gyorgy [54]		x					x		x	x							x	
2004	Iliescu [79]		x							x	x		x			x			
2004	Iliescu [139]		x							x			x						
2004	Jiménez [78]	x					x	x		x		x							

Table 5.5 (continued)

		Specificity of the particular system						Physico-chemical characterization techniques used									Testing		
		Laser type																	
				Nd:YAG															
Year	Author(s)	ArF	KrF	SHG	THG	FHG	Modifications	FTIR	Raman	XRD	SEM	EDS	TEM	AFM	RBS/SIMS	XPS/AES	Mechanical	In – vitro	In – vivo
2004	Jiménez [78]	x						x		x						x	x		
2004	Nelea [140]		x							x	x		x				x		
2004	Nelea [99]		x				x										x		
2004	Nistor [141]			x	x						x		x				x		
2004	Pelletier [142]		x				x										x		
2004	Pelletier [143]		x				x										x		
2004	Pelletier [144]		x				x										x		
2004	Pelletier [145]		x				x										x		
2004	Socol [80]		x							x			x					x	
2005	Beltrano [146]			x					x	x	x								
2005	Bigi [112]		x							x	x	x						x	
2005	Blind [48]				x					x	x			x	x		x		
2005	Borrajo [147]	x						x		x						x			
2005	Ferro [51]			x						x	x						x		
2005	Fernández-Pradas [77]			x					x	x				x	x	x			
2005	Katto [50]		x					x		x	x					x			
2005	Kim [148]		x							x									
2005	Kusunoki [83]	x								x									
2005	Mihailescu [149]		x										x			x		x	
2005	Solla [90]	x					x	x		x		x							
2006	Peraire [118]	x									x								x
2006	Seydlova [111]		x							x	x							x	
2006	Suda [55]			x				x		x						x			

surfaces (Ti-s and PLDs) after 12 weeks of implantation. This experiment seems to indicate that the chemical effect of the HA coatings in promoting bone response has a greater contribution than topography.

With regard to bone bonding, and in agreement with the fact that surface roughness gives higher shear strength due to mechanical interlocking, the two grit-blasted surfaces resulted in higher values than their smooth counterparts (Ti-g versus Ti-s, PLDg versus PLDs). Surprisingly, the plasma-sprayed coating did not improve bonding compared to grit-blasted titanium owing to cohesion failure on shear loading. Despite these plasma-sprayed coatings yielding the highest percentage of bone contact in this experiment, under shear loading in an orthopedic device the debonding of the osseointegrated coating from the implant can end up catastrophically; the metallic implant would become loose, and revision would be necessary. The highest mean shear strength was obtained for the PLD coating on the grit-blasted surface, but both PLD-coated samples (grit-blasted and smooth) improved bone bonding with regard to their corresponding uncoated counterparts, substantiating the histomorphometric findings. In agreement with the 6-month rabbit tibia results, after implantation for 12 weeks in dog jaws large areas of the nearly intact PLD coating were observed by SEM.

It is interesting to compare the bone response to the ArF laser-deposited coatings (PLDg), after implantation during 24 weeks in rabbit tibias [118] and during half of this time (12 weeks) in dog jaws [119]. The percentage of bone apposition on the laser-deposited coating has been higher and more differentiated from the other materials in the rabbit than in the dog despite the facts that: (1) in the rabbit tibia, the implants were in contact with both cortical and trabecular bone; and (2) alveolar bone from dog jaw is dense and in general regenerates faster than trabecular bone. Thus, one would expect faster osseointegration in the dog jaw. Generally, it is assumed that in the longer term all biocompatible materials implanted in the body tend to osseointegrate, and the difference in bone response between diverse materials is likely to disappear. In fact, for sputtered coatings, Mohammadi et al. [121, 122] found less differentiation between coated and uncoated materials in a long-term study (9 months) than in the short-term investigation (up to 6 weeks) after implantation in cortical and trabecular bone of rabbits. This result is in opposition to our findings, wherein after the longer implantation time the PLD coating showed more significantly differentiated bone apposition with regard to the reference material than in the shorter experiment, where bone was still remodeling. Concerning the differences in response between trabecular and cortical bone, Mohammadi et al. found that trabecular bone differentiated better between the different materials than cortical bone, in agreement with our findings.

5.8 Conclusions and Prospects for Applications

We have presented a synthesis of the considerable effort performed by various research groups to optimize the deposition conditions for diverse thin CaP coatings. Great effort has also been dedicated to understanding the processes that occur as the material is transported from target to substrate, in search of scientific bases for optimizing the coatings beyond empirical work.

It has been demonstrated that PLD can produce thin, dense, well adhering coatings with extraordinary controlled chemistry and crystallinity. A number of advantages of the PLD technique have become clear.

- Conditions for congruent deposition have been established. Various CaP phases with and without diverse substitutions and morphologies can be deposited, so the degree of resorption may be adapted to a specific medical application.

- Coatings with graded composition, or graded crystallinity can readily be produced.
- Film thickness can be well controlled simply by turning the laser on and off.
- The use of the laser as the external energy source results in an extremely clean process compared to plasma spraying.
- The droplets or particulates in the film can be avoided by using the ArF laser wavelength or minimized using other lasers by proper selection of the processing parameters. However, some medical applications may profit from the rougher morphology granted by the presence of particulates on the film
- The possibility of coating is not limited to metal substrates, but polymer surfaces can also be coated via either a pretreatment or modifications of the PLD technique.
- *In vitro* and *in vivo* testing has verified similar or better osseointegration than the commercial available plasma sprayed coatings but with improved adhesion properties, without risk of delamination or detachment of the coating, as can be the case with the plasma-spray technique.

The technique is thus sufficiently mature for an industrial scale-up on the one hand and the start of clinical tests with real implants on the other hand. Commercial dental implants and orthopedic spine screws have been coated with the ArF laser, demonstrating the uniformity of the coating thickness around the corners and sidewalls of implant devices.

Even if the technique is a line-of-sight technique, there is no technological limitation to PLD coating of large areas. The laser can be rastered across the target surface, or the implant can be rotated/moved inside an industrial deposition chamber [123] to reach all parts of the implant. Despite these significant advantages, industrial uptake of PLD has not yet taken place to our knowledge. Thus, activity has been confined to the research environment, although some small and medium-sized enterprises have been involved in some of the developments. In our opinion, there seem to be two main reasons for the delay in industrial involvement: the price of lasers and the vacuum requirement. However, one can speculate that as UV laser (excimer and solid state) development proceeds, the price of these processing tools will decrease, allowing their wider introduction into the industrial environment. Moreover, as the processing complexity of medical device production increases, vacuum technology will take its place in this production branch.

Acknowledgments The work performed at the University of Vigo could not have been possible without the valuable contributions of present and past coworkers: J.L. Arias, M.B. Mayor, F. García, E. Jiménez, J. Pou, S. Chiussi, P. González, J. Serra, J.P. Borrajo, S. Liste, E. Solla, M. Pérez-Amor, C. Peraire, D. Bernal, and A. Arañó. I would like to express my gratitude to all of them. Some fruitful discussions with F. Driessens have stimulated our activities. P. Kitajlowicz has technically helped with the manuscript. Financial support of CICYT (MAT93-0271, DPI2000-0393-P4-04 MAT2003-09277-C03-01), UE CRAFT (BRE2.CT94.1533), MINER (PATI 665/95), Xunta de Galicia (INFRA93, INFRA94-58, INFRA96-ED405A-50 and C. Educación 200612), and the University of Vigo is acknowledged.

References

1. H. M. Smith and A.F. Turner, *Appl. Opt.* **4** (1965) 147.
2. D. Dijkkamp, *Appl. Phys. Lett.* **51** (1987) 619.
3. M. Jarcho, *Clin. Orthop.* **157** (1981) 259.
4. R. Z. Legeros, *Adv. Dent. Res.* **2** (1988) 164.
5. K. De Groot, in "Bioceramics of Calcium Phosphate" edited by De Groot K. (CRC Press, Boca Raton, FL, USA, 1983) p. 100.
6. R. G. T. Geesink, K. De Groot, and C. P. A. T. Klein, *J. Bone Joint Surg.* **70-B** (1988) 17.
7. R. D. Bloembaum and J. A. Dupond, *J. Arthroplast.* **8** (1993) 195.
8. J. D. Bobyn, E. S. Mortimer, A. H. Glassman, C. A. Engh, J. E. Miller, and C. E. Brooks, *Clin. Orthop.* **261** (1992) 196.
9. W. L. Jaffe and D. F. Scott, *J. Bone Joint Surg.* **78-A** (1996) 1918.
10. M. Okazaki, J. Takahashi, H. Kimura, and T. Aoba, *J. Biomed. Mater. Res.* **16** (1982) 851.
11. M. J. Filiaggi, R. M. Pilliar, and N. A. Coombs, *J. Biomed. Mater. Res.* **27** (1993) 191.
12. X. S. Zhang, P. A. Revell, S. L. Evans, M. A. Tuke, and P. J. Gregson, *J. Biomed. Mater. Res.* **46** (1999) 279.
13. X. Zheng, M. Huang, and C. Ding, *Biomaterials* **21** (2000) 841.
14. M. P. Ferraz, J. C. Knowles, J. Olsen, F. J. Monteiro, and J. D. Santos, *Biomaterials* **21** (2000) 813.
15. P. Ducheyne, W. Van Raemdonck, J. C. Heughebaert, and M. Heughebaert, *Biomaterials* **7** (1986) 97.
16. M. Yoshinari, Y. Ohtsuka, and T. Dérand, *Biomaterials* **15** (1994) 529.
17. J. A. Jansen, J. G. Wolke, S. Swann, J. P. Van Der Waerden, and K. De Groot, *Clin. Oral Implants Res.* **4** (1993) 28.
18. W. R. Lacefield, *Ann. NY Acad. Sci.* **523** (1988) 72.
19. P. Li, *J. Biomed. Mater. Res.* **66A** (2003) 79.
20. C. M. Cotell, D. B. Chrisey, K. S. Grabowski, and J. A. Sprague, *J. Appl. Biomater.* **3** (1992) 87.
21. P. Baeri, L. Torrisi, N. Marino, and G. Foti, *Appl. Surf. Sci.* **54** (1992) 210.
22. G. Sardin, J. Palau, M. Varela, J. Esteve, and J. L. Morenza, in "Hydroxyapatite and related materials" edited by Brown P. W. and Constantz B. (CRC press, 1994) p. 225.
23. R. K. Singh, F. Qian, V. Nagabushnam, R. Damodaran, and B. M. Moudgil, *Biomaterials* **15** (1994) 522.
24. P. Serra, J. Palau, M. Varela, J. Esteve, and J. L. Morenza, *J. Mater. Res.* **10** (1995) 473.
25. M. Jelínek, V. Olsan, L. Jastrabík, V. Studnicka, V. Hnatowicz, J. Kvítek, V. Havránek, T. Dostálová, I. Zergioti, A. Petrakis, E. Hontzopoulos, and C. Fotakis, *Thin Solid Films* **257** (1995) 125.
26. V. N. Bagratashvili, E. N. Antonov, E. N. Sobol, V. K. Popov, and S. M. Howdle, *Appl. Phys. Lett.* **66** (1995) 2451.
27. B. E. Tucker, G. H. Nancollas, C. M. Cottell, R. C. Y. Auyeung, and M. Spector, *Biomaterials* **17** (1996) 631.
28. S. Hontsu, M. Nakamori, H. Tabata, J. Ishii, and T. Kawai, *Jpn. J. Appl. Phys.* **35** (1996)
29. O. Guillot-Noël, R. Gómez-San Román, J. Perriére, J. Hermann, V. Craciun, C. Boulmer-Leborgne, and P. Barboux, *J. Appl. Phys.* **80** (1996) 1803.
30. C. K. Wang, J. H. Chern Lin, C. P. Ju, H. C. Ong, and R. P. H. Chang, *Biomaterials* **18** (1997) 1331.
31. J. L. Arias, M. B. Mayor, F. J. García-Sanz, J. Pou, B. León, M. Pérez-Amor, and J. C. Knowles, *J. Mater. Sci. : Mater. Med.* **8** (1997) 873.
32. J. M. Fernández-Pradas, G. Sardin, L. Cléries, P. Serra, C. Ferrater, and J. L. Morenza, *Thin Solid Films* **317** (1998) 393.
33. V. Craciun, I. W. Boyd, D. Craciun, P. Andreazza, and J. Perriere, *J. Appl. Phys.* **85** (1999) 8410.

34. C. M. Cotell, *Appl. Surf. Sci.* **69** (1993) 140.
35. L. Torrisi, *Thin Solid Films* **237** (1994) 12.
36. L. Torrisi and R. Setola, *Thin Solid Films* **227** (1993) 32.
37. E. N. Antonov, V. N. Bagratashvili, V. K. Popov, E. N. Sobol, S. M. Howdle, C. Joiner, K. G. Parker, T. L. Parker, A. A. Doktorov, V. B. Likhanov, A. I. Volozhin, S. S. Alimpiev, and S. M. Nikiforov, *J. Biomed. Optics* **3** (1998) 423.
38. R. Kelly and A. Miotello, in "Pulsed Laser Deposition of Thin Films" edited by Chrisey D. B. and Hubler G. H. (John Wiley & Sons, New York, 1994) p. 55.
39. D. B. Geohegan, in "Pulsed Laser Deposition of Thin Films" edited by Chrisey D. B. and Hubler G. H. (John Wiley & Sons, New York, 1994) p. 115.
40. J. S. Horwitz and J. A. Sprague, in "Pulsed Laser Deposition of Thin Films" edited by Chrisey D. B. and Hubler G.H. (John Wiley & Sons, New York, 1994) p. 229.
41. B. Feddes, A. M. Vredenberg, M. Wehner, J. C. G. Wolke, and J. A. Jansen, *Biomaterials* **26** (2005) 1645.
42. H. Zeng, W. R. Lacefield, and S. Mirov, *J. Biomed. Mater. Res.* **50** (2000) 248.
43. F. J. García-Sanz, M. B. Mayor, J. L. Arias, J. Pou, B. León, and M. Pérez-Amor, *J. Mater. Sci.: Mater. Med.* **8** (1997) 861.
44. J. M. Fernández-Pradas, L. Clériés, G. Sardin, and J. L. Morenza, *Biomaterials* **23** (2002) 1989.
45. J. L. Arias, PhD thesis (University of Vigo, Spain, 2000).
46. E. Masetti, M. Jelínek, and C. Grivas, *Proc. SPIE* **2965** (1996) 128.
47. J. M. Fernández-Pradas, PhD thesis (University of Barcelona, Spain, 1999).
48. O. Blind, B. Dailey, L. Jordan, and L. H. Klein, *Dent. Mater.* **21** (2005) 1017.
49. J. L. Arias, F. J. García-Sanz, M. B. Mayor, S. Chiussi, J. Pou, B. León, and M. Pérez-Amor, *Biomaterials* **19** (1998) 883.
50. M. Katto, K. Kurosawa, A. Yokotani, S. Kubodera, A. Kameyama, T. Higashiguchi, T. Nakayama, and M. Tsukamoto, *Appl. Surf. Sci.* **248** (2005) 365.
51. D. Ferro, J. V. Rau, S. M. Barinov, R. Teghil, and A. Latini, *Biomaterials* **26** (2005) 805.
52. M. P. Ferraz, F. J. Monteiro, D. Giao, B. León, P. González, S. Liste, J. Serra, J. Arias, and M. Pérez-Amor, *Key Eng. Mater.* **254–256** (2004) 347.
53. E. L. Solla, J. P. Borrajo, P. González, J. Serra, S. Chiussi, B. León, and J. García-López, *Appl. Surf. Sci.* **253** (2006) 8282.
54. E. Gyorgy, G. Socol, M. Iliescu, I. N. Mihailescu, P. Toricelli, J. Werckman, I. Mayer, and A. Bigi, *J. Biomed. Mater. Res. A* **71A** (2004) 353.
55. Y. Suda, H. Kawasaki, T. Ohshima, S. Nakashima, S. Kawazoe, and T. Toma, *Thin Solid Films* **506–507** (2006) 115.
56. P. Serra and J. L. Morenza, *Thin Solid Films* **335** (1998) 43.
57. P. Serra and J. L. Morenza, *Appl. Surf. Sci.* **127–129** (1998) 662.
58. P. Serra, J. M. Fernández-Pradas, G. Sardin, and J. L. Morenza, *Appl. Surf. Sci.* **109–110** (1997).
59. P. Serra, L. Clériés, and J. L. Morenza, *Appl. Surf. Sci.* **96–98** (1996) 216.
60. P. Serra, J. M. Fernández-Pradas, J. Navarro, and J. L. Morenza, *Appl. Phys. A* **69** (1999)
61. J. L. Arias, M. B. Mayor, J. Pou, B. León, and M. Pérez-Amor, *Appl. Surf. Sci.* **186** (2002) 448.
62. J. L. Arias, M. B. Mayor, J. Pou, B. León, and M. Pérez-Amor, *Appl. Surf. Sci.* **208–209** (2003) 57.
63. D. G. A. Nelson and J. D. B. Featherstone, *Calcif. Tiss. Int.* **34** (1982) 69.
64. R. Z. Legeros, O. R. Trautz, J. P. Legeros, and E. Klein, *Bull. Soc. Chim.(Fr.)* **special issue** (1968) 1712.
65. H. Zeng and W. R. Lacefield, *Biomaterials* **21** (2000) 23.
66. J. L. Arias, M. B. Mayor, J. Pou, B. León, and M. Pérez-Amor, *Appl. Surf. Sci.* **154** (2000) 434.

67. E. N. Antonov, V. N. Bagratashvili, L. I. Krotova, V. K. Popov, M. Ball, S. Downes, D. M. Grant, S. M. Howdle, and W. J. Lo, *Key Eng. Mater.* **192–195** (2001) 107.
68. J. M. Fernández-Pradas, L. Clèries, P. Serra, G. Sardin, and J. L. Morenza, *Appl. Phys. A* **72** (2001) 613.
69. P. Serra and J. L. Morenza, *J. Appl. Phys.* **85** (1999) 3289.
70. J. M. Fernández-Pradas, G. Sardin, and J. L. Morenza, *Appl. Phys. A* **76** (2003) 251.
71. J. L. Arias, M. B. Mayor, J. Pou, B. León, and M. Pérez-Amor, *Vacuum.* **67** (2002) 653.
72. M. B. Mayor, J. Arias, S. Chiussi, F. Garcia, J. Pou, B. León, and M. Pérez-Amor, *Thin Solid Films* **317** (1998) 363.
73. E. Jiménez, J. L. Arias, B. León, and M. Pérez-Amor, *Thin Solid Films* **453–454** (2004) 422.
74. J. Arends and W. L. Jongebloed, *Recl. Trav. Chim. Pays-Bas* **100** (1981) 3.
75. M. B. Mayor, PhD thesis (University of Vigo, Spain, 2000).
76. R. Z. Legeros and J. P. Legeros, in "An introduction to bioceramics" edited by Hench L.L. and Wilson J. (World Scientific, 1993) p. 139.
77. J. M. Fernández-Pradas, M. V. García-Cuenca, and J. L. Morenza, *Appl. Phys. A* **80** (2005) 325.
78. E. Jiménez, J. L. Arias, B. León, and M. Pérez-Amor, *Key Eng. Mater.* **254–256** (2004) 415.
79. M. Iliescu, J. Werckmann, V. Nelea, I. N. Mihailescu, G. Socol, A. Bigi, and B. Bracci, *Thin Solid Films* **453–454** (2004) 157.
80. G. Socol, F. Miroiu, I. N. Mihailescu, P. Torricelli, B. Bracci, A. Bigi, M. Iliescu, and J. Werckmann, *Biomaterials* **25** (2004) 2539.
81. E. N. Antonov, V. N. Bagratashvili, V. K. Popov, M. D. Ball, D. M. Grant, S. M. Howdle, and C. A. Scotchford, *J. Mater. Sci. : Mater. Med.* **14** (2003) 151.
82. S. Hontsu, T. Matsumoto, J. Ishii, M. Nakamori, H. Tabata, and T. Kawai, *Thin Solid Films* **295** (1997) 214.
83. M. Kusunoki, M. Kawasima, H. Nishikawa, K. Morimoto, T. Hayami, S. Hontsu, and T. Kawai, *Jpn. J. Appl. Phys. 2* **44** (2005)
84. E. N. Antonov, V. N. Bagratashvili, L. I. Krotova, and V. K. Popov, in Proceedings of the 13th International Symposium on Ceramics in Medicine, edited by Giannini S. and Moroni A. (Trans Tech Publications, Bologne, Italy, 2001).
85. M. D. Ball, S. Downes, C. A. Scotchford, E. N. Antonov, V. N. Bagratashvili, V. K. Popov, W. J. Lo, D. M. Grant, and S. M. Howdle, *Biomaterials* **22** (2001) 337.
86. J. P. Borrajo, J. Serra, S. Liste, P. González, S. Chiussi, B. León, and M. Pérez-Amor, *Appl. Surf. Sci.* **248** (2005) 355.
87. V. Nelea, H. Pelletier, M. Iliescu, J. Werckmann, V. Craciun, I. N. Mihailescu, C. Ristoscu, and C. Ghica, *J. Mater. Sci. : Mater. Med.* **13** (2002) 1167.
88. M. Katto, M. Nakamura, T. Tanaka, and T. Nakayama, *Appl. Surf. Sci.* **197–198** (2002) 768.
89. M. Katto, M. Nakamura, T. Tanaka, T. Matsutani, M. Kuwata, and T. Nakayama, *Surf. Coat. Tech.* **169–170** (2003) 712.
90. E. L. Solla, J. P. Borrajo, P. González, J. Serra, S. Liste, S. Chiussi, B. León, and M. Pérez-Amor, *Appl. Surf. Sci.* **248** (2005) 360.
91. P. J. Burnett and D. S. Rickerby, *Thin Solid Films* **157** (1988) 233.
92. Y. Yang and J. L. Ong, *J. Biomed. Mater. Res. A* **64** (2003) 509.
93. L. Clèries, E. Martínez, J. M. Fernández-Pradas, G. Sardin, J. Esteve, and J. L. Morenza, *Biomaterials* **21** (2000) 967.
94. J. M. Fernández-Pradas, L. Clèries, Martínez E., G. Sardin, J. Esteve, and J. L. Morenza, *Biomaterials* **22** (2001) 2171.
95. J. L. Arias, M. B. Mayor, J. Pou, B. León, M. Pérez-Amor, and Y. Leng, *Biomaterials* **24** (2003) 3403.
96. J. M. Fernández-Pradas, M. V. García-Cuenca, L. Clèries, G. Sardin, and J. L. Morenza, *Appl. Surf. Sci.* **195** (2002) 31.

97. C. G. Zhang, M. F. Cheng, Y. Leng, P. Tong, and J. Y. Chen, in Biomedical Materials Research in the Far East (III), edited by Zhang Z. and Ikada Y. (Kobushi Kantokai Inc, Kyoto, 1997).
98. V. Nelea, H. Pelletier, P. Mille, V. Craciun, I. N. Mihailescu, M. Iliescu, and J. Werckmann, *Appl. Surf. Sci.* **208–209** (2003) 638.
99. V. Nelea, H. Pelletier, P. Mille, and D. Muller, *Thin Solid Films* **453–454** (2004) 208.
100. L. Cléries, J. M. Fernández-Pradas, G. Sardin, and J. L. Morenza, *Biomaterials* **19** (1998) 1483.
101. L. Cléries, J. M. Fernández-Pradas, G. Sardin, and J. L. Morenza, *Biomaterials* **20** (1999) 1401.
102. J. L. Arias, J. Pou, B. León, C. Peraire, and A. Arañó, in Transactions – 7th World Biomaterials Congress, edited by Howlett R. (Australian Society for Biomaterials Inc., Sydney, 2004).
103. C. Peraire, A. Rovira, A. Araño, B. Mayor, J. L. Arias, J. Pou, and B. León, Report (EU CRAFT project: BRE2.CT94.1533, 1997).
104. T. L. Parker, K. G. Parker, S. M. Howdle, E. N. Antonov, V. N. Bagratashvili, V. K. Popov, E. Sobol, and C. J. Roberts, *Cell Eng.* **1** (1996) 91.
105. L. Cléries, J. M. Fernández-Pradas, and J. L. Morenza, *J. Biomed. Mater. Res.* **49** (2000) 43.
106. J. D. De Bruijn, J. E. Davies, and C. A. Van Blitterswijk, *J. Biomed. Mater. Res.* **29** (1995) 89.
107. J. E. Davies, *Anat. Rec.* **245** (1996) 426.
108. J. Morgan, K. R. Holtman, J. C. Keller, and C. M. Stanford, *Implan. Dent.* **6** (1996) 264.
109. H. Matsuoka, H. Akiyama, Y. Okada, H. Ito, C. Shigeno, J. Konishi, T. Kokubo, and T. Nakamura, *J. Biomed. Mater. Res.* **47** (1999) 176.
110. L. Himmlová, T. Dostálová, M. Jelínek, J. Bártová, V. Pesáková, and M. Adam, *Proc. SPIE* **3564** (1998) 221.
111. M. Seydlova, Z. Teuberova, T. Dostálová, B. Dvorankova, K. Smetana, M. Jelínek, T. Kocourek, and W. Mróz, *J. Appl. Phys.* **99** (2006) 014905.
112. A. Bigi, B. Bracci, L. Sturba, F. Cuisinier, R. Elkaim, M. Fini, P. Torricelli, I. Mayer, I. N. Mihailescu, and G. Socol, *Biomaterials* **26** (2005) 2381.
113. C. M. Cotell, J. A. Conklin, R. C. Y. Auyeung, S. S. Wong, C. M. Klapperich, and M. Spector, *Mater. Res. Soc. Symp. Proc.* **414** (1996) 171.
114. T. Dostálová, M. Jelínek, L. Himmlová, and C. Grivas, *Proc. SPIE* **3593** (1999) 81.
115. T. Dostálová, L. Himmlová, M. Jelínek, and C. Grivas, *Laser Phys.* **8** (1998) 182.
116. M. Jelínek, T. Dostálová, L. Himmlová, C. Grivas, and C. Fotakis, *Mol. Cryst. Liq. Cryst. Sci. Tech. A Mol. Cryst. Liq. Cryst.* **374** (2002) 599.
117. T. Dostálová, L. Himmlová, M. Jélinek, and C. Grivas, *J. Biomed. Optics* **6** (2001) 239.
118. C. Peraire, J. Arias, D. Bernal, J. Pou, B. León, A. Arañó, and W. Roth, *J. Biomed. Mater. Res.* **77A** (2006) 370.
119. C. Peraire, A. Arañó, A. Arsuaga, B. Assenza, A. Borrell, A. Padrós, J. L. Arias, J. Pou, and B. León, Final report (EU CRAFT Project: BRE2. CT94. 1533, 1997).
120. D. Lew, A. A. Marino, J. M. Startzell, and J. C. Keller, *J. Oral Maxillofac. Surg.* **52** (1994) 952.
121. S. Mohammadi, M. Esposito, L. Emanuelsson, and P. Thomsen, in Transactions- 7th World Biomaterials Congress, edited by Howlett R. (Australian Society for Biomaterials Inc., Sydney, 2004).
122. S. Mohammadi, M. Esposito, L. Emanuelsson, and P. Thomsen, in Transactions- 7th World Biomaterials Congress, edited by Howlett R. (Australian Society for Biomaterials Inc., Sydney, 2004).
123. J. A. Greer, in "Pulsed Laser Deposition of Thin Films" edited by Chrisey D. B. and Hubler G. H. (John Wiley & Sons, Inc., New York, 1994) p. 293.

124. J. M. Fernández-Pradas, L. Cléries, E. Martínez, G. Sardin, J. Esteve, and J. L. Morenza, *Appl. Phys. A* **A71** (2000) 37.
125. S. Hontsu, J. Ishii, M. Nakamori, N. Kato, T. Matsumoto, H. Tabata, and T. Kawai, *Jpn. J. Appl. Phys. 2* **37** (1998)
126. L. L. Hench and J. Wilson, in "An Introduction to Bioceramics" edited by Hench L. L. and Wilson J. (World Scientific, Singapore, 1993) p. 1.
127. E. N. Antonov, V. N. Bagratashvili, V. K. Popov, E. N. Sobol, and S. M. Howdle, *Spectrochimica Acta Part A* **52A** (1996) 123.
128. E. N. Antonov, V. N. Bagratashvili, V. K. Popov, E. N. Sobol, M. C. Davies, S. J. B. Tendler, C. J. Roberts, and S. M. Howdle, *Biomaterials* **18** (1997) 1043.
129. F. García, J. L. Arias, B. Mayor, J. Pou, B. León, M. Pérez-Amor, I. Rehman, J. Knowles, S. Best, and W. Bonfield, *J. Biomed. Mater. Res.* **43** (1998) 69.
130. M. B. Mayor, J. L. Arias, F. J. García-Sanz, S. Chiussi, J. Pou, B. León, and M. Pérez-Amor, *Biomaterials* **11** (1998) 209.
131. P. Serra and J. L. Morenza, *Appl. Phys. A* **67** (1998) 289.
132. V. Craciun, D. Craciun, P. Andreazza, J. Perriere, and I. W. Boyd, *Appl. Surf. Sci.* **138** (1999) 587.
133. L. Cléries, J. M. Fernández-Pradas, and J. L. Morenza, *Biomaterials* **21** (2000) 1861.
134. W. J. Lo, D. M. Grant, B. S. Welsh, M. D. Ball, S. M. Howdle, E. N. Antonov, V. N. Bagratashvili, and V. K. Popov, *J. Biomed. Mater. Res.* **50** (2000) 536.
135. V. Nelea, H. Pelletier, P. Mille, A. Cornet, C. Ristoscu, C. Chiritescu, I. N. Mihailescu, and C. Ghica, *Appl. Surf. Sci.* **168** (2000) 127.
136. H. Zeng and W. R. Lacefield, *J. Biomed. Mater. Res.* **50** (2000) 239.
137. V. Nelea, H. Pelletier, D. Muller, N. Broll, P. Mille, C. Ristoscu, and I. N. Mihailescu, *Appl. Surf. Sci.* **186** (2002) 483.
138. P. N. De Aza, J. M. Fernández-Pradas, and P. Serra, *Biomaterials* **25** (2004) 1983.
139. M. Iliescu, J. Werckmann, V. Nelea, and I. N. Mihailescu, *Surf. Coat. Tech.* **187** (2004) 131.
140. V. Nelea, C. Morosanu, M. Iliescu, and I. N. Mihailescu, *Appl. Surf. Sci.* **228** (2004) 346.
141. L. C. Nistor, C. Ghica, V. S. Teodorescu, S. V. Nistor, M. Dinescu, D. Matei, N. Frangis, N. Vouroutzis, and C. Liutas, *Mater. Res. Bull.* **39** (2004) 2089.
142. H. Pelletier, V. Nelea, P. Mille, and D. Muller, *J. Mater. Sci.* **39** (2004) 4185.
143. H. Pelletier, V. Nelea, P. Mille, and D. Muller, *J. Mater. Sci.* **39** (2004) 3605.
144. H. Pelletier, V. Nelea, P. Mille, and D. Muller, *Nucl. Instr. and Meth. in Phys. Res. B* **216** (2004) 269.
145. H. Pelletier, V. Nelea, P. Mille, and D. Muller, *Nucl. Instr. and Meth. in Phys. Res. B* **216** (2004) 275.
146. J. Beltrano, L. Torrisi, and D. Margarone, *Radiation Effects and Defects in Solids* **160** (2005) 545.
147. J. P. Borrajo, J. Serra, S. Liste, P. González, S. Chiussi, B. León, and M. Pérez-Amor, *Appl. Surf. Sci.* **248** (2005) 355.
148. H. Kim, R. P. Camata, Y. K. Vohra, and W. R. Lacefield, *J. Mater. Sci. : Mater. Med.* **16** (2005) 961.
149. I. N. Mihailescu, G. Socol, F. Miroiu, P. Torricelli, A. Bigi, I. Mayer, M. Iliescu, J. Werckmann, F. Cuisinier, R. Elkaim, and G. Hildebrand, *Appl. Surf. Sci.* **248** (2005) 344.

Chapter 6
Ion Beam Techniques for Thin Calcium Phosphate Coating Production

Masao Yoshinari

Abstract Calcium phosphate (CaP) coatings produced by the plasma-spraying method show frequent fractures and dissolution in their coatings as well as at the titanium interface after implantation, leading to peeling off of the coating due to the thick, porous, nonuniform, poorly adherent CaP layer. These peeled fragments of a certain size may induce phagocytosis by macrophages, leading to inflammation. Therefore, it is necessary to develop coatings that are defect-free and strongly adherent to titanium substrates. Such coatings must allow rapid osteogenesis and thereafter complete resorption in the host tissues so they may be eventually entirely replaced by bone tissue. CaP coatings should not be thicker than absolutely necessary to facilitate osteogenesis (remodeling of bones) at sites of resorption of old bone. The thin CaP coatings produced by ion beam techniques have inherent properties, such as fewer defects in the coatings themselves and superior adhesion between the coatings and underlying metals, that offer several advantages: They prevent fractures in CaP ceramics; they do not change the surface topography, which has a marked effect on cell behavior; and they enable immobilization of functional proteins and drugs. This chapter describes the ion beam technique, mechanical properties of the coatings, change in bond strength and solubility by heat treatment, mechanism for debonding of CaP coatings, and biological responses.

6.1 Introduction

Calcium phosphate (CaP) coatings produced by the plasma-spraying method often develop fractures, in the coating itself and at the titanium interface, after implantation. This is supposed to result from the comparatively thick (30–200 μm), porous, nonuniform (crystalline, surrounded by an amorphous mass), poorly adherent quality of the CaP layer (Fig. 6.1a). Such deterioration may

M. Yoshinari (✉)
Oral Health Science Center and Department of Dental Materials Science,
Tokyo Dental College, Chiba 261-8502, Japan
e-mail: yasinari@tdc.ac.jp

B. León, J.A. Jansen (eds.), *Thin Calcium Phosphate Coatings for Medical Implants*,
DOI 10.1007/978-0-387-77718-4_6, © Springer Science+Business Media, LLC 2009

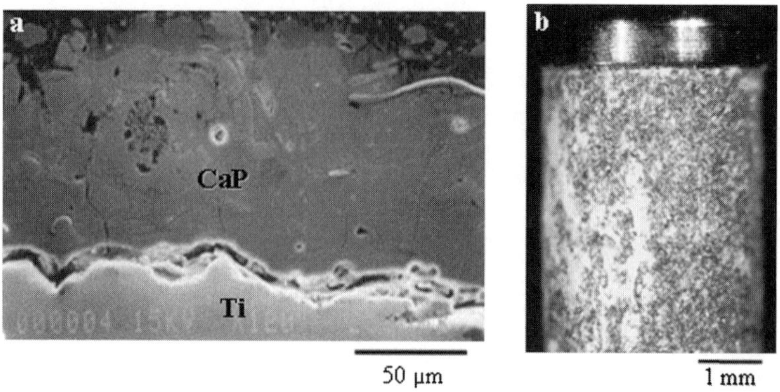

Fig. 6.1 Calcium phosphate (*CaP*) coatings produced by a plasma-spraying method. (**a**) Scanning electron micrograph (SEM) of a cross section. *Ti*, titanium. (**b**) Optical micrograph of the surface after soaking in 0.9% NaCl solution at pH 6.0 for 30 weeks

also lead to disintegration of the coating itself and detachment of the coating at the titanium interface. (Fig. 6.1b). If large enough, such fragmentation may induce phagocytosis and subsequent inflammation. Therefore, it is necessary to develop coatings that are defect-free and strongly adherent to titanium substrates. Such coatings must allow rapid osteogenesis and subsequent absorbance of coatings by host tissues so they may be eventually entirely replaced by bone tissue. CaP coatings should be no thicker than absolutely necessary to facilitate osteogenesis (remodeling of bones) at sites of resorption of old bone.

Thin CaP coatings produced by ion beam techniques have inherent properties, such as fewer defects in the coatings themselves and superior adhesion between the coating and underlying metal, that offer several advantages: They prevent fractures in CaP coatings; they do not change the surface topography, which has a marked effect on cell behavior; and they enable immobilization of functional proteins and drugs.

6.2 Ion Beam Technique

Recent progress in the semiconductor industry has seen the development of thin film formation techniques that use charged particles, such as electrons and ions, in a cold plasma atmosphere. This approach is superior in that it is environmentally pollution-free, it yields safe products, and good quality control can be maintained, thereby ensuring defect-free films. In this process, substrates and targets are placed in a vacuum chamber, a vacuum is created, and the coating materials are then deposited onto the substrates in a cold plasma atmosphere.

Figure 6.2 shows the formation of a CaP coating with both the plasma-spraying method and ion beam techniques. The fundamental difference between the plasma-spraying method and an ion beam technique, known as a

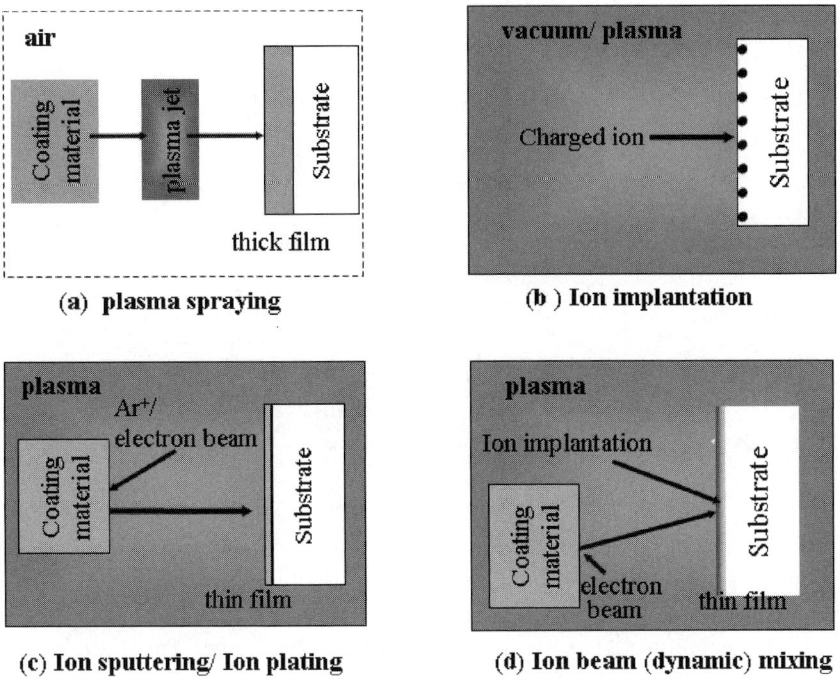

Fig. 6.2 CaP coating formation with plasma spraying method (**a**) and ion beam techniques (**b–d**)

dry process [1], is that with the latter it is carried out under a high vacuum or in a cold plasma atmosphere. There are various ion beam techniques, including ion implantation [2], ion sputtering (IS) [3–5] , ion plating (IP) [6], and ion beam dynamic mixing (IBDM) [7], all of which produce a thin, homogeneous, adherent CaP coating.

With the calcium ion implantation method, the titanium (Ti) surface is modified by high energy irradiation with Ca ions at an acceleration energy of around 20 keV and an ion-beam current density of 50 mA/cm^2. In this case, the assist gas for the implantation is krypton [8].

With the IS and IP methods, an evaporant such as hydroxyapatite (HA) is sputtered with Ar ions and evaporated with electron beams, and a negative voltage of several hundred to several thousand volts is applied to the metal substrate. A plasma state is produced as a result of glow discharge, leading to ionization of the evaporant. The generated ions or clusters are accelerated in an electric field and impinge at high energy on the surface of the metal substrates. The IBDM method, a combination of ion implantation and IP, offers the advantages of excellent adhesion due to a calcium ion-implanted layer, a high deposition rate, and production of transparent thin films that are more defect-free than those obtained with conventional thin film deposition techniques.

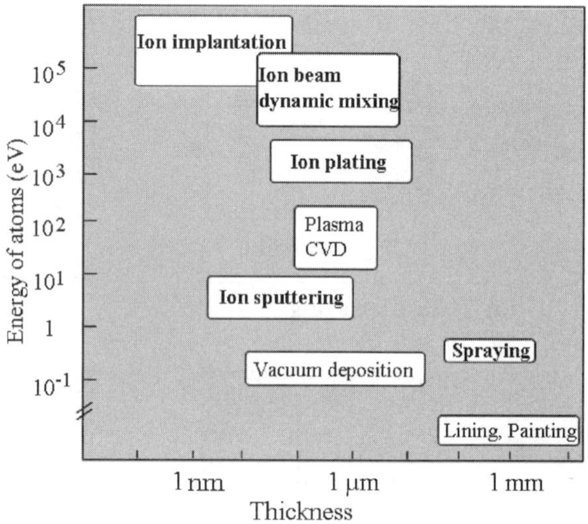

Fig. 6.3 Relation between film thickness and energy of atoms, which is related to adherence of coatings. *CVD*, chemical vapor deposition

Figure 6.3 shows the relation between film thickness and energy of atoms, which is related to the adherence of coatings, in various coatings produced by ion beam techniques. The figure indicates that the thinner the coatings, the higher the degree of adherence. Figure 6.4a shows a commercially available Brånemark implant and CaP-coated implant by the IBDM method, the latter showing a slight color change due to the thin coating layer. Figure 6.4b,c shows

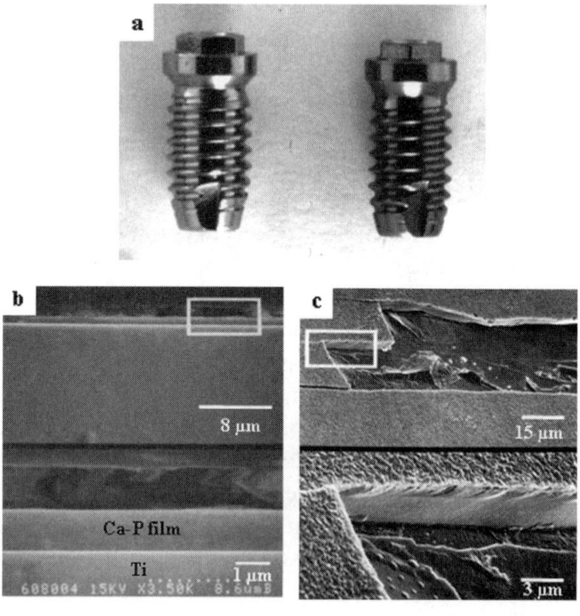

Fig. 6.4 **a** Brånemark implant (*left*) and CaP-coated implant by ion beam dynamic mixing (IBDM) method (*right*). **b** Scanning electron microscopy (SEM) images of cross sections of CaP coatings produced by IBDM. **c** SEM images of ion plating (IP) coatings after bending test. Lower images in **b** and **c** show higher magnification of the areas shown in the rectangles in the upper micrographs

a cross-sectional view of CaP coatings produced by IBDM [7] and by IP [6] after the bending test (Fig. 6.4c). Thin, defect-free films can be seen in the coating, which is adhered to the Ti substrate.

6.3 Coating Characterization

With the Ca ion implantation method, the modified layer is about 7 to 12 nm thick and consists of CaO, $CaTiO_3$, and TiO_2 [2]. The Ca/P ratio in the coatings produced by ion beam techniques have a reported range of 1.6 to 2.6 for IS coatings [9–13], 1.7 to 1.8 for IP coatings [6], and 1.5 to 2.3 for IBDM coatings [7] using an electron probe microanalysis (EPMA). In general, CaP coatings produced by the ion beam method have a slightly higher Ca/P ratio than stoichiometric HA. The composition of the coating is different from that of the target material, depending on the type of coating system and parameters

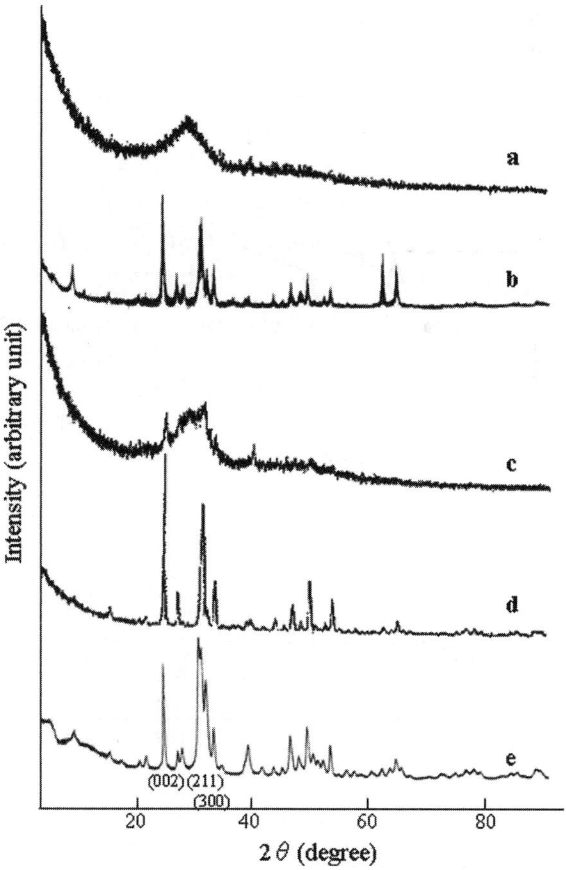

Fig. 6.5 Thin x-ray diffraction (XRD) profiles. *a*, as-deposited coating; *b*, furnace-heated at 500°C for 4 hours; *c*, *d*, rapid heating with infrared radiation at 500°C (*c*) and 700°C (*d*); *e*, HA powder as evaporant for coating

used for deposition. The evaporated HA may decompose into Ca and PO_4 during the coating process. The composition of the deposited film seems to depend mainly on evaporation velocity and the ionization pressure of each atom or molecule. The evaporation velocity and ionization potential of Ca have comparatively high values-1 $\times$ 10^3 kg/m^2·s (1200°C) and 10.5 eV, respectively-but those of PO_4 remain to be determined.

Although as-deposited coatings were confirmed to be amorphous by thin x-ray diffraction (XRD) analysis, postdeposition heat treatment was reported to result in a change in crystallinity [6, 7, 14–19]. The diffraction pattern of heat-treated coatings showed mainly HA, with a preferential orientation of the c-axis (002) (Fig. 6.5) [18]. Fourier transform infrared (FTIR) analysis revealed absorption of OH^- and PO_4^{3-} in both as-deposited and heat-treated coatings [19]. The binding energies of P2p, Ca2p3/2, and O1s obtained from coated specimens were close to those of bulk HA, according to XPS analysis [7].

6.4 Mechanical Properties of Thin Coatings (Composites with Ceramics and Metals)

The mechanical properties of Ca-ion implanted and thin CaP-coated Ti, such as proof stress and modulus of elasticity, are the same as those of Ti substrates, as the modified layers are extremely thin compared to the thickness of the substrates.

With composite materials that combine brittle ceramics as a coating and metals as a substrate, it is of major importance to minimize the thickness of the ceramic layer. Table 6.1 shows the mechanical and physical properties of the substrates (SUS316, Ti) and coating materials (alumina, HA). Table 6.2 shows the maximum deflection without breakage of alumina and HA at thicknesses of 1 mm and 10 μm, respectively [20]. These data were calculated by the following equation for a three-point bending test at a span length of 30 mm (Fig. 6.6a) using the specific values listed in Table 6.1.

$$\delta = \sigma l^2/6hE$$

Table 6.1 Mechanical and physical properties of substrates (SUS316, Ti) and coating materials (Alumina, Hydroxyapatite)

Substrate/coating material	Proof stress (MPa)	Elastic modulus (GPa)	Thermal expansioncoefficient (× 10–6/K)
Stainless steel (SUS316)	300	180	16
Ti (grade 2)	350	100	8
Alumina	500–1000	350–400	5–8
Hydroxyapatite	100–200	35–120	10–13

Table 6.2 Maximum deflection (mm) without breakage of ceramics in three-point bending test (Span length 30 mm)

Coating material	Maximum deflection, by the thickness of the coating	
	1 mm	10 μm
Alumina	0.19–0.38	19–38
Hydroxyapatite	0.13–0.25	13–25

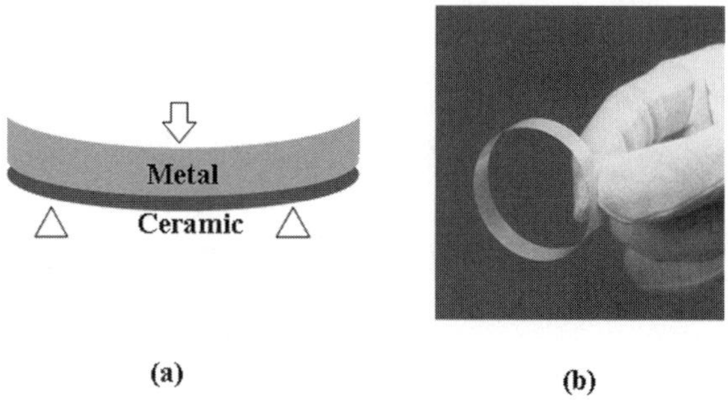

Fig. 6.6 **a** Three-point bending test. **b** Example of thin ceramic with great capacity for bending without breakage

where δ is the deflection at the center; l is the span length; σ is the proof stress; h is the thickness; and E is the elastic modulus. It can be seen that a ceramic layer of not more than 10 μm in thickness yields a huge radius of maximum flexion without breakage (Fig. 6.6b). Thus, reducing the thickness of the ceramic layer offers the advantage of optimizing the beneficial properties of the metal substrates.

Thin CaP coatings produced by ion beam techniques demonstrate high bond strength to Ti substrates, as they have fewer defects than, and offer superior adhesion to, those produced by conventional plasma-spraying methods.

6.5 Change in Bond Strength and Solubility by Heat Treatment

The tensile bond strength of as-deposited coatings to Ti substrates has been reported to be 38 to 45 MPa with ion beam sputter deposition [3], more than 53 MPa with magnetron sputtering [4], and above 59 MPa with IBDM [7]. Unfortunately, as-deposited coatings are amorphous (Fig. 6.5a, XRD analysis), resulting in films that easily dissolve in body fluids [18]. This renders them inappropriate for biomedical use.

As-deposited coatings crystallize during heat treatment using a conventional electric furnace (Fig. 6.5b), leading to decreased solubility [14, 18, 19]. Such coatings, however, tend to crack easily, resulting in a reduction in bond strength [14], especially after soaking in body fluid [7, 18]. Therefore, a suitable heat treatment is required that offers control of the solubility of the CaP coating without weakening its adhesion to the Ti substrate.

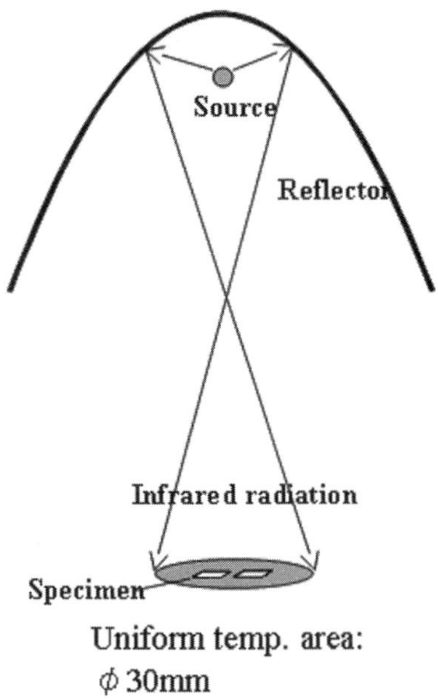

Fig. 6.7 Rapid heating with infrared radiation. Defocused radiation technique allows uniform temperature over an area 30 mm in diameter

It has been reported that rapid, homogeneous, comparatively low-temperature heating at 600° to 700°C, such as defocused infrared radiation (Fig. 6.7), allows control of CaP solubility and ensures adherence of both IS and IBDM coatings [18, 19]. Figure 6.8 shows scanning electron microscopy (SEM) images of furnace-heated coatings before and after immersion for 35 days in simulated body fluid (SBF). Cracks are observed in the coatings after immersion in SBF (Fig. 6.8b). Among those rapid-heated with infrared radiation at 400°C (Fig. 6.9a), the coatings disappeared, and many precipitates appeared on the Ti substrate after immersion in SBF. No apparent change was observed in the coatings rapidly heated at 600°C due to limited dissolution of coatings (Fig. 6.9b). However, many cracks were observed on the coatings rapidly heated at 800°C (Fig. 6.9c).

Figure 6.10 shows the change in film thickness of IBDM coatings relative to originally 1.0 μm thick deposited coatings after soaking in SBF. The as-deposited coatings almost completely disappeared after 1 day. Furnace-heated coatings decreased in thickness depending on the duration of immersion, and there was a large standard deviation after 5 weeks of immersion that may have been caused by partial peeling of the coatings. The coatings rapidly heated with infrared radiation at 400°C (IR400) almost disappeared after 1 week, whereas those at IR600 and IR800 retained approximately 60% and 55% of their thickness, respectively, after 5 weeks of immersion. This tendency is presumably correlated with the crystallinity of the coatings. The IR800 specimens, however, showed large standard deviations after 1 and 5 weeks of immersion due to partial peeling of the coatings.

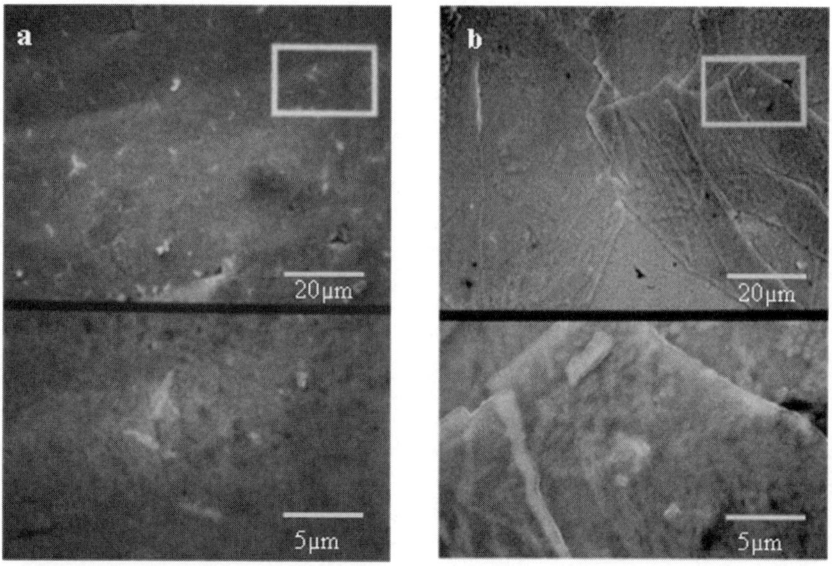

Fig. 6.8 SEM of coatings (furnace-heated at 500°C for 1 hour) as heat-treated (**a**) and after immersion in simulated body fluid (SBF) for 35 days (**b**). Lower images in **a** and **b** show higher magnification of the areas shown in the rectangles in the upper micrographs

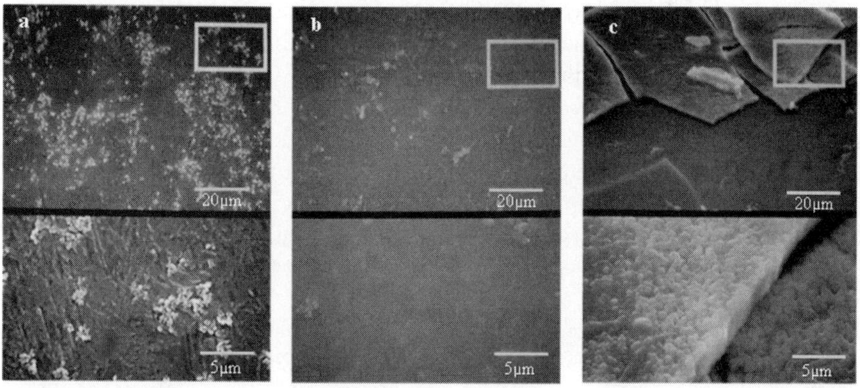

Fig. 6.9 SEM of annealed coatings achieved by rapid heating with infrared radiation at 400°C (**a**), 600°C (**b**), and 800°C (**c**) after immersion in SBF for 35 days. Lower images in **a**, **b**, and **c** show higher magnification of the areas shown in the rectangles in the upper micrographs

Table 6.3 shows the change in tensile bond strength between coatings and Ti substrate after immersion in SBF [7, 18]. It also shows the change in surface morphology associated with dissolution or cracking of the coatings. As-deposited coatings and rapid-heated coatings at 400°C with infrared radiation dissolved within a couple of days. Cracks were observed in the coatings with

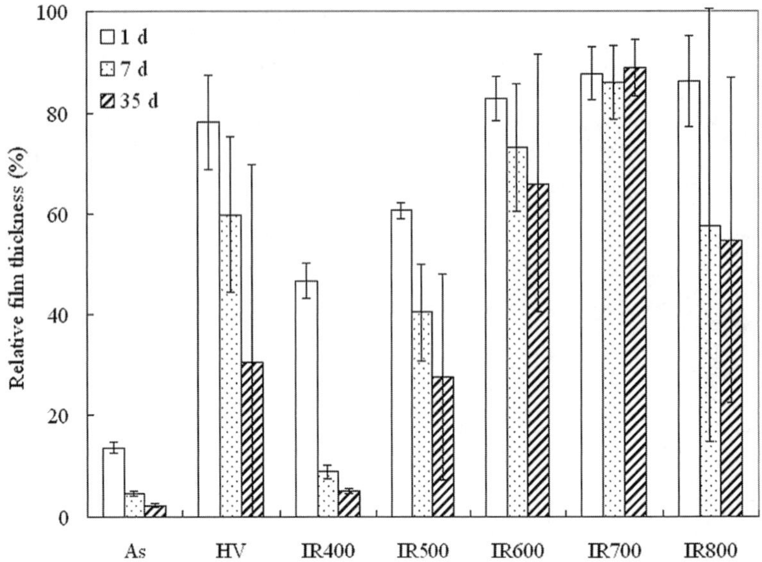

Fig. 6.10 Change in film thickness of coatings relative to the as-deposited (*As*) thickness of approximately 1.0 μm in SBF. *HV*, furnace-heated coatings

furnace heating at 500°C and rapid heating at 800°C. Rapid heating at 600° and 700°C yielded high bond strength. These results indicate that high temperatures and long duration are unnecessary to obtain crystallinity in thin coatings.

Dissolution of coated film and/or precipitation of CaP from the solution on the surface appear to occur simultaneously. With HA, the SBF solution is supersaturated with Ca and P, so precipitation should be the major reaction if HA is crystallized completely. However, dissolution is often observed in CaP coatings. Dissolution is dependent on the crystallinity, grain size, and density of CaP films. Low crystallinity, small grain size, lower density, and the presence of impurities such as CO^{3-} result in higher solubility [21–24].

Table 6.3 Change in bond strength (MPa) between coatings and Ti substrate after immersion in SBF for 35 days. Tensile bond strength was measured in specimens showing no change in surface morphology

	Before immersion	After immersion
As-deposited	59.0 (10.5)	Dissolved
Furnace heated at 500°C for 1 h	46.3 (17.0)	Cracked
Infrared radiation (rapid heating)		
400°C	59.6 (13.0) *	Dissolved
500°C	55.7 (6.9) *	Peeled partially
600°C	60.2 (13.8) *	44.9 (9.6)
700°C	57.8 (9.6) *	48.4 (11.7)
800°C	35.5 (15.4)	Cracked

* Cohesive failure in epoxy glues used for bonding test

Reduction in bond strength is observed in heat-treated specimens. This appears to be a result of internal stresses caused by a change in film density and the formation of titanium oxides and Ti-P compounds due to diffusion of elements. This has an adverse influence on the bond between the CaP coating and the Ti substrate [3].

The behavior of the elements involved in the debonding mechanism at the CaP coating–Ti interface after heat-treatment has been studied [18]. The results of XPS analyses of the interface between the coating and the Ti substrate (depth profile of Ti substrates in which CaP coatings were removed by epoxy glue) are shown in Fig. 6.11a. The intensities of the P^{3-} states of the furnace-heated and 800°C rapid-heated specimens were larger than those of as-deposited or 600°C rapid-heated specimens, and the intensities of the Ca2p spectrum decreased in the furnace-heated and 800°C rapid-heated specimens. In addition, there were no marked differences in the Ti-oxidation state (TiO_2) among the specimens. These results suggest that too much growth of Ti–P compounds and decreased thickness of Ca-implanted layers is a major reason for cracks due to debonding of coatings. According to the binary phase diagram, the Ti–Ca system has neither solid solutions nor intermetallic compounds. In contrast, the Ti–P system has many intermetallic compounds such as Ti_3P_4, Ti_3P, Ti_5P_3, and

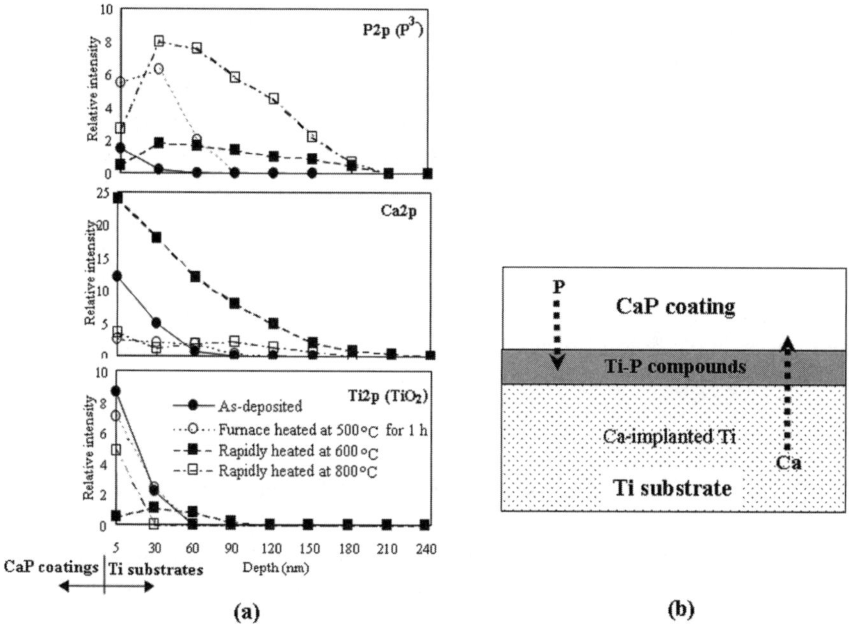

Fig. 6.11 **(a)** XPS depth profiles of titanium (Ti) substrates in which Ca-P coatings were removed by epoxy glue. **(b)** Diffusion of P and Ca and creation of many Ti-P compounds at the interface that leads to debonding of CaP coating if too much thermal energy is applied to CaP-coated Ti

Ti_2P. Therefore, if too much thermal energy is applied to CaP-coated Ti, P diffuses toward the Ti substrate, creating many Ti–P compounds at the interface; this results in cracks in the coatings due to debonding, and the Ca diffuses out of the Ti substrate (Fig. 6.11b). Titanium oxide is not thought to play a dominant role in bonding between thin CaP coatings and Ti substrates.

6.6 Biological Responses

6.6.1 In Vitro *Cell Behavior of Thin CaP Coatings*

It has been reported that CaP coatings prepared with IS and IBDM promote differentiation and expression in osteogenic cells, and that bone formation proceeds faster on CaP surfaces than on Ti substrates [25, 26]. Dissolution characteristics appear to be the key to understanding cell behavior in relation to CaP coatings. It has been suggested that, first, CaP dissolves, thereby increasing local concentrations of Ca and P in the microenvironment. This step is then followed by reprecipitation of Ca and P and the formation of a bone-like mineral layer [27]. It is suggested that the formation of this bone-like mineral layer promotes adhesion of the extracellular matrix (ECM), thus providing a suitable substrate for cell attachment as well as the functional differentiation of resident osteoblasts or committed osteoblast precursors.

The behavior of cultured osteogenic cells is affected by the crystallinity of the CaP bulk or thin CaP coatings using IS methods [28–32]. It is hypothesized that crystallinity determines the dissolution characteristics of the deposited coating, which in turn can influence its osteogenic capacity. Cells on the crystalline coating exhibit the highest expression of the osteogenic differentiation marker osteocalcin and yield the highest amounts of calcification of cell cultures, followed by Ti substrates. Calcification may be related to the abundant deposition of collagen fibrils. In contrast, no proliferation or differentiation of rat bone marrow (RBM) cells has been seen on amorphous coatings [28]. Evidently, the high level of dissolution with amorphous coatings inhibits RBM cell proliferation and differentiation [28].

6.6.2 In Vivo *Bone Behavior of Thin CaP Coatings*

When osteogenesis occurs at a site where old bone is absorbed (bone remodeling), the CaP coatings should be not thicker than necessary. It was reported that thin CaP coatings produced by the IS method were comparable to plasma-sprayed HA coatings with respect to bone formation and ultimate interfacial strength [33]. In a study of TiO_2-grit-blasted and CaP-coated implants using the IS method, the CaP coatings showed improved initial fixation and healing response when implanted into the trabecular bone of a goat [34–36]. In addition, histological examination indicated that more new bone activity was observed around CaP-coated implants using the IBDM method after 27 days of implantation [25]. The influence of thin CaP coatings and surface roughness on trabecular bone response was also investigated in the femoral condyles of rabbits [37]. CaP coatings were produced by the IBDM method and subjected to rapid heating with infrared radiation at 700°C. Twelve weeks after implantation, the highest percentage of bone contact was found around the CaP-coated implants, suggesting that a thin CaP coating enhances the implant–bone response during the healing phase. Furthermore, bone response to titanium implants treated with a thin CaP coating was evaluated by inserting them into edentulous areas in the mandibular molar region of beagle dogs [38]. Four weeks after implantation, a higher percentage of bone contact was found around the thin CaP-coated implants than around untreated titanium implants. These data suggest that a thin coating of CaP produced by ion beam techniques effectively promotes osteogenesis around implants.

With regard to the thickness of CaP coatings, 1 μm thick heat-treated CaP sputter coatings on roughened titanium implants appear to be of sufficient thickness to display bioactive properties [39]. The bone response toward CaP sputter-coated implants with different thicknesses and crystallinities (i.e., 0.1 μm and 2.0 μm amorphous and 0.1 μm and 2.0 μm crystalline) was also examined [40, 41]. The results showed that sputtered crystalline CaP-coated implants with an ultra-thin 0.1 μm thickness were associated with improved bone response in comparison with uncoated titanium implants after both short- and long-term implantation. No further improvement in bone response was observed with 2 μm thick coatings. In addition, it is suggested that once early osseointegration is achieved, biodegradation of thin CaP coatings is not detrimental for bone–coating–implant fixation and does not compromise the final bone responses [29, 30, 42]. These studies clearly indicate that ion beam techniques are viable alternatives to plasma spraying for application of CaP coatings to implants.

6.6.3 Immobilization of Bisphosphonates Through Thin CaP Coatings

Immobilization of osteogenesis-promoting drugs on thin CaP coatings is a promising new approach to achieve rapid osseointegration and improvement of the bone bed at the bone tissue/implant interface. In the treatment of osteoporosis, bisphosphonates and simvastatins have been reported to stimulate bone formation [43] and to increase expression of bone morphogenetic protein-2 (BMP-2), respectively [44].

Bisphosphonates not only work as potent inhibitors of osteoclastic bone resorption but also exert a direct effect on osteoblasts [45]. It was reported that bisphosphonates could be immobilized on titanium implants through thin CaP

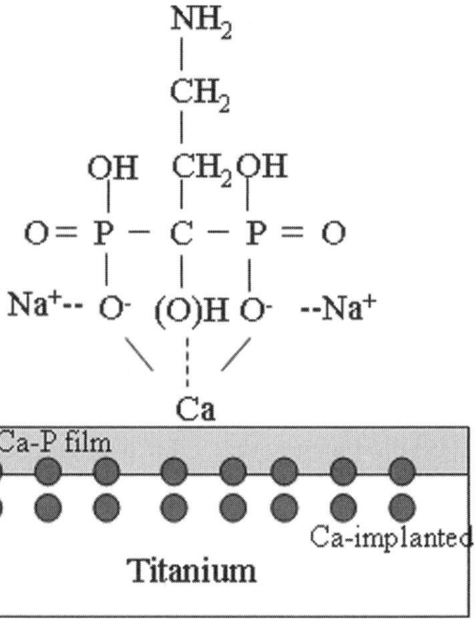

Fig. 6.12 Possible structure of immobilization of bisphosphonates (pamidronate disodium) to Ti through thin Ca-P coatings

coatings [38, 46]. The reason for this may be their marked affinity to CaPs. X-ray photoelectron spectroscopy (XPS) and FTIR analyses revealed that titanium surfaces modified with thin CaP coatings allowed immobilization of bisphosphonate and that such surfaces revealed physiologically active functional groups of bisphosphonate origin (Fig. 6.12).

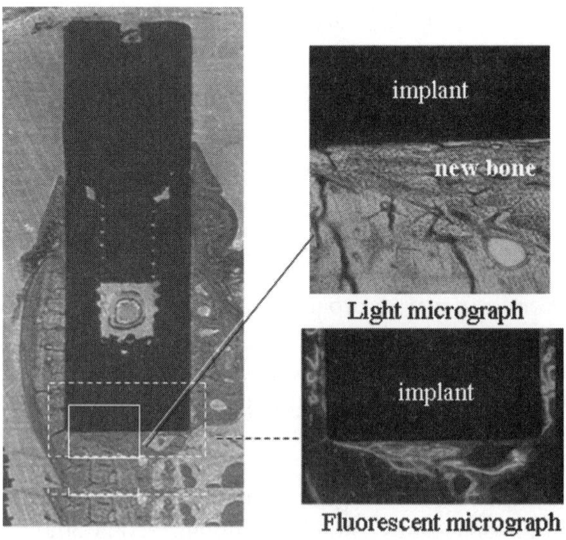

Fig. 6.13 Light and fluorescence micrographs of the bisphosphonate-coated Ti implant–bone interface 12 weeks after implantation in a beagle dog (*See* Color Insert)

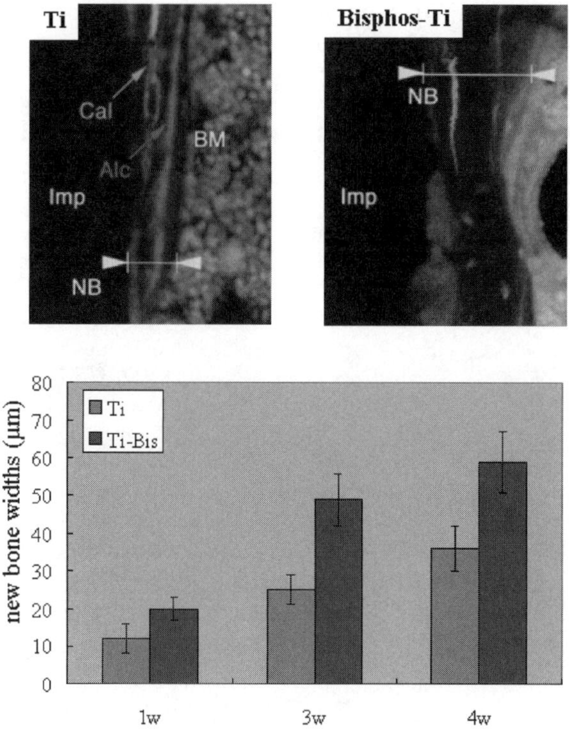

Fig. 6.14 *Top* Confocal laser scanning microscopy. *Cal*, calcein (1 week); *Alc*, alizarin complexone (3 weeks); *BM*, bone marrow; *Imp*, implant; *NB*, new bone. *Bottom* New bone width of Ti and bisphosphonate-immobilized implants in Wistar rats (*See* Color Insert)

Alkaline phosphatase expression activity and bone-like nodule formation in RBM cells showed a greater increase on plates with immobilized bisphosphonate than on as-received titanium, indicating that bisphosphonate immobilization has no toxic effect on osteoblasts and that it provides a favorable microenvironment for osteogenesis [26]. In an *in vivo* test using beagle dogs, fluorescence was widely observed in newly formed bone tissue around bisphosphonate-immobilized implants, and the ratio of bone contact to the bisphosphonate-immobilized implants was significantly higher than around other implants at 12 weeks [38] (Fig. 6.13). In addition, confocal laser scanning microscopy revealed that bone formation significantly increased around bisphosphonate-immobilized implants compared with pure titanium implants [47] (Fig. 6.14).

6.7 Critical Assessment of Prospective Use

Ion beam techniques in a cold plasma atmosphere are promising methods for creating thin, defect-free CaP coatings that can be strongly adherent to titanium substrates. In addition, these CaP coatings enable immobilization of bisphosphonates, and bisphosphonate-immobilized surfaces promote osteogenesis around implants. It is necessary to clarify the optimal thickness and solubility of CaP coatings for biomedical use.

Appendix: Significant references for this chapter

Reference	Technique	Evaluation, significance
2	Ion implantation	Ca ions, 10^{17}ions/cm^2, Ti substrate
3	Single-beam IS	Post annealing: 600°C in air for 1 hour, XRD, solubility, bond strength
4	Magnetron IS	EPMA. XRD, Bond strength, *in vitro*, *in vivo*
5	IS	Fluorapatite, in situ annealing, post annealing, XRD, TEM
6	Radiofrequency IP	EPMA, XRD, XPS, bond strength, dissolution
7	IBDM	Post annealing, XRD, XPS, FTIR, bond strength, dissolution
8	Ion implantation	Histologic study, rat tibia
9	Magnetron IS	Dissolution, XRD, FTIR
18	IBDM	Post annealing, rapid heating, dissolution, bonding mechanism, EPMA, XRD, XPS
19	Magnetron IS	Post annealing, rapid heating, dissolution, EPMA, XRD, FTIR
20	Elecrophoretic deposition	Crystallinity, XRD, FTIR
25	IBDM	Cell culture, magnetron IS, histologic study, rabbit femur
26	Ion implantation, IBDM	Ca ions, bisphosphonate, cell culture, ALP activity
33	IS	Post annealing, crystallinity, XRD, FTIR
34	Magnetron IS	Surface roughness, film thickness, torque test, goat
35	Magnetron IS	Surface topography, film thickness, histologic study, goats
37	IBDM	Surface topography, histologic study, rabbit femur
38	IBDM	Post annealing, rapid heating, bisphosphonate, histologic study, dogs, mandible
39	Magnetron IS	Thickness, post annealing, crystallinity, histologic study, rabbits
47	Ion implantation	Ca ions, bisphosphonate, histologic study, rat tibia

Ti, titanium; IS, ion sputtering; XRD, x-ray diffraction; XPS, x-ray photoelectron spectroscopy; IP, ion plating; EPMA, electron probe microanalysis; TEM, transmission electron microscopy; FTIR, Fourier transform infrared spectroscopy; IBDM, ion beam dynamic mixing; ALP, alkaline phosphatase

References

1. M. Yoshinari, Y. Oda, T. Inoue and M. Shimono, *Metallurgical and Materials Transactions A* **33** (2002) 511.
2. T. Hanawa, H. Ukai and K. Murakami, *J. Electron Spectrosc.* **63** (1993) 347.
3. J.L. Ong , L.C. Lucas, W.R. Lacefield and E.D. Rigney, *Biomaterials* **13** (1992) 249.

4. J.A. Jansen, J.G.C. Wolke, J.P.C.M. van der Waerden and K. de Groot, *Clin. Oral Impl. Res.* **4** (1993) 28.
5. T.S. Chen and W.R. Lacefield, *J. Mater. Res.* **9** (1994) 1284.
6. M. Yoshinari, K. Ozeki and T. Sumii, *Bull. Tokyo Dent. Coll.* **32** (1991) 147.
7. M. Yoshinari, Y., Ohtsuka and T. Derand, *Biomaterials* **15** (1994) 529.
8. T. Hanawa, Y. Kamiura, S. Yamamoto, T. Kohgo, A. Amemiya, H. Ukai, K. Murakami and K. Asaoka, *J. Biomed. Mater. Res.* **36** (1997) 131.
9. J.G. Wolke, K. van Dijk, H.G. Schaeken, K. de Groot and J.A. Jansen, *J. Biomed. Mater. Res.* **28** (1994) 1477.
10. J.L. Ong, G.N. Raikar and T.M. Smoot, *Biomaterials* **18** (1997) 1271.
11. J.L. Ong and L.C. Lucas, *Biomaterials* **19** (1998) 455.
12. Y. Yang, C.M. Agrawal, K-H. Kim, H. Martin, K. Schulz, J.D. Bumgardner and J.L. Ong., *J. Oral Implantol.* **XXIX** (2003) 270.
13. J.E.G. Hulshoff, K. van Dijk, J.E. De Ruijter, F.J.R. Rietveld, L.A. Ginsel and J.A. Jansen, *J. Biomed. Mater. Res.* **40** (1998) 464.
14. J.L. Ong and L.C. Lucas, *Biomaterials* **15** (1994) 337.
15. K. van Dijk, H.G. Schaeken, J.G.C. Wolke and J.A. Jansen, *Biomaterials* **17** (1996) 405.
16. Y. Yang, K-H. Kim, C.M. Agrawal and J.L. Ong, *Biomaterials* **24** (2003) 5131.
17. Y. Yang, K.-H. Kim, C.M. Agrawal and J.L. Ong, *J. Dent. Res.* **82** (2003) 833.
18. M. Yoshinari, Y. Watanabe, Y. Ohtsuka and T. Derand, *J. Dent. Res.* **76** (1997) 1486.
19. M. Yoshinari, T. Hayakawa, J.C.G. Wolke, K. Nemoto and J.A. Jansen, *J. Biomed. Mater. Res.* **37** (1997) 60.
20. M. Yoshinari, *Bull. Tokyo Dent. Coll.* **30** (1989) 51.
21. P. Ducheyne, W.V. Raemdonck, J.C. Heughebaert and M. Heughebaert, *Biomaterials* **7** (1986) 97.
22. P. Ducheyne and J.M. Cuckler, *Clin. Orthop.* **276** (1992) 102.
23. U. Saalfeld, N. M. Meenen, T. T. Jüres and H. Saalfeld, *Biomaterials* **15** (1994) 905.
24. S.R. Radin and P. Ducheyne, *J. Biomed. Mater. Res.* **28** (1994) 1303.
25. M. Yoshinari, B. Klinge and T. Derand, *Clin. Oral Impl. Res.* **7** (1996) 96.
26. M. Yoshinari, Y. Oda, H. Ueki and S. Yokose, *Biomaterials* **22** (2001) 709.
27. R.Z. LeGeros and I. Orly in "The bone biomaterial interface" (University of Toronto Press, Toronto, 1991) p. 76
28. P. J. ter Brugge and J.A.Jansen, *J. Biomed. Mater. Res.* **60** (2002) 70.
29. S.H. Maxian, J.P. Zawadsky and M.G. Dunn, *J. Biomed. Mater. Res.* **27** (1993) 111.
30. J.L. Ong, D.L. Carnes and A. Sogal, Int. *J. Oral Maxillofac. Implants* **12** (1999) 217.
31. D.R. Villarreal, A Sogal and J L. Ong, *J. Oral Implantol.* **XXIV** (1998) 67.
32. Y. Yang, J.D. Bumgardner, R. Cavin, D.L. Carnes and J.L. Ong, *J. Dent. Res.* **82** (2003) 449.
33. Y. Yang, K-H. Kim and J.L. Ong, *Biomaterials* **26** (2005) 327.
34. S. Vercaigne, J.G.C. Wolke, I. Naert and J.A. Jansen, *Clin. Oral Implant. Res.* **11** (2000) 305.
35. S. Vercaigne, J.G.C. Wolke, I. Naert and J.A. Jansen, *Clin. Oral Implant. Res.* **11** (2000) 314.
36. T. Hayakawa, M. Yoshinari, K. Nemoto, J.G.C. Wolke and J.A. Jansen, *Clin. Oral Implant. Res.* **11** (2000) 296.
37. T. Hayakawa, M. Yoshinari, H. Kiba, H. Yamamoto, K. Nemoto and J.A. Jansen, *Biomaterials* **23**(2002) 1025.
38. M. Yoshinari, Y. Oda, T. Inoue, K. Matsuzaka and M. Shimono, *Biomaterials* **23** (2002) 2879.
39. J.G.C. Wolke, J.P.C.M. van der Waerden, H.G. Schaeken and J.A. Jansen, *Biomaterials* **24** (2003) 2623.
40. S. Mohammadi, M. Esposito, J. Hall, L. Emanuelsson, A. Krozer and P. Thomsen, *Clin. Implant Dent. Relat. Res.* **5** (2003) 241.

41. S. Mohammadi, M. Esposito, J. Hall, L. Emanuelsson, A. Krozer and P. Thomsen, Int. *J. Oral Maxillofac. Implants* **19** (2004) 498.
42. K. de Groot, J.G.C. Wolke and J.A. Jansen, *J. Oral Implantol.* **XX** (1994) 232.
43. H. Fleisch in "Bisphosphonates in bone disease" (Academic press, San Diego, 2000), p.27
44. G. Mundy, R. Garrett, S. Harris, J. Chan, D. Chen, G. Rossini, B. Boyce, M. Zhao and G. Gutierrez., *Science* **286** (1999) 1946.
45. N. Giuliani, M. Pedrazzoni, G. Negri, G. Passeri, M. Impicciatore and G.G. Irasole, *Bone* **22** (1998) 455.
46. M. Yoshinari, K. Matsuzaka, T. Inoue, Y. Oda and M. Shimono, *Materials Transactions* **43** (2002) 2494.
47. H. Kajiwara T. Yamaza, M. Yoshinari, T. Goto, S. Iyamade, I. Atsuta, A.M. Kido and T. Tanaka, *Biomaterials* **26** (2005) 581.

Chapter 7
Calcium Phosphate Coating Produced by a Sputter Deposition Process

Joo L. Ong, Yunzhi Yang, Sunho Oh, Mark Appleford, Weihui Chen, Yongeing Liu, Kyo-Han Kim, Sangwon Park, Jeol Bumgardner, Warren Haggard, C. Mauli Agrawal, David L. Carner, and Namsik Oh

Abstract The properties of implant surfaces play critical roles in inducing a biological response. In the case of dental and orthopedic implants, deposition of calcium phosphate (CaP) coatings on these implant surfaces are often employed as means of enhancing implant osseointegration with the bone. Although most implants are coated using a plasma spraying process, sputtering is currently being accepted by some implant vendors as one of the means for depositing thin CaP coatings on dental and orthopedic implants. Acceptance of the sputtering technology and recent research are indications that the sputtering process is promising and has potential for eliminating some of the problems associated with the plasma-spraying process. This chapter discusses some of the various modes of sputtering, properties of thin CaP coatings, and the biological responses to these coatings *in vitro* and *in vivo*. The limitations and strengths of the sputtering process are also addressed.

7.1 Introduction

Biological fixation is defined as the process by which prosthetic components are firmly bonded to host bone by ongrowth or ingrowth without the use of bone cement [1–3]. Since the late 1960s, the use of biological or cementless fixation using bioactive calcium phosphate (CaP) coatings has been proposed as an alternative to cemented fixation of load-bearing orthopedic implants. CaP materials, such as hydroxyapatite (HA), are found in the inorganic portion of bones and teeth, rendering these materials highly biocompatible. However, CaP materials are ceramics that have traditionally been known for their poor mechanical properties, particularly due to their brittle behavior. As a result, the rationale for use of CaP coatings, such as hydroxyapatite (HA), originated from the desire to combine the strength of titanium (Ti) with a bioactive HA

J.L. Ong (✉)
Department of Biomedical Engineering, University of Texas at San Antonio, One UTSA Circle, San Antonio, TX 78249, USA
e-mail: anson.ong@utsa.edu

B. León, J.A. Jansen (eds.), *Thin Calcium Phosphate Coatings for Medical Implants*, DOI 10.1007/978-0-387-77718-4_7, © Springer Science+Business Media, LLC 2009

coating [4–8]. In fact, HA coatings have continuously been reported to enhance clinical success since Furlong and Osborn's first clinical trials [9], with three current studies reporting a less than 2% failure rate during a mean follow-up study of 10 years [6, 10, 11].

The current commercial process used by many vendors to deposit CaP or HA coatings on metallic implants is reported to be plasma spraying or arc plasma spraying [12, 13]. At the present time, minimal requirements for HA coatings have been described in the U.S. Food and Drug Administration (FDA) guidelines as well as in the International Organization for Standardization guidelines [14, 15]. Although continuous improvements in plasma-spraying technology and indications of clinical success with the use of plasma-sprayed HA-coated implants have been reported, their use has initiated substantial controversy in the field of dental and orthopedic implantology. Reported problems have included variations or poor coating–metal adhesion strength, nonuniformity in coating thickness among vendors, alteration in structural and chemical properties during the coating process, and nonuniformity in coating density [3–9, 16, 17]. As shown in Fig. 7.1, failure of the plasma-sprayed HA coating was observed at 12 weeks' implantation and 1 year' loading in a dog's mandible after pullout testing. Fracture was observed at the Ti–HA coating interface as well as within the coating. As a result of the poor coating–metal adhesion strength, there is controversy over the benefits and success of HA-coated implants. However, problems observed with plasma-sprayed HA-coated implants are not shortcomings inherent in the rationale for HA coating but, rather, in the plasma-spray technology currently used for depositing HA coatings on implant surfaces.

Aside from the inherent coating technology, there is no standard guideline for producing HA coatings on implant surfaces. Investigations have suggested that all HA coatings are not the same, and variations in coating properties have attributed to many conflicting animal and clinical observations [4–6]. Findings

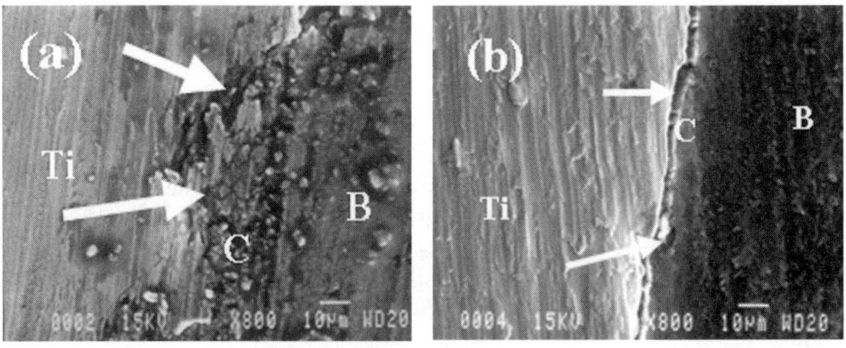

Fig. 7.1 Scanning electron microscopy (SEM) photomicrographs of a fractured interface. **a** Plasma-sprayed hydroxyapatite (HA) coating after 12 weeks of implantation. **b** Plasma-sprayed HA coating after 1 year of loading. *C*, coating; *B*, bone; *Ti*, titanium substrate. *Arrows* indicate cracks at the coating–metal interface after pullout testing

of plasma-sprayed HA-coated implants suggesting promotion of early implant stability are not universal, and these equivocal findings likely stem from the fact that HA coatings are poorly characterized. Typical plasma-sprayed HA coatings have been reported to consist primarily of partially dehydrated HA, with amorphous CaP and other more soluble CaP phases such as tricalcium phosphate (TCP) produced during the high-temperature deposition process. In addition, the crystallinity for plasma-sprayed HA coatings produced under a normal deposition process is approximately 65%, even though the plasma-spraying technology has the capability of producing coatings with crystallinity in the range of 30% to 70%. At the extreme, some implant vendors (e.g., Zimmer Dental, Carlsbad, CA, USA) have increased their HA coating crystallinity beyond 70% on their implant surfaces.

The ratio of HA to TCP has been reported to be crucial for bone regeneration. It is known that CaP phases as well as coating crystallinity affected the dissolution rate of an HA coating. An increase in amorphous and TCP phases predispose the coatings to higher dissolution rates. In addition, the formation of bone apatite-like minerals is promoted in the presence of dissolved calcium and phosphorus ions localized in the pericellular environment. Similarly, the presence of high Ca ion concentration is known to induce apoptosis of bone-forming cells and the formation of osteoclasts. As shown in Fig. 7.2 and by other investigators [18, 19], reduced cell viability and osteoblast differentiation were observed as a result of rapid dissolution. As an example of the effect of coating dissolution on bone responses *in vivo*, Fig. 7.3 shows bone formation to be highly dependent on coating crystallinity [20]. As indicated in the figure,

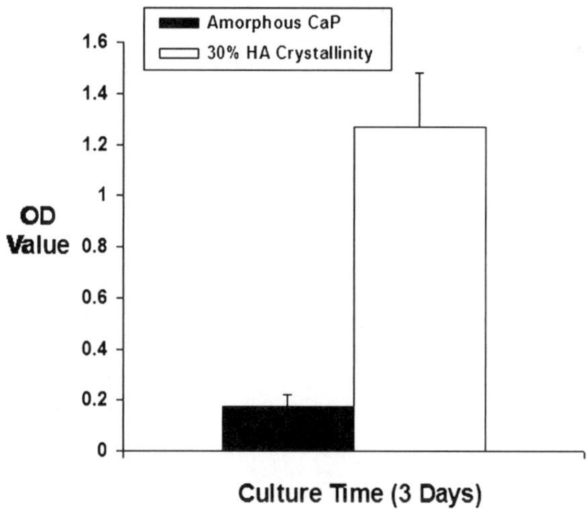

Fig. 7.2 Cell viability of ATTC CRL 1486 human embryonic palatal mesenchymal cells, an osteoblast precursor cell line, as measured by [3-(4, 5-dimethylthiazol-2-yl)-5-(3-carboxymethoxyphenyl)-2-(4-sulfophenyl)-2H-tetrazolium, inner salt] (MTS) assay

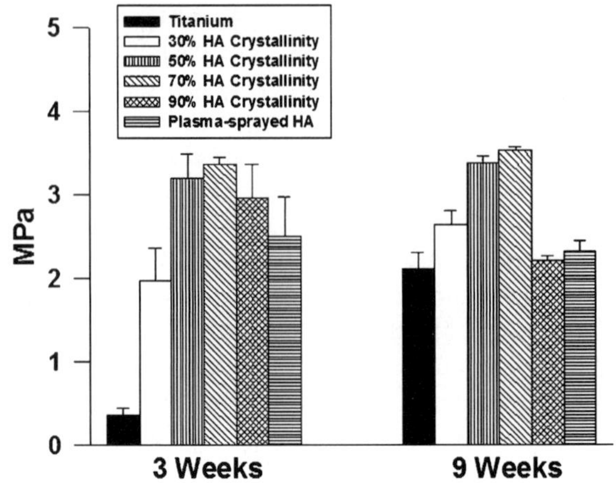

Fig. 7.3 Push-out strength at the implant–bone interface using a rat femur model

bone–implant interfacial strength was significantly affected by varying the HA coating crystallinity. These studies suggested a further need to investigate coating crystallinity that would result in optimum dissolution properties and ultimately provide maximum bone–implant interfacial strength. Given the vast number of deposition processes [21–64], as shown in Table 7.1, this chapter focuses on sputtering technology.

Table 7.1 Hydroxyapatite coating produced using various deposition technologies

Technique	Thickness	Advantages	Disadvantages	Refs.
Thermal spraying	30–200 μm	High deposition rates; low cost	Line of sight technique; high temperatures induce decomposition; rapid cooling produces amorphous coatings	[21–30]
Sputter coating	0.5–3.0 μm	Uniform coating thickness on flat substrates; dense coating	Line of sight technique; expensive, time-consuming; produces amorphous coating	[31–39]
Pulsed laser deposition	0.05–5.00 μm	Coating with crystalline and amorphous; coating with dense and porous	Line of sight technique	[40–42]

Table 7.1 (continued)

Technique	Thickness	Advantages	Disadvantages	Refs.
Dynamic mixing method	0.05–1.30 μm	High adhesive strength	Line of sight technique; expensive; produces amorphous coating	[43]
Dip coating	0.05–0.50 mm	Inexpensive; coating applied quickly; can coat complex substrates	Requires high sintering temperatures; thermal expansion mismatch	[44–48]
Sol-gel	< 1 μm	Can coat complex shapes; low processing temperatures; relatively inexpensive as coating is very thin	Some processes require controlled atmosphere processing; expensive raw materials	[49–52]
Electrophoretic deposition	0.1–2.0 mm	Uniform coating thickness; rapid deposition rates; can coat complex substrates	Difficult to produce crack-free coatings; requires high sintering temperatures	[53–60]
Biomimetic coating	< 30 μm	Low processing temperatures; can form bone-like apatite; can coat complex shapes; can incorporate bone growth stimulating factors	Time-consuming; requires replenishment and constant pH of simulated body fluid	[61–63]
Hot isostatic pressing	0.2–2.0 mm	Produces dense coatings	Cannot coat complex substrates; high temperature required; thermal expansion mismatch; elastic property differences; expensive; removal/ interaction of encapsulation material	[64]

7.2 Sputtering Technique

Sputtering is a reported physical phenomenon since 1952 and has developed into a thin film deposition technique [65, 66]. The process operates at room temperature but in a vacuum environment. In general, sputtering involves the erosion of target materials from a surface. The eroded target material is largely driven by momentum exchange as a result of collisions between high energy gaseous ions generated using plasma or ion guns and atoms from the target surface. The high energy gaseous ions, accelerated by high voltage, bombard and collide with atoms on the target surface. As a result, the atoms or occasionally entire molecules of the target material are then ejected and transported to the substrate surface, subsequently resulting in a thin film that forms mechanical interlocking and chemical bonding with diverse substrates.

There are several modes of sputtering that are generally classified into radiofrequency (RF) magnetron sputtering [67, 68], RF diode sputtering [69, 70], direct current (DC) magnetron sputtering [71], ion-beam sputtering [72, 73], and reactive DC sputtering [74]. The selection of a sputtering mode for a specific experiment is dependent on the electrical conductivity of the coating materials. Because HA is an electrically insulating material, DC sputtering cannot be used as a deposition process. This is because the HA target serves as a cathode, attracting positively charged ions, and the insulating nature of HA determines the accumulation of these charges on the HA surfaces. Consequently, fluxes of ions and electrons to the surface are equalized, regardless of the negative potential applied to the cathode. As this equalization occurs, the sheath voltage across the HA target falls, and no voltage remains to drive the discharge. As a result, the DC discharge during the deposition process rapidly diminishes.

In contrast to a DC source, RF sputtering utilizes an alternating current (AC) source. A representative RF magnetron sputtering process is shown in Fig. 7.4. Typically, RF sputtering employs a sinusoidal wave generator operating at 13.56 MHz. The use of a matching network and a controller allows the RF supply to match the generator output impedance to the impedance of the cathode and anode. During RF sputtering, positive charges accumulate on the HA target surface during one cycle and are neutralized by electron bombardment during the next half-cycle. The potential alternates with a period

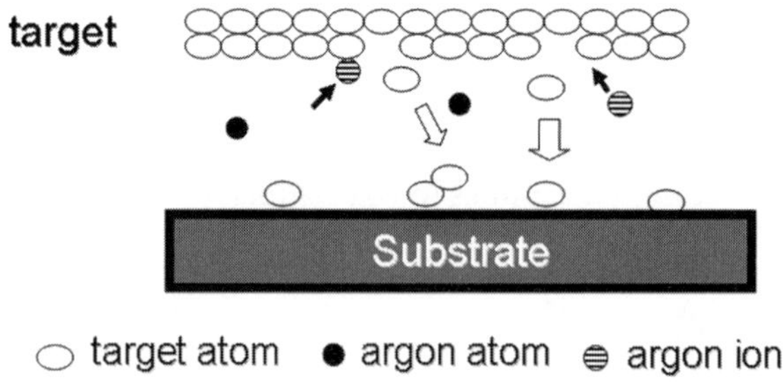

Fig. 7.4 Sputtering process

that is shorter than the time it takes for positive ions to travel from the edge of the plasma sheath back to the target surface. This provides the capability of the much faster electrons to respond to the alternating fields.

The efficiency of RF magnetron sputtering is further enhanced by creating a magnetic field above and parallel to the target surface. The magnetic field allows redirection of free electrons to the target surface before they are lost to the anode. As a result, collision of electrons with argon carrier molecules is increased, thereby enhancing the discharging effectiveness. As a result of its increased discharge effectiveness, the RF magnetron sputtering is one of the preferred thin film coating processes for depositing a wide range of materials, including HA ceramics. Despite the advantage of having a higher discharge, however, production of the desired thin film with optimal coating properties requires control of the coating parameters. In addition to the target composition, it is known that the coating properties are affected by the ionized gas pressure [75], the substrate temperature [76], and the voltage across the various sheaths [77].

7.3 Physicochemical Properties of Sputtered Coatings

It was reported that the mechanical strength of polycrystalline HA ceramics at room temperature depended on the grain size [78]. As finer grain size results in higher strength, it is desirable for HA to have fine grain microstructures. In addition, it is also known that the compressive strength of HA ceramics is dependent on the density and the porosity of the ceramics, which in turn is dependent on the sintering temperature and time. The strength of 100% dense synthetically prepared polycrystalline HA was reported to be similar to human tooth enamel [78]. Furthermore, a concurrent decrease in strength was reported when apatites were degraded in strongly acidic (pH 2.0) solutions [78].

The sputtering process was reported to produce highly dense, uniform, continuous coatings that have high coating–substrate bonding strength [8]. As shown in Fig. 7.5, nano-sized crystals of 100 to 200 nm were also observed within the sputtered HA coatings [79]. In addition, the surface morphology and roughness of sputtered HA coatings was reported to be dependent on the annealing temperature and time, and these changes were attributed to changes in the crystal structure and residual stress [35, 39, 53, 54, 79, 80].

The sputtering process can also produce amorphous coatings [35, 39, 79, 80]. Because it is critical to maintain the integrity of HA coatings, controlling the heat-treatment temperatures and heating environment results in conversion of amorphous coatings to HA coatings of different degrees of crystallinity (Table 7.2). In addition, changes in the most intense x-ray diffraction peak between postdeposited heat-treated HA coatings and HA target suggested differences in structural orientation of the crystallites. As indicated by a single x-ray diffraction peak at 32.9° (2θ), poorly crystallized HA coatings were observed after the 450°C

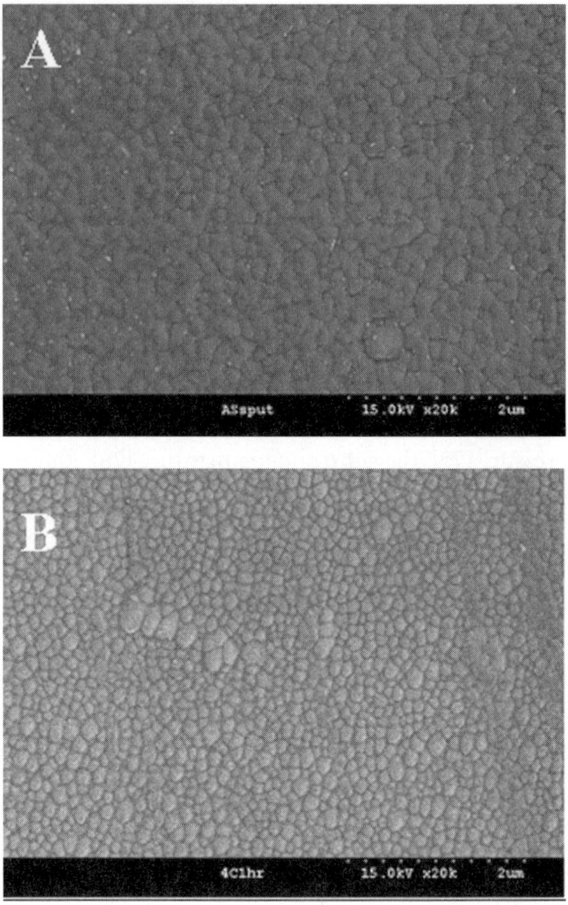

Fig. 7.5 Representative SEM micrographs. **A** Amorphous CaP (X20K). **B** HA coating after a 400°C heat treatment (X20K)

postdeposition heat treatments in the absence of water vapor. This single peak observed for the poorly crystallized HA coatings suggests that crystal growth initially began at the [300] crystal plane. The most intense peak remained at 32.9° (2θ) for the HA coatings heat treated at 450°C in the presence of water vapor and coatings heat-treated at 500°C and 600°C in the presence and absence of water vapor. It thus implies that the [300] plane was the preferred growth plane in the initial heat-treated sputtered HA coatings.

Table 7.2 also indicates a significant increase in coating crystallinity as the heating temperature was increased from 450°C to 500°C in the absence of water vapor. Interestingly, the amorphous-to-crystalline phase transformation temperature was also reported at approximately 500°C postdeposition heat treatment for plasma-sprayed HA coatings [81]. Moreover, in comparison to coatings heat-treated at 450°C in the absence of water vapor, a significant increase in coating crystallinity was reported for sputtered coatings heat-treated in the

Table 7.2 Crystallinity of sputtered hydroxyapatite after various postdeposition heat treatments

	Crystallinity (%)	
Treatment	Without water vapor	With water vapor
As-sputtered coating	0	0
350°C	0	2.5 ± 0.5
400°C	1.9 ± 0.4	2.8 ± 0.6
450°C	2.0 ± 1.0	68.0 ± 2.0
500°C	62.0 ± 2.0	65.0 ± 1.0
600°C	67.0 ± 2.0	66.0 ± 8.0

presence of water vapor [79]. This suggested that the presence of water vapor during postdeposition heat treatments plays an important role in increasing HA crystallinity [82–84]. Using high resolution transmission electron microscopy (TEM), a higher annealing temperature caused HA to undergo densification, increased the grain size or crystallinity, and improved crystal perfection by minimizing the number, or preventing the formation, of crystal void defects [85]. An increase in coating crystallinity after heat treatments at 450°C (in the presence of water), 500°C (in the presence and absence of water), and 600°C (in the presence and absence of water) was confirmed by scanning electron microscopy (SEM) images showing brittle fractures on these coatings, suggesting crystal growth [80].

In general, the sputtering rate, or film growth, is also known to be dependent on the target composition. Sputtering of a multicomponent target, such as HA or superconducting oxides, often resulted in coating stoichiometry that was different from the bulk target [86, 87]. A minimum of about 1000 Å or more of the multicomponent target needs to be removed before the coating reflects the stoichiometry of the bulk target [88]. Components of the target such as hydroxide, oxygen, and hydrogen may not be completely transferred to the substrates owing to the low environmental pressure in the chamber. As a result, the composition of the coating may differ from that of the target material, depending on the type of sputtering system and the deposition parameters. The surface Ca/P ratios for the sputtered HA coatings have been reported to range from 1.6 to 2.6 [89–93]. The difference in the Ca/P ratio between the HA target and the sputtered coatings has been attributed to the preferential deposition of Ca ions and a possible significant loss of P ions, which may be pumped away before reaching the substrate [88]. Other investigators have also reported the loss of phosphorus ions, suggesting a weaker bonding of P ions to the growing film; they are thus more readily sputtered away by incoming ions or electrons [63]. As an indication of coating thickness, a representative cross section of the CaP coating on slide glass substrate is shown in Fig. 7.6. Aside from target composition, coating thickness is dependent on the sputtering time. Figure 7.7 shows the effect of sputtering time on the deposition of TiO_2 coatings, with the thickness of the coatings increasing with time.

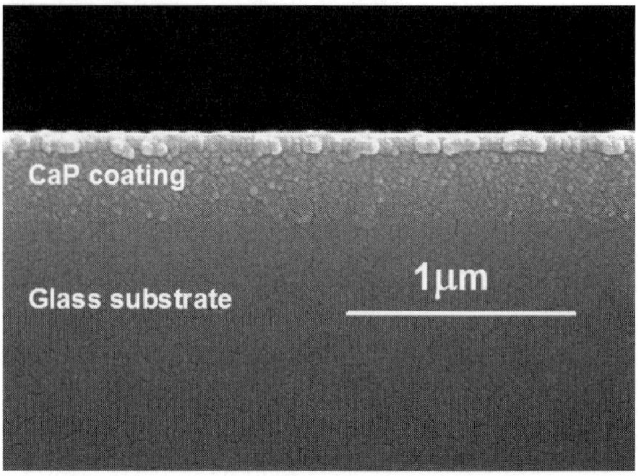

Fig. 7.6 Representative SEM micrograph of a continuous, dense as-sputtered calcium phosphate (CaP) coating on glass substrate. The as-sputtered CaP coating was observed to consist of nano-particles approximately 5 nm in diameter and in the range of 50 to 100 nm in diameter in the subsurface and surface, respectively

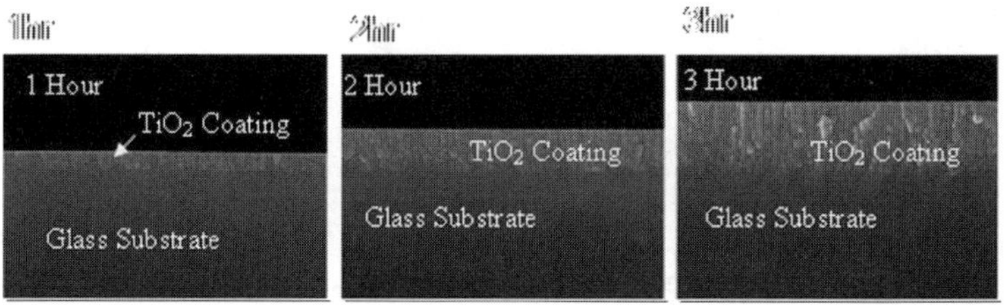

Fig. 7.7 Representative SEM micrographs of fractured TiO_2 coating with respect to three sputtering times

Additionally, coating roughness was suggested to be dependent on substrate topography. Topographical features, with a resolution on the order of 0.1 Å, have been investigated using atomic force microscopy (AFM) [94]. Contact mode scans on a representative CaP coating on a Ti surface is shown in Fig. 7.8. The columnar features, ranging from 40 to 80 nm above an otherwise flat surface, are observed in Fig. 7.8; the tallest columnar feature is approximately 120 nm high. The mean cross-sectional area of the columns is about $6 \pm 3 \times 10^4$ nm^2. The growth mode may be imposed on the coating by the surface morphology of the Ti substrate, and as such the cross-sectional areas of the columns represent the underlying microscopic roughness of the surface. This limitation in film growth is reported to be affected by the angle of the incident beam to the target during the deposition process [95]. Studies of other materials have also suggested that the arrival of sputtered materials from one direction, condensing with little adatom movement, may have contributed to the columnar growth [96]. Thus, by altering the direction of the beam relative to the target, a different direction of film growth may be achieved.

Another property of interest to the biomedical community is the coating–substrate interface. The average adhesion strength data for the sputtered coatings is reported to be approximately 38 MPa [73]. Annealing was observed to affect the mechanical integrity of the coating–substrate interface, with the

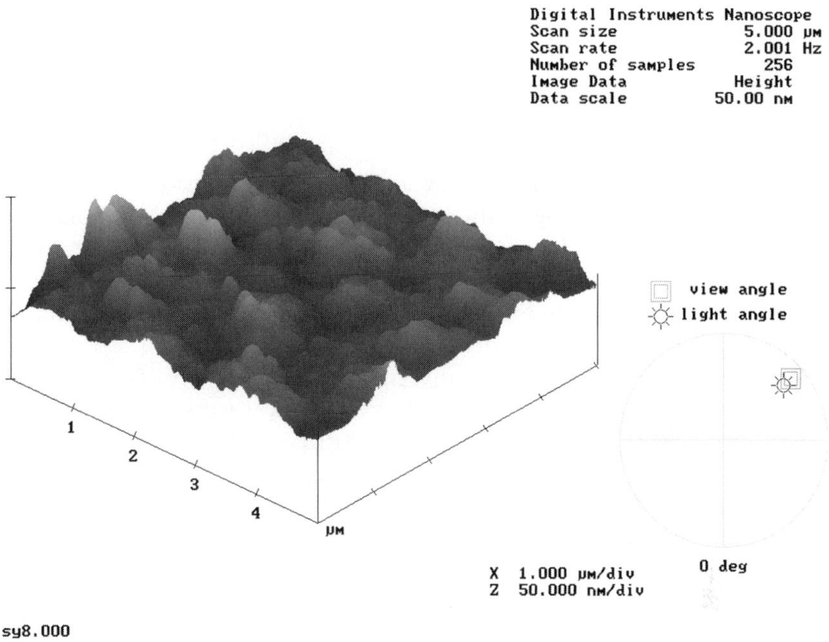

Fig. 7.8 Atomic force microscopy (AFM) images of CaP coating

coating–substrate adhesion strength depending on the types of annealing and the surface condition. Annealing followed by either quenching or furnace cooling coatings on passivated Ti surfaces resulted in a reduction in strength. The strength for the quenched and furnace cooled coatings were 17.9 and 9.0 MPa, respectively [73]. However, annealing followed by quenching on the nonpassivated Ti surfaces resulted in an adhesion strength of 45.8 MPa. Differences in the adhesion strength after annealing were attributed to differences in substrate treatments. Because passivation enhances the thickness of the oxide film and growth of a lateral oxide layer within the existing oxide occurs during annealing [97], the presence of this lateral oxide layer was reported to have caused localized weakening in the existing oxide. With a thinner oxide layer present on the nonpassivated Ti surfaces prior to annealing, the higher strength observed after quenching indicates that the surface condition of the substrate is critical for maintaining the mechanical integrity of the coating–substrate interface.

7.4 Dissolution

Among many factors affecting dissolution, the solubility of the CaP coating is dependent on its chemical composition [98–101]. In general, all CaP coatings and ceramics are degradable, with the following order of relative solubility

$$ACP \gg DCP > TTCP > \alpha\text{-}TCP > \beta\text{-}TCP \gg HA$$

where ACP is amorphous calcium phosphate, DCP is monetite ($CaHPO_4$), TTCP is tetracalcium phosphate ($Ca_4P_2O_9$), TCP is tricalcium phosphate [$Ca_3(PO4)_2$], and HA ishydroxyapatite [$Ca_{10}(PO_4)_6(OH)_2$].

The solubility of the coatings is also dependent on the degree of crystallinity or amorphous content in the coating [102]. As observed, the amorphous coatings completely dissolved more rapidly than coatings that were annealed. Increasing heat treatment temperatures are expected to increase the crystallinity of the coatings. As shown in Fig. 7.9, greater release of P ions was observed for sputtered HA coatings heat-treated at 400°C than for sputtered HA coatings heat-treated at 600°C [91]. Additionally, significantly more P ions were released from non-heat-treated HA coatings than from heat-treated coatings. The released P ions were reported to bind with hydrogen ions in solution to form HPO_4 and H_2PO_4, thereby buffering the falling pH and decreasing the dissolution rate [103]. Neuman and Neuman reported that extremely small crystals are not restrained by interionic attraction of the ions [104]; therefore, it would not be surprising that the amorphous as-sputtered coatings dissolved rapidly.

Microporosity is another major factor influencing HA degradation. It has been reported that dense CaP ceramics displayed no significant degradation within a year of study [105]. Solubility is also affected by the powder weight to liquid volume ratio and the pH of the solution [63]. Decreasing the solution's pH was reported to result in an increase in HA solubility [106]. It was also reported that crystal defects, such as impurities, vacancies, or dislocation, have an effect on

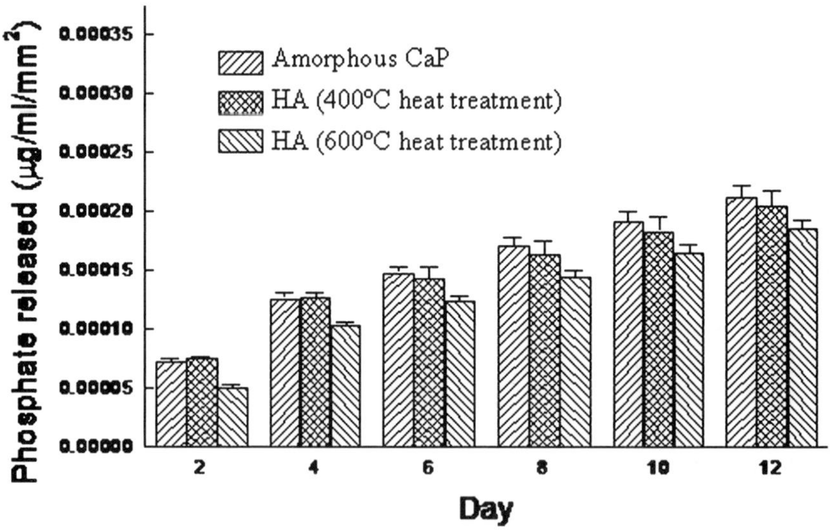

Fig. 7.9 Release of phosphorus ions from sputtered-HA coating after different deposition heat treatments following immersion in solution

the diffusion phenomenon, thereby influencing the dissolution rate [107]. Chemical reactivity of solids was known to vary inversely to their crystalline perfection and crystal dimension [108]. As the solubility of HA coatings can be increased by a variety of factors, there are many ways to decrease it. One way to decrease solubility is to increase crystal growth and thus halt the decrease in solubility after achieving growth to some critical crystal size [104]. Other researchers have suggested substitution of ions, such as fluorine for hydroxyl ions, to cause lower solubility [107, 109]. The incorporation of sodium and carbonate ions have been reported to lower the resistance to solubility significantly [110].

In addition to changes in coating crystallinity and phase composition, dissolution of the coatings is influenced by the quantity and structure (interconnected or isolated) of porosity in the coating. A high porosity level, especially if the porosity is interconnected, results in a higher dissolution rate of the coating. Interestingly, past reports have indicated a much lower dissolution rate for 100% amorphous plasma-sprayed coatings compared to HA coatings having 40% amorphous and 60% crystallinity [111]. This was attributed to the fact that the coating parameters were changed to yield a highly melted, highly fluid material with little or no porosity during the production of 100% amorphous plasma-sprayed coatings. Additionally, inhibition of HA and CaP coatings solubility was observed with residual compression, whereas the promotion of solubility was reported with tensile stress [112]. As such, coating solubility was suggested to be influenced by the coating's stress status [112, 113].

The solubility of HA coatings was reported to decrease with decreasing porosity, decreasing surface area, and decreasing particle size [114, 115]. As reported in other investigations, the solubility of HA coatings can also be influenced by over- or undersaturation of the solution with respect to the ionic species (e.g., OH^-, Ca^{2+}, PO_4^{3-}, F^-) and the presence of proteins and amino acids in solution [116–119]. Sputtered HA coatings were reported to release significantly more P ions in the presence of fibronectin compared to coatings immersed in the absence of protein [91]. Precoating Ti surfaces with albumin was reported to modify the morphology, composition, and crystallinity of the coating, whereas preadsorption of fibronectin on Ti surfaces was reported to inhibit CaP layer formation [120]. It was suggested that some organic macromolecules such as amino acids and proteins have a high binding affinity for Ca and P ions on HA or CaP surfaces, thereby inhibiting the growth and formation of CaP [121–125].

7.5 *In Vitro* and *In Vivo* Biological Evaluation

Although HA and CaP coatings are considered biocompatible materials, they are not biologically inert. Isolated human bone cells were reported to ingest synthetic CaP granules, suggesting the participation of bone cells in the degradation of CaP coatings [126]. An increase in intracellular Ca ions after intralysosomal dissolution was also observed [127]. A consequence of this dissolution process includes increases in ^{3}H-uridine, leucine, and proline incorporation in bone cell cultures [126]. The presence of Ca is speculated to regulate the initiation of messenger ribonucleic acid (mRNA) transcription and protein synthesis. As such, the presence of Ca ions is a precursor of cellular differentiation.

Because the solubility of HA and CaP coatings is governed by the crystallinity, phase composition, and quantity and structure (interconnected or isolated) of porosity, control of these parameters affects Ca and P ion release. As such, altering the HA or CaP solubility profile can influence biological responses [128, 129]. As an example, nano-sized HA was suggested to be more biocompatible than micro-sized HA owing to the fact that bone contains nano-sized apatites [130]. Other investigators have reported the attachment and spreading of human osteoblast cells *in vitro* on nano-sized HA [131].

7.5.1 In Vitro *Study*

Cell culture studies on sputtered HA surfaces have indicated significantly less cellular proliferation than on Ti surfaces [132]. In addition, TEM analysis of cells cultured on HA-coated surfaces revealed the presence of extracellular matrix (ECM), with collagen fibers embedded in crystallized, needle-shaped structures. Although integrin expression during the initial cell–material interactions was unaffected by the surface characteristics of HA-coated or Ti surfaces, sputtered HA coatings were reported to promote the differentiation and expression of osteogenic cells [93, 133]. Moreover, more rapid formation of bone occurs on HA surfaces than on Ti surfaces. In addition, it was also observed that the response of osteogenic cells was affected by the crystallinity of sputtered HA coatings [93, 134 137].

With respect to bone resorption, it was reported that sputtered HA coatings did not support chemotaxis, proliferation, or colony formation of osteoclast precursor cells *in vitro* [138]. Although sputtered coatings may promote osteoblast formation, the inhibition of osteoclast activities was observed to be enhanced by HA crystallinity [138]. This observation was in agreement with other studies indicating that the presence of Ca ions on HA coatings may inhibit osteoclastic bone-resorbing activity by increasing cytoplasmic free Ca levels in osteoclasts [139–142].

The response of cell types other than bone cells has been investigated on sputtered HA and CaP surfaces. In the attempt to control bacterial adhesion to HA and CaP surfaces, co-sputtering of HA and silver (Ag) has been reported [143]. Figure 7.10 shows significantly less adhesion of *Staphylococcus aureus* on co-deposited Ag and HA surfaces than on Ti and sputtered HA surfaces. Interestingly, no significant difference in osteoblast cell viability was observed on Ag-HA surfaces when compared to sputtered-HA surfaces, suggesting that

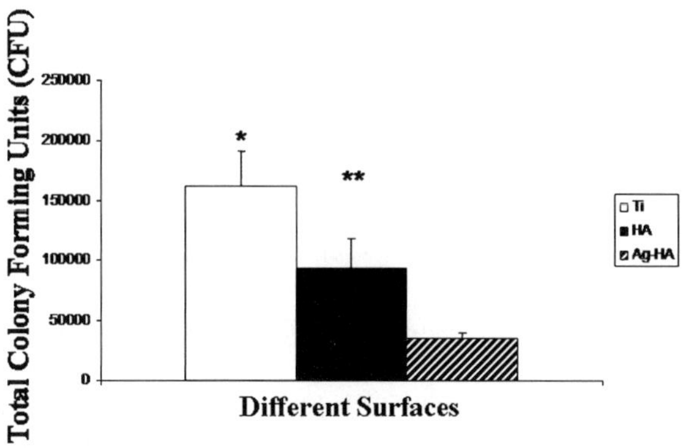

Fig. 7.10 Adhesion of *Staphylococcus aureus* to co-sputtered Ag-HA, sputtered HA, and Ti surfaces after a 24-hour incubation. Asterisk (*) indicates significant difference

co-sputtered Ag-HA surfaces can be used as viable coatings not only to improve bone formation but also as antibacterial coatings.

7.5.2 In Vivo *Study*

Because *in vivo* evaluation is an important phase in the development of new implant materials and designs [2], HA-coated implants have been evaluated in a wide variety of animal models, such as rats [144–147], rabbits [148, 149], dogs [150–153], sheep [154, 155], goats [156–158], and pigs [159]. Placing a number of small devices in the animal's intramedullary canal [160, 161], cortical bone (transcortical) [162–164], or subcutaneous sites [142] are common for evaluating tissue adaptation to the implant. Table 7.3 shows significantly greater bone contact for sputtered HA implants with no heat treatment than for heat-treated HA and Ti implants after 3 weeks of implantation in the dog mandible. At 12 weeks, the bone contact of non-heat-treated HA implants remained significantly higher that that of heat-treated HA and Ti implants. These values were similar to those obtained in other studies reporting a mean direct bone contact

Table 7.3 Bone contact length at 3 and 12 weeks after implantation

Sample	Bone contact length (%)
At 3 weeks	
Ti implant (control)	33.7 ± 0.8
Amorphous CaP	50.3 ± 4.2
HA implants after heat treatment	30.3 ± 6.7
At 12 weeks	
Ti implant (control)	53.1 ± 7.5
Amorphous CaP	70.4 ± 1.6
HA implants after heat treatment	58.2 ± 4.5

Ti, titanium; CaP, calcium phosphate; HA, hydroxyapatite

of 69% between mineralized bone and Ti implants after 12 weeks implantation in a dog mode [165]. Other investigators indicated bone–Ti and bone–HA contact of 60% and 76%, respectively, after 6 months of implantation [166]. These studies suggested that the bone contact length on the sputtered HA implants after heat treatment is similar to that of plasma-sprayed HA coatings at 12 weeks.

As shown in Fig. 7.11, sputtered HA implants with and without heat treatment were observed to have greater pullout strength than Ti implants. At 3 weeks after implantation, the mean pullout strength value for the non-heat-treated HA implants was statistically greater than that for the heat-treated HA implants. Additionally, the pullout strengths of HA implants (non-heat-treated and heat-treated) were statistically greater than the mean pullout strength of the Ti implants. The high pullout strength for HA implants after 3 weeks of implantation was attributed to the increase in bone contact length and the increased rate of bone growth on the implant surfaces.

After 12 weeks' implantation, no statistical difference in mean pullout strength values between HA-coated and Ti implants was observed. Interestingly, the mean pullout strength value for the heat-treated HA and the Ti implants at 12 weeks was not statistically different from the non-heat-treated HA implants at 3 weeks. As shown in Fig. 7.12, the pullout force of the sputtered HA implants was similar to the pullout force of the plasma-sprayed

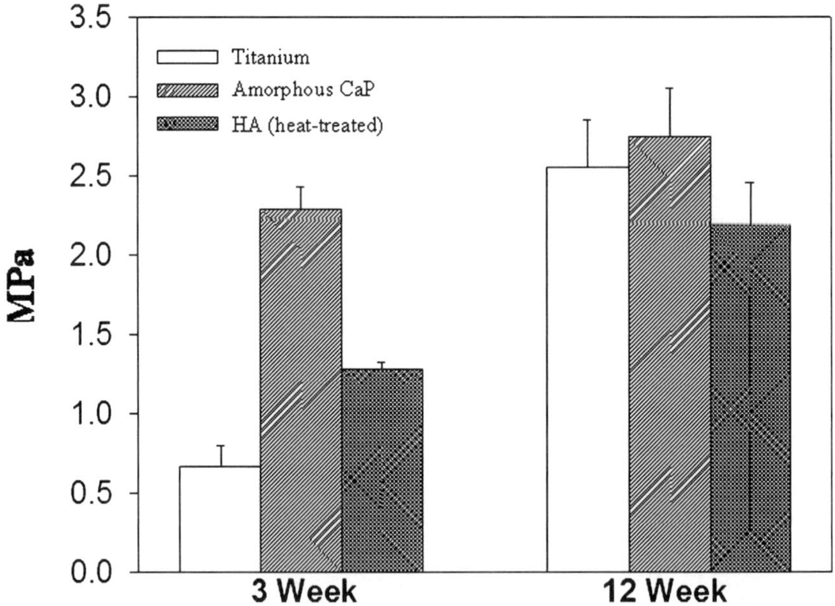

Fig. 7.11 Ultimate interfacial strength of sputtered HA coating (with and without heat treatment) and titanium implants (control) after 3 and 12 weeks of implantation. Results are the mean, and the error bars represent one standard error

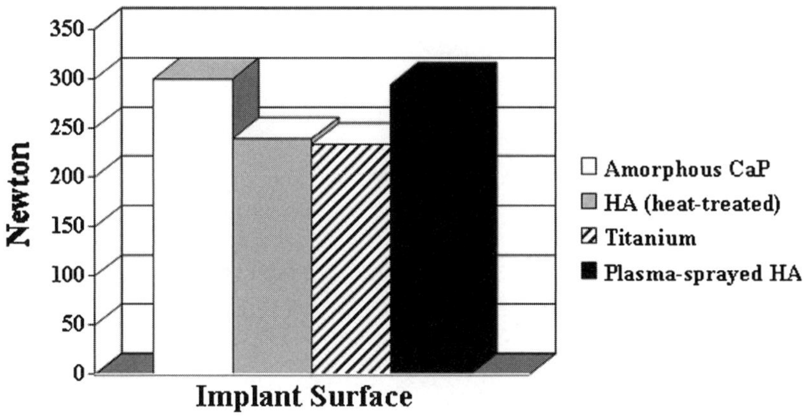

Fig. 7.12 Ultimate interfacial force of sputtered HA-coated implants (with and without heat treatment), titanium implants (control), and plasma-sprayed HA-coated implants after 12 weeks of implantation. Results are the mean, and the error bar represents one standard error

HA implants after 12 weeks' implantation, suggesting that the sputtered thin HA coatings were comparable to the thick plasma-sprayed HA implants with respect to implant fixation. These observations were consistent with other reports indicating improved initial fixation and healing response for sputtered CaP coatings implanted into trabecular bone of the goat [132, 134, 167]. These studies, together with other reported studies, suggested that once early osseointegration was achieved biodegradation of the HA coatings would be nondetrimental to bone–coating–implant fixation [7, 168, 169].

It has been postulated that the solubility of HA coatings may play a role in the bioactivity of the coatings, and this bioactivity could lead to a higher rate of early bone tissue formation. The *in vivo* cellular response has been suggested to be compromised by highly crystallized HA ceramics, indicating that some amorphous or more soluble phases in the coatings would be desirable and would result in a more stable interface with the biological environment [170]. Other investigators have suggested that dissolution of the HA coating may produce solution-mediated events affecting biocomponents circulation [171], bone cell activity, organic matrix deposition, and mineral precipitation and resorption [172, 173].

7.6 Conclusion

In general, this chapter has indicated that the sputtering process can be universally utilized to deposit metallic and inorganic materials. Table 7.4 shows some of the significant CaP research pertaining to characterization and biological responses. The advantages of the sputtering process over other coating processes include the production of dense coatings that are highly uniform and

Table 7.4 Significant papers on sputtering

		Coating characterizations							Biological testing	
Year	Authors	XPS	AES	Contact Angle	SEM	FTIR	XRD	Mechanical	*In vitro*	*In vivo*
2006	Chen [143]						x		x	
1999	Ding [32]				x	x	x	x		
2003	Ding [31]				x		x	x		
1998	Hulshoff [93]				x				x	
1991	Lacefield [87]				x		x			
1993	Li [76]						x			
2001	Massaro [34]				x		x		x	
2007	Ohtsu [68]				x					x
1991	Ong [86]									
1992	Ong [73]				x		x	x		
1994	Ong [35]					x	x	x		
1994	Ong [36]					x				
1995	Ong [92]	x				x	x		x	
1997	Ong [90]	x		x		x	x			
1998	Ong [89]		x							
2002	Ong [174]							x		x
2003	Stover [138]								x	
1995	Van Dijk [38]				x	x	x			
1996	Van Dijk [39]					x	x			
1994	Wolke [37]						x			
2003	Wolke [33]				x		x			x
2003	Yang [80]				x	x	x			
2003	Yang [79]					x	x			
2003	Yang [91]	x		x		x	x			
2003	Yang [137]				x		x		x	

continuous, and these coatings have been reported to have significantly higher coating–metal interfacial bonding strength compared to plasma-sprayed coatings [4, 5]. In addition to its highly adhesive bond strength, the sputtered coatings contain nano-sized crystals [5]. Despite a film thickness of $\leq 2\ \mu m$ for the sputtered coatings, evidence from animal studies have suggested an equivalent bone–implant contact length and interfacial strength for these coatings when compared to plasma-sprayed coatings at 12 weeks prior to loading [174]. Although studies reported in this chapter have indicated the sputtering process to be a viable alternative to plasma spraying for the application of HA coatings on dental and orthopedic implant surfaces, a need for optimizing HA and CaP properties to induce maximum bone formation is suggested for future studies.

New, promising techniques for coating medical devices are continuously being investigated. Although the sputter process is currently not a popular technology for the modification of dental and orthopedic implant surfaces when compared to plasma spraying, the sputtering technology is slowly being accepted by some implant vendors. For instance, thin HA sputter-coated implant systems are currently being sold by BioComp Industries BV (Vught, The Netherlands) and Biocon (Boston, MA, USA). Acceptance of the sputtering technology and recent research is an indication that the sputtering process is promising and has potential for eliminating some of the problems associated with the plasma-spraying process. Although it has been generally accepted that sputtered HA and CaP coatings improve bone strength and the initial osseointegration rate, optimal coating properties required to achieve maximum bone response are yet to be determined. Current problems with the sputtering of HA coatings include the need for annealing to crystallize the coatings. Additionally, because sputtering is a line-of-sight process, uniform deposition of HA coatings on cylindrical implants may be a problem. Future investigations of the sputtering process must include improvements in the coating process. There should be more clinical trials to optimize coating properties, to continue the preclinical research to provide additional understanding of bone responses to coated-implant surfaces of different properties, and to explore the possibility of coupling sputtered HA and CaP coatings with growth factors.

In conclusion, sputtering is a viable alternative deposition process that should continue to be developed to replace plasma-spraying of HA and CaP coatings on dental and orthopedic implants.

Acknowledgments Part of the study presented in this chapter was funded by grants from the National Institute of Health (grants 1RO1AR46581 and 1S10RR016879-01).

References

1. W.L. Jaffe, and D.F. Scott, *J. Bone Joint Surg.* **78A** (1996) 1918.
2. K.A. Thomas, *Orthopedics* **17** (1994) 267.
3. P. Ducheyne, and J.M. Cuckler, *Clin. Orthop. Rel. Res.* **276** (1992) 102.

4. R.G.T. Geesink, *Clin. Orthop. Rel. Res.* **395** (2002) 53.
5. L.I. Havelin, L.B. Engesaeter, B. Espehaug, O. Furnes, S.A. Lie, and S.E. Vollset, *Acta Orthop. Scand.* **71** (2000), 337.
6. J.A. D'Antonio, W.N. Capello, M.T. Manley, and R. Geesink, *Clin. Orthop. Rel. Res.* **393** (2001) 101.
7. K. De Groot, J.G.C. Wolke, and J.A. Jansen, *J. Oral Implantol.* **20** (1994) 232.
8. Y. Yang, J.L. Ong, and K. Bessho, in *Biomaterials in Orthopedics*, edited by M.J. Yaszemski, D.J. Trantolo, K.-U. Lewandrowski, V. Hasirci, D.E. Altobelli, and D.L. Wise (Marcel Dekker, Inc., New York, 2004) p. 401.
9. R.J. Furlong, and J.F. Osborn, *J. Bone Joint Surg.* **73B** (1991) 741.
10. W.N. Capello, J.A. D'Antonio, M.T. Manley, and J.R. Feinber, *Clin. Orthp. Rel. Res.* **355** (1998) 200.
11. J.A. D'Antonio, W.N. Capello, M.T. Manley, and J. Feinberg, *Clin. Orthp. Rel. Res.* **344** (1997) 124.
12. J.L. Ong, and C.N. Chan, *Crit. Rev. in Biomed. Eng.* **28** (1999) 667.
13. H. Herman, *MRS Bulletin* **12** (1988) 60.
14. F.D.A., (Food and Drug Administration, Washington, DC, 1992) p. 1.
15. I.S.O. 13779-2:2000 (International Organization for Standardization, Switzerland, 2000).
16. J.E. Lemons, *Clin. Orthp. Rel. Res.* **235** (1988), 220.
17. W.R. Lacefield, in *Bioceramics: Material Characteristics versus In Vivo Behavior*, edited by P. Ducheyne, J.E. Lemons (The New York Academy of Science, New York, 1988) p. 72.
18. Z. Meleti, I.M. Shapiro, and C.S. Adams, *Bone* **27** (2000) 359.
19. C.S. Adams, K. Mansfield, R.L. Perlot, and I.M. Shapiro, *J. Bio. Chem.* **276** (2001) 20316.
20. S. Oh, E. Tobin, Y. Yang, D. Carnes, and J.L. ONG, *J. Oral Maxillofac Implants* **20** (2005) 726.
21. K.A. Gross, and C.C. Berndt, *J. Biomed. Mater. Res.* **39** (1998) 580.
22. K.A. Gross, C.C. Berndt, and H. Herman, *J. Biomed. Mater. Res.* **39** (1998) 407.
23. H. Li, K.A. Khor, and P. Cheang, *Biomaterials* **23** (2002) 85.
24. Y. Yang, and J.L. Ong, *J. Biomed. Mater. Res.* **64** (2003) 509.
25. Z. Zyman, J. Weng, X. Liu, X. Zhang, and Z. Ma, *Biomaterials* **14** (1993) 225.
26. S. Tao, H. Ji, and C. Ding, *J. Biomed. Mater. Res.* **52** (2000) 572.
27. J. Weng, X. Liu, X. Zhang, Z. Ma, X. Ji, and Z. Zyman, *Biomaterials* **14** (1993) 578.
28. J. Chen, J.G.C. Wolke, and K. De Groot, *Biomaterials* **15** (1994) 396.
29. Z. Zyman, J. Weng, X. Liu, X. Li, and X. Zhang, *Biomaterials* **15** (1994) 151.
30. C.M. Roome, and C.D. Adam, *Biomaterials* **16** (1995) 691.
31. S.-J. Ding, *Biomaterials* **24** (2003) 4233.
32. S.-J. Ding, C.-P. Ju, and J.-H.C. Lin, *J. Biomed. Mater. Res.* **44** (1999) 266.
33. J.G.C. Wolke, J.P.C.M. van der Waerden, H.G. Schaeken, and J.A. Jansen, *Biomaterials* **24** (2003) 2623.
34. C. Massaro, M.A. Baker, F. Cosentino, P.A. Ramires, S. Klose, and E. Milella, *J. Biomed. Mater. Res. (Appl. Biomater.)* **58** (2001) 651.
35. J.L. Ong, and L.C. Lucas, *Biomaterials* **15** (1994) 337.
36. J.L. Ong, L.C. Lucas, G.N. Raikar, J.J. Weimer, and J.C. Gregory, *Col. and Surf.* **87** (1994) 151.
37. J.G.C. Wolke, K. van Dijk, H.G. Schaeken, K. De Groot, and J.A. JANSEN, *J. Biomed. Mater. Res.* **28** (1994) 1477.
38. K. van Dijk, H.G. Schaeken, J.G.C. Wolke, C.H.M. Maree, F.H.P.M. Habraken, J. Verhoven, and J.A. Jansen, *J. Biomed. Mater. Res.* **29** (1995) 269.
39. K. van Dijk, H.G. Schaeken, J.G.C. Wolke, and J.A. Jansen, *Biomaterials* **17** (1996) 405.
40. L. Cleries, E. Martinez, J.M. Fernandez-Pradas, G. Sardin, J. Esteve, and J.L. Morenza, *Biomaterials* **21** (2000) 967.

41. J.M. Fernandez-Pradas, L. Cleries, E. Martinez, G. Sardin, J. Esteve, and J.L. Morenza, *Biomaterials* **22** (2001) 2171.
42. H. Zeng, and W.R. Lacefield, *J. Biomed. Mater. Res.* **50** (2000) 239.
43. M. Yoshinari, Y. Ohshiro, and T. Derand, *Biomaterials* **15** (1994) 529.
44. W. Weng, and J.L. Baptisa, *Biomaterials* **19** (1998) 125.
45. J. Choi, D. Bogdanski, M. Koller, S.A. Esenwein, D. Muller, G. Muhr, and M. Epple, *Biomaterials* **24** (2003) 3689.
46. D. Shi, G. Jiang, and J. Bauer, *J. Biomed. Mater. Res. (Appl. Biomater.)* **63** (2002) 71.
47. G. Jiang, and D. Shi, *J. Biomed. Mater. Res. (Appl. Biomater.)* **43** (1998) 77.
48. A.A. Campbell, L. Song, X.S. Li, B.J. Nelson, C. Bottoni, D.E. Brooks, and E.S. Dejong, *J. Biomed. Mater. Res. (Appl. Biomater.)* **53** (2000) 400.
49. P. Li, K. De Groot, and T. Kokubo, *J. Sol-gel Sci. Technol.* **7** (1996) 27.
50. M. Manso, M. Langlet, C. Jimenez, and J.M. Martinez-Duart, *Biomol. Eng.* **19** (2002) 63.
51. D. Liu, Q. Yang, and T. Troczynski, *Biomaterials* **23** (2002) 691.
52. C.S. Chai, , K.A. Gross, and B. Ben-Nissan, *Biomaterials* **19** (1998) 2291.
53. P. Ducheyne, W. van Raemdonck, J.C. Heughebaert, and M. Heughebaert, *Biomaterials* **7** (1986) 97.
54. Y. Han, K. Xu, J. Lu, and Z. Wu, *J. Biomed. Mater. Res.* **45** (1999) 198.
55. Y. Han, T. Fu, J. Lu, and K. Xu, *J. Biomed. Mater. Res.* **54** (2001) 96.
56. X. Zhu, K. Kim, and Y. Jeong, *Biomaterials* **22** (2001) 2199.
57. L.A. De Sena, M.C. De Andrade, A.M. Rossi, and G.D.A. Soares, *J. Biomed. Mater. Res.* **60** (2002) 1.
58. J. Ma, C. Wang, and K.W. Peng, *Biomaterials* **24** (2003) 3505.
59. X. Nie, A. Leyland, A. Matthews, J.C. Jiang, and E.I. Meletis, *J. Biomed. Mater. Res.* **57** (2001) 612.
60. M. Manso, C. Jimenez, C. Morant, P. Herrero, and J.M. Martinez-Duart, *Biomaterials* **21** (2000) 1755.
61. P. Habibovic, F. Barrere, C.A. van Bliterswijk, K. De Groot, and P. Layrolle, *J. Am. Ceramic Soc.* **85** (2002) 517.
62. A.L. Oliveira, C. Elvira, R.L. Reis, B. Vazquez, and J. San Roman, *J. Mater. Sci.: Mater. in Med.* **10** (1999) 827.
63. P. Li, C. Ohtsuki, T. Kokubo, K. Nakanishi, and N. Soga, *J. Am. Ceramic Soc.* **75** (1992) 2094.
64. H. Wie, H. Hero, and T. Solheim, *Inter. J. Oral Maxillofac. Implants* **13** (1998) 837.
65. A.W. Warner, and C.D. Stockbridge, *J. Appl. Phys.* **34** (1963) 437.
66. K.L. Chopra, in *Thin Film Phenomena*, (Krieger Pub Co, Florida, 1979).
67. M. Nakamura, I. Sugimoto, and H. Kuwano, *J. Intelligent Mater. Systems and Structure* **5** (1994) 315.
68. N. Ohtsu, K. Sato, A. Yanagawa, K. Saito, Y. Imai, T. Kohgo, A. Yokoyama, K. Asami, and T. Hanawa, *J. Biomed. Mater Res.* **82A** (2007) 304.
69. G. Sobe, H. Schreiber, G. Weise, and A. Heinrich, *Contributions to Plasma Phys.* **33** (2006), 325.
70. J.V. Anguita, M. Thwaites, B. Holton, P. Hockley, S. Rand, and S. Haughton. *Plasma Process. Polym.* **4** (2007) 48.
71. K.P. Mohanchandra, K.K. Ho, and G.P. Carman, *J. Intelligent Mater. Systems and Structures* **15** (2004) 387.
72. B.L. Barthell, T.A. Archuleta, and R. Kossowsky, *Mater. Res. Soc. Symp. Proc.* **110** (1989) 709.
73. J.L. Ong, L.A. Harris, L.C. Lucas, W.R. Lacefield, and D. Rigney, *Biomaterials* **13** (1992) 249.
74. Y. Mizokawa, O. Komoda, T. Miyasato, S. Hasegawa, M. Tokumura, and S. Kanamura, *Electronics Commun. Japan (Part II: Elecronics)* **70** (2007), 40.
75. S.H. Han, H.J. Kim, I.K. Kang, and J.J. Lee, *J. Mat. Sci.* **28** (1993) 3267.
76. Y. Li, W.V. Youdelis, B.S. Chao, and H. Yamauchih, *J. Vac. Sci. Technol.* **A11** (1993) 2771.
77. C.M. Horwitz, *J. Vac. Sci. Technol.* **A1** (1983) 60.

78. W. Raja Rao, and R.F. Boehm, *J. Dent. Res.* **53** (1974) 1351.
79. Y. Yang, K.-H. Kim, C.M. Agrawal, and J.L. Ong, *J. Dent. Res.* **82** (2003) 833.
80. Y. Yang, K.-H. Kim, C.M. Agrawal, and J.L. Ong, *Biomaterials* **24** (2003) 5131.
81. Z.E. Erkmen, *J. Biomed. Mater. Res. (Appl. Biomater.)* **48** (1999) 861.
82. J. Chen, W. Tong, Y. Cao, J. Feng, and X. Zhang, *J. Biomed. Mater. Res.* **34** (1997) 15.
83. Y. CAO, J. Weng, J. Chen, J. Feng, Z. Yang, and X. Zhang, *Biomaterials* **17** (1996) 419.
84. W. Tong, J. Chen, Y. Cao, L. Lu, J. Feng, and X. Zhang, *J. Biomed. Mater. Res.* **36** (1997) 242.
85. G. Daculsi, R.Z. Legeros, J.P. Legeros, and D. Mitre, *J. Appl. Biomater.* **2** (1991) 147.
86. J.L. Ong, L.A. Harris, L.C. Lucas, W.R. Lacefield, and D. Rigney, *J. Am. Ceramic Soc.* **74** (1991) 2301.
87. W.R. Lacefield, E.D. Rigney, L.C. Lucas, J. Ong, and J.B. Gantenberg, in *Ceramics in Substitutive and Reconstructive Surgery*, edited by P. Vincenzini (Elsevier Science Publishers B.V., New York, 1991) p. 167.
88. P.C. Zalm, in *Handbook of Ion Beam Processing Technology*, edited by J.J. Cuomo, S.M. Rossnagel, H.R. Kaufman (Noyes Publications, Park Ridge, NJ, 1989) p. 78.
89. J.L. Ong, and L.C. Lucas, *Biomaterials* **19** (1998) 455.
90. J.L. Ong, G.N. Raikar, and T.M. Smoot, *Biomaterials* **18** (1997) 1271.
91. Y. Yang, C.M. Agrawal, K.-H. Kim, H. Martin, K. Schulz, J.D. BUMGARDNER, and J.L. ONG, *J. Oral Implantol.* **29** (2003) 270.
92. J.L. Ong, L.C. Lucas, G.N. Raikar, C.W. Prince, in Encyclopedia of Biomaterials and Bioengineering Materials, Part A: Materials, Volume 2, edited by D.L. Wise, D.E. Altobelli, E.R. Schwartz, M. Yaszemski, J.D. Gresser, D.J. Trantolo (Marcel Dekker, Inc., New York, 1995) p. 1565.
93. J.E.G. Hulshoff, K. van Dijk, J.E. De Ruijter, F.J.R. Rietveld, L.A. Ginsel, and J.A. Jansen. *J. Biomed. Mater. Res.* **40** (1998) 464.
94. D. Rugar, and P.K. Hansma, *Phys. Today* **43** (1990) 43.
95. J.A. Thornton, in "Deposition Technologies for Films and Coatings: Developments and Applications," edited by R.F. Bunshah, et. al. (Noyes Publications, Park Ridge, N.J., 1982) p. 170.
96. J.A. Thornton, *Ann. Rev. Mater. Sci.* **7** (1977) 239.
97. F.A. Golightly, F.H. Scott, and G.C. Wood, *Oxid. Metals* **10** (1976) 163.
98. P.K. Bajpai, and H.A. Benhuzzi, *J. Biomed. Mater. Res.* **22** (1988) 1245.
99. A. Barroug, J. Fastrez, J. Lemaitre, and P.G. Rouxhet, *J. Col. Interf. Sci.* **189** (1997) 37.
100. A. Barroug, J. Lemaitre, and P.G. Rouxhet, *Col. Surf.* **37** (1989) 339.
101. A. Barroug, and M.J. Glimcher, *J. Ortho. Res.* **20** (2002) 274.
102. R.Z. Legeros, J.R. Parsons, G. Daculsi, F. Driessens, D. Lee, S.T. Liu, S. Metsger, D. Peterson, and M. Walker, in *Bioceramics: Material Characteristics versus In Vivo Behavior*, edited by P. Ducheyne and J.E. Lemons (The New York Academy of Science, New York, 1988) p. 268.
103. R.Z. Legeros, *Clin. Orthop. Rel. Res.* **395** (2002) 81.
104. W.F. Neuman, and M.W. Neuman, in *The Chemical Dynamics of Bone Mineral* (University of Chicago Press, Chicago, 1958) p. 1.
105. P. Griss, M. Winter, G. Heimke, and K. Sawai, in *First World Biomaterials Congress*, Baden, Austria, 1980, Abstract 4.10.5.
106. H. Monma, S. Ueno, and T. Kanazawa, *J. Chem. Technol. Biotechnol.* **31** (1981) 15.
107. W. van Raemdonck, P. Ducheyne, and P. De Meester, in *Metal and Ceramic Biomaterials. Vol. II: Strength and Surface*, edited by P. Ducheyne, G.W. Hastings (CRC Press Inc., Boca Raton, Florida, 1984) p. 143.
108. N.C. Blumenthal, F. Beth, and A.S. Posner, in *25th Annual Meeting of the Orthopaedics Research Society*, San Francisco, 1979, p. 119.
109. G.S. Ingram, *Bull. Soc. Chim. Fr.* (1968) 1841.
110. F.C.M. Driessens, J.W.E. van Dijk, and J.M.P.M. Borggreven, *Cal. Tis. Res.* **26** (1978) 127.
111. S.H. Maxian, J.P. Zawadsky, and M.G. Dunn, *J. Biomed. Mater. Res.* **27** (1993) 111.

112. Y. Han, K. Xu, and J. Lu, *J. Biomed. Mater. Res.* **55** (2001) 596.
113. V. Sergo, O. Sbaizero, and D.R. Clarke, *Biomaterials* **18** (1997) 477.
114. R. Z. Legeros, *Clin. Mater.* **14** (1993) 65.
115. L. Sun, C.C. Berndt, K.A. Khor, H.N. Cheang, and K.A. Gross, *J. Biomed. Mater. Res.* **62** (2002) 228.
116. F.C.M. Driessens, M.G. Boltong, I. Khairoun, E.A.P. Maeyer, M.P. Ginebra, R. Wenz, J.A. Planell, and R.M.II. Verbeeck, in *Biomaterials Engineering and Devices: Human Applications, Volume 2*, edited by D.L. Wise (Human Press, Inc., Totowa, NJ, 2000) p. 253.
117. F.C.M. Driessens, and R.M.H. Verbeeck, in *Biominerals* (CRC Press, Boca Raton, FL, 1990). P. 37.
118. A.P. Serro, A.C. Fernandes, and B. Sasamago, *J. Biomed. Mater. Res.* **49** (2000) 345.
119. N.C. Blumenthal, *Clin. Orthp. Rel. Res.* **247** (1989) 279.
120. K. Wikiel, E.M. Burke, J.W. Perich, E.C. Reynolds, and G.H. NANCOLLAS, *Arch. Oral Biol.* **39** (1994) 715.
121. H.B. Wen, J.R. De Wijn, C.A. van Blitterswijk, and K. De Groot, *J. Biomed. Mater. Res.* **46** (1999) 245.
122. A.L. Boskey, M. Maresca, W. Ullrich, S.B. Doty, W.T. Butler, and C.W. Prince, *Bone Mineral* **22** (1993) 147.
123. C. Chen, A.L. Boskey, and L.C. Rosenberg, *Calcif. Tissue Inter.* **36** (1984) 285.
124. H. Gilman, and D.W.L. Hukins, *J. Inorg. Biochem.* **55** (1994) 21.
125. J.R. Long, J.L. Dindot, H. Zebroski, and S. Kiihne, *Proc. Natl. Sci. U.S.A.* **95** (1998) 12083.
126. M. Gregoire, I. Orly, and J. Menanteau, *J. Biomed. Mater. Res.* **24** (1990) 165.
127. R.W. Evans, H.S. Cheung, and D.J. Mccarty, *Calcif. Tissue Inter.* **36** (1984) 645.122.
128. J. T. Krauser, *Dent. Clin. North Amer.* **33** (1989) 879.
129. M.H. Zablotsky, *Dent. Clin. North Amer.* **36** (1992) 117.
130. R. A. Young, *Clin. Orthop. Rel. Res.* **113** (1975) 249.
131. T. J. Webster, C. Ergun, R. H. Doremus, R. W. Siegel, and R. Bizios, *Biomaterials* **21** (2000) 1803.
132. D. Perozzollo, W.R. Lacefield, and D.M. Brunette, *J. Biomed. Mater. Res.* **56** (2001) 494.
133. P.J. ter Brugge, and J.A. Jansen, *Biomaterials* **23** (2002) 3269.
134. S.H. Maxian, T. Di Stefano, M.C. Melican, M.L. Tiku, and J.P. ZAWADSKY, *J. Biomed. Mater. Res.* **40** (1998) 171.
135. J.L. Ong, D.L. Carnes, and A. Sogal, *Inter. J. Oral Maxillofac. Implants* **12** (1999) 217.
136. D.R. Villarreal, A. Sogal, and J.L. Ong, *J. Oral Implantology* **24** (1998) 67.
137. Y. Yang, J.D. Bumgardner, R. Cavin, D.L. Carnes, and J.L. Ong, *J. Dent. Res.* **82** (2003) 449.
138. R.E. Stover, Y. Yang, C. Brambila, E. Boland, D. Carnes, and J.L. Ong, *J. Dent. Res.* **82: Spec. Iss. B** (2003) Abstract # 0262.
139. T. Kameda, H. Mano, Y. Yamada, H. Takai, N. Amizuka, M. Kobori, N. Izumi, H. Kawashima, H. Ozawa, K. Ikeda, A. Kameda, Y. Hakeda, and M. Kumegawa, *Biochem. Biophys. Res. Commun.* **245** (1998) 419.
140. M. Zaidi, J. Kerby, C.L.H. Huang, A.S.M.T. Alam, H. Rathod, T.J. Chambers, and B.S. Moonga, *J. Cell. Physiol.* **149** (1991) 422.
141. O.A. Adebanjo, V.S. Shankar, M. Pazianas, A. Zaidi, B. Simon, C.L.H. Huang, and M. Zaidi, *Biochem. Biophys. Res. Commun.* **199** (1994) 742.
142. H. Ohgushi, M. Okumura, T. Yoshikawa, K. Inoue, N. Senpuku, and S. Tamai, *J. Biomed. Mater. Res.* **26** (1992) 885.
143. W. Chen, Y. Liu, H.S. Courtney, M. Bettenga, C.M. Agrawal, J.D. Bumgardner, and J.L. Ong, *Biomaterials* **27** (2006) 5512.
144. J.L. Ong, K. Bessho, R. Cavin, and D.L. Carnes, *J. Biomed. Mater. Res.* **59** (2002) 184.

145. T. Shirota, K. Donath, Y. Matsui, K. Ohno, and K. Michi, *J. Oral Implantol.* **20** (1994) 307.
146. S.J. Renon, M.B. Guglielmotti, A.D.L. Torre, and R.L. Cabrini, *Clin. Oral Implant Res.* **12** (2001) 468.
147. J.D. Brujin, C.A. van Blitterswijk, and J.E. Davies, *J. Biomed. Mater. Res.* **29** (1995) 88.
148. G. Darimont, R. Cloots, E. Heinen, L. Seidel, and R. Legrand, *Biomaterials* **23** (2002) 2569.
149. H. Kanitani, Y. Tomotake, R. Wigianto, N. Kawamoto, and T. Ichikawa, *J. Oral Implantol.* **26** (2000) 250.
150. D.E. Steflik, S.L. White, G.R. Parr, A. Sisk, S.P. Schoen, F.T. Lake, and P.J. Hanes, *J. Oral Implantol.* **19** (1993) 199.
151. S.D. Cook, *J. Oral Implantol.* **20** (1994) 292.
152. A.A. Comut, H.P. Weber, S. Shortkroff, F.Cui, and M. Spector, *Clin. Oral Implant Res.* **12** (2001) 433.
153. S.A. Hacking, M. Tanzer, E.J. Harvey, J.J. Krygier, and J.D. Bobyn, *Clin. Orthop. Rel. Res.* **405** (2002) 24.
154. B. Sanden, C. Olerud, C. Johansson, and S. Larsson, *Spine* **26** (2001) 2673.
155. T.J. Gao, T.S. Lindholm, B. Kommonen, P. Ragni, A. Paronzini, and T.C. Lindholm, *Biomaterials* **16** (1995) 1175.
156. J.E.G. Hulshoff, and J.A. Jansen, *Clin. Oral Implant Res.* **8** (1997) 393.
157. S. Vercaigne, J.G.C. Wolke, I. Naert, and J.A. Jansen, *Clin. Oral Implant Res.* **11** (2000) 305.
158. S. Vercaigne, J.G.C. Wolke, I. Naert, and J.A. Jansen, *Clin. Oral Implant Res.* **11** (2000) 314.
159. D. Buser, R.K. Schenk, S. Steinemann, J.P. Fiorellini, C.H. Fox, and H. Stich, *J. Biomed. Mater. Res.* **25** (1991) 889.
160. P. Ducheyne, L.L. Hench, A. Kagan, M. Martens, A. Bursens, and J.C. Mulier, *J. Biomed. Mater. Res.* **14** (1980) 225.
161. D.P. Rivero, J. Fox, A.K. Skipor, R.M. Urban, and J.O. Galante, *J. Biomed. Mater. Res.* **22** (1988) 191.
162. R.G.T. Geesink, K. De Groot, and C.P.A.T. Klein, *Clin. Orthp. Rel. Res.* **225** (1987) 147.
163. K.A. Thomas, S.D. Cook, J.F. Kay, and M. Jarcho, *J. Biomed. Mater. Res.* **21** (1987) 1395.
164. S.D. Cook, K.A. Thomas, J.F. Kay, and M. Jarcho, *Clin. Orthp. Rel. Res.* **230** (1988) 303.
165. K. Gotfredsen, L. Nimb, R. Hjörting-Hansen, J.S. Jensen, and A. Holmén, *Clin. Oral Implants Res.* **3** (1992) 77.
166. M. Gottlander, T. Albrektsson, and L.V. Carlsson, *Inter. J. Oral Maxillofac Implants* **7** (1992) 485.
167. R. Z. Legeros, and I. Orly, in *The Bone-Biomaterial Interface*, edited by J.E. Davies (University of Toronto Press, Toronto, 1991) p.76.
168. S.H. Maxian, J.P. Zawadsky, and M.G. Dunn, *J. Biomed. Mater. Res.* **27** (1993) 717.
169. J.G.C. Wolke, J.M.A. De Blieck-Hogervorst, W.J.A. Dhert, C.P.A.T. Klein, and K. De Groot, *J. Thermal Spray. Technol.* **1** (1992) 75.
170. C.A. van Bitterswijl, H. Leenders, J. V.D. Brink, Y. Bovell, J. Flach, J. De Bruijn, and K. De Groot, in *Transactions of the 16th Annual Meeting of the Society for Biomaterials*, Birmingham, AL., April 1993 (Society for Biomaterials, MN, 1993) p. 337.
171. C. Mangano, E.G. Bartolucci, and C. Mazzocco, *Inter. J. Oral Maxillofac. Implants* **18** (2003) 23.
172. T. Fujui, and M. Ogino, *J. Biomed. Mater. Res.* **18** (1984) 845.
173. L.L. Hench, in *Bioceramics: Material Characteristics versus In Vivo Behavior*, edited by P. Ducheyne, J.E. Lemons (New York Academy of Science, New York, 1988) p. 54.
174. J.L. Ong, K. Bessho, and D.L. Carnes, *Inter. J. Oral Maxillofac. Implants* **17** (2002) 581.

Chapter 8
Silicon-Substituted Hydroxyapatite Thin Films

Eng San Thian and Serena M. Best

Abstract There have been numerous interests in the development of hydroxyapatite (HA) coatings on metallic orthopedic implants to maintain mechanical strength while exploiting the excellent biological properties of HA. The addition of silicon (Si) to HA has been demonstrated to enhance the rate of bone repair processing. Magnetron sputtering is a physical vapor deposition technique with the ability to achieve dense, well adhered thin coatings. This chapter describes the synthesis and characterization of Si-substituted HA thin coatings on a titanium substrate, giving good physical, chemical, and biological characteristics for bone ingrowth.

8.1 Introduction

Calcium phosphates, particularly hydroxyapatite (HA)-$Ca_{10}(PO_4)_6(OH)_2$-have attracted considerable interest regarding the development of bone-related implants owing to similarities in their composition with bone mineral [1–3]. HA is bioactive and as such has an ability to encourage direct bone apposition, which distinguishes it from many other metallic or polymeric biomaterials [4]. Although new bone forms directly on the surface of HA, the rate at which this mechanism proceeds can be slow relative to some bioactive glasses and glass ceramics [5]. This effect inevitably results in the need for a long postoperative rehabilitation program. Because HA has the ability to undergo a series of anionic or cationic substitutions, a potential way to enhance the bone healing process is to produce HA with a chemical composition resembling that of bone mineral.

Silicon (Si) is of particular interest as it has long been recognized to be associated with the mineralization of calcified tissues [6–9]. Carlisle [6] reported that Si levels of up to 0.5 wt% were observed using electron probe microanalysis in the nonmineralized osteoid regions of the bones of young mice and rats.

E.S. Thian (✉)
Department of Materials Science and Metallurgy, University of Cambridge, Pembroke Street, Cambridge, CB2 3QZ, UK
e-mail: est23@cam.ac.uk, E.S. Thian.02@cantab.net

B. León, J.A. Jansen (eds.), *Thin Calcium Phosphate Coatings for Medical Implants*, DOI 10.1007/978-0-387-77718-4_8, © Springer Science+Business Media, LLC 2009

These results were later confirmed by Landis and coworkers [10], who detected Si in the long bones of embryonic chicks and young rats using secondary ion mass spectrometry. Both sets of results showed that Si is an essential element during early bone mineralization.

Glass-ceramics [11] and silica-based glasses [12] were then developed and subsequently introduced and used extensively in a number of biomedical applications. Significant up-regulation of osteoblast proliferation and gene expression were noted when exposed to released Si^{4+} ions from bioactive glasses [13, 14]. These bioactive materials also tend to form an immediate new hydroxy-carbonate apatite layer on the surface when exposed to an aqueous environment, demonstrating a rapid bone regeneration rate. The formation of a silica-rich surface layer due to dissolution of silicon facilitates apatite phase nucleation [15]. However, this benefit seems to be dose-dependent as a low level of bioavailable Si is capable of inducing mineralized nodule formation, whereas high levels of bioavailable Si could contribute to apoptosis (cell death) [16, 17].

Based on all these studies, the benefit of delivering a small amount of Si^{4+} ions to the skeletal site is evident. This effect was studied extensively *in vitro* [18, 19] and *in vivo* [20–22] using dense Si-substituted HA (SiHA). The results have demonstrated that in addition to the increase in the rate of bone apposition the quality of bone repair was improved and an ordered bone structure was obtained. Therefore, there is logic in the development of novel SiHA coatings as they are likely to offer the potential for enhanced bioactivity.

8.2 Production of SiHA Coatings

The aim of this section is to provide a detailed overview of the production and characterization of SiHA thin films via magnetron co-sputtering at room temperature. The application of this technique to incorporate Si into the HA is novel, as it allows the establishment of dense, uniform, well adhered thin coatings, with the possibility of adding controlled levels of Si. In 2004, Porter et al. [23] reported co-deposition of SiHA coatings on titanium (Ti) substrates. Different Si contents in the films were obtained by varying the substrate's distance relative to the Si target. However, at that stage, detailed characterization of the physical, chemical, and biological properties of thin SiHA coatings was not performed.

There now follows a detailed description of a method to produce Si-containing calcium phosphate (CaP) thin films. Thian et al. [24, 25] reported a systematic way to produce these films. Deposition of SiHA coatings was performed using a custom-built sputter deposition system (Fig. 8.1). Commercially pure Si and slip-cast phase-pure sintered HA were used as sputtering targets. Commercially pure Ti was used as substrate. For each deposition run, a constant flow of high purity argon (Ar) gas was supplied to the chamber, bringing the working pressure to 0.6 Pa. A sputtering time of 4 hours was used. The coating composition was controlled by the relative discharge power supplied to each target. A radiofrequency (RF) (13.56 MHz) power of 60 W was

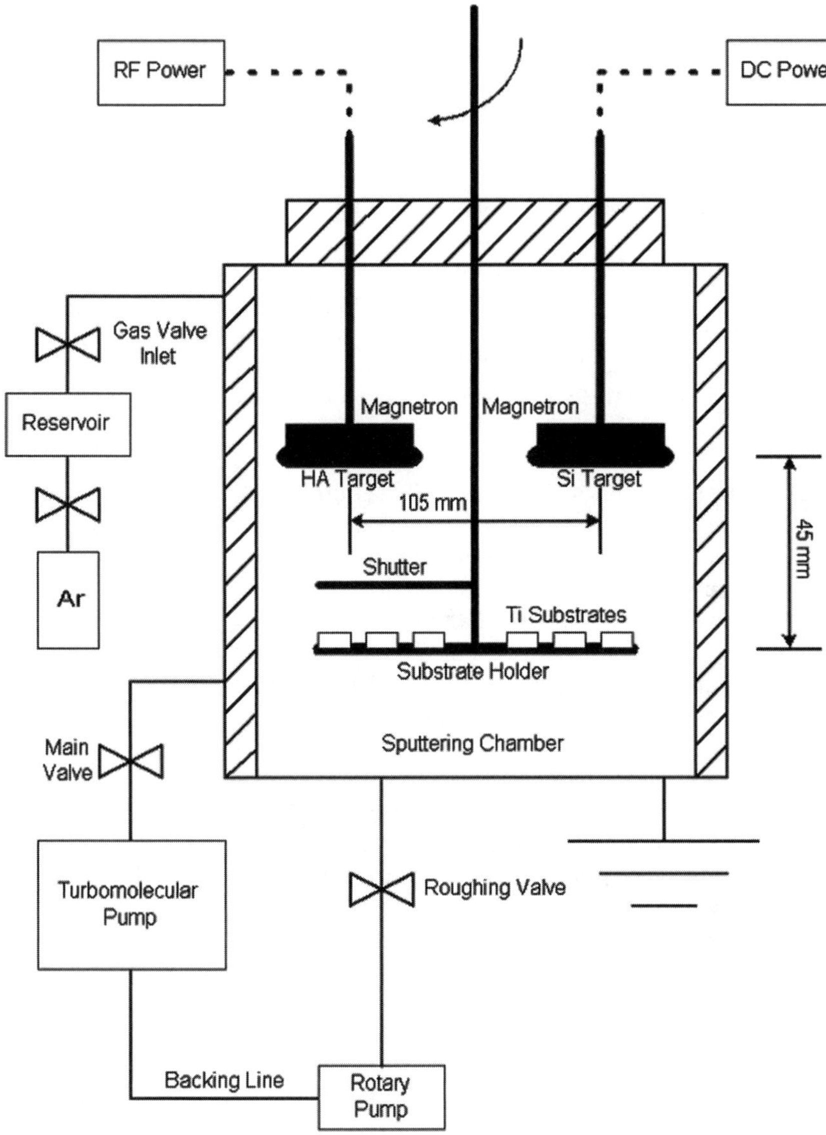

Fig. 8.1 Magnetron co-sputtering system. From [25], with permission

supplied to the HA target, and three direct current (DC) powers of 3, 9, and 15 W were supplied to the Si target to achieve coatings with three varying Si contents. Some of the as-deposited films were annealed for 3 hours under a water vapor-Ar atmosphere in a tube furnace.

Following the successful production of sputtered SiHA coatings, there have been few other reports on the preparation of SiHA coatings. Hijon et al. [26] produced SiHA film with a thickness 0.6 μm on titanium alloy substrates using a sol-gel technique. Si contents up to 2.8 wt% were obtained, and the bioactive property of these films was enhanced by the presence of Si. Solla et al. [27] demonstrated that SiHA coatings could be obtained by a pulsed laser deposition (PLD) technique as analyses revealed that Si was incorporated into the HA structure.

8.3 Physicochemical Characterization of SiHA Coating

Thian et al. [25] produced SiHA thin coatings 0.7 μm thick with varying Si compositions (0.8, 2.2, and 4.9 wt%) using magnetron co-sputtering at room temperature. The Si content in the film increased with increasing DC power, and the RF power remained at 60 W.

Annealing induced the conversion of amorphous (defective, nanocrystalline) coatings into single-phase polycrystalline coatings with major peak positions matching that of HA [Joint Committee on Powder Diffraction Standards (JCPDS) #9-432] as indicated in x-ray diffraction (XRD) scans. There was no evidence of secondary phases such as tricalcium phosphate, tetracalcium phosphate, or calcium oxide present in the coatings. With increasing Si level, these lattice plane reflections became broad and less intense.

Thian et al. [25] also reported that a broad absorption band at 1038 cm^{-1}, associated with the presence of ν_3 phosphate (P–O) stretching mode, was the only main feature observed in the infrared (IR) spectrum for the as-deposited coating. Annealing led to several changes in the spectra, with four typical absorption bands for HA being observed: one at 3571 cm^{-1}, which was associated with the stretching mode of hydroxyl (O–H); the second ν_3 P–O stretching mode, centered at 1089 cm^{-1}, became sharp and more intense; the third at 1038 cm^{-1}, which was also assigned to ν_3 P–O stretching mode; and the fourth at 962 cm^{-1}, which was assigned to ν_1 P–O stretching mode. An additional band at 935 cm^{-1} suggested the incorporation of Si into the HA, which resulted in changes in the chemical bonding and symmetry of P–O groups [28]. It was noted that the band intensities corresponding to O–H and P–O (most noticeably at 962 cm^{-1}) decreased as the Si content increased.

All these changes signified the formation of a well crystallized HA phase after annealing. This phenomenon is in agreement with the results of several reported studies [29–31] in which annealing resulted in a significant increase in the coating's crystallinity.

Substitution of Si^{4+} ions into the HA structure resulted in a change in the crystallite size and unit cell parameters of the annealed films [25]. With increasing Si addition from 0.8 to 4.9 wt%, the crystallite size of SiHA (L_{001}, obtained using the Scherrer equation) decreased from 50 nm to 19 nm. Results for the measurement of crystallite size are in agreement with those of bulk SiHA, for which Si incorporation inhibited grain growth, the effect being more significant as the level of Si increased [32, 33]. Thus, it could be expected that increased Si concentration would cause HA crystals to be more soluble, releasing more calcium (Ca^{2+}) and phosphorus (P^{5+}) ions into the culture medium. This action would result in rapid reprecipitation and development of a newly formed CaP-rich layer, with features similar to the mineral phase found in bone, hence providing an ideal site for the osteoblast cells to attach, grow, and form new bone [34]. This phenomenon is demonstrated later in the chapter.

Both the unit cell parameters' axes increased with Si substitution (*a*- from 0.9436 to 0.9466 nm and *c*- from 0.6915 to 0.6956 nm), following the trend in bulk SiHA as described by Kim et al. [35]. These findings are logical because the ionic radius of Si^{4+} (0.042 nm) is larger than that of P^{5+} (0.035 nm).

Although the addition of Si increased the unit cell parameters and reduced the crystallite size, the x-ray data showed insignificant changes in the relative peak intensities. Such changes are normally expected when there is an atomic substitution but are not expected in this case, as Si and P are adjacent in the Periodic Table (and differ by only 1 atomic number); moreover, the Si level is relatively low (< 5 wt%).

From the physical and chemical viewpoints, the addition of Si to HA resulted in a stoichiometric apatite coating. It appears that Si^{4+} ions are structurally incorporated into the HA lattice in solid solution, not segregated as a second phase. The phosphate tetrahedra were replaced by the silicate tetrahedra in the HA structure, reflected in a decrease in infrared (IR) P–O intensity with increasing substitution of Si. Thus, the mechanism in which substitution of Si into the HA lattice $[Ca_{10}(PO_4)_{6-x}(SiO_4)_x(OH)_{2-x}\Box_x]$, as proposed by Gibson et al. [28], appears to be confirmed by the reduction in the IR O–H peak intensity at 3571 cm^{-1} with increasing Si concentration. The compensation of the extra negative charge introduced by the SiO_4^{4-} anions is resolved by the formation of anionic vacancies of the OH^- site.

The amount of substituted Si in SiHA films that can be controlled using magnetron co-sputtering, as observed in this study, is of particular interest. It appears that substituted Si levels as high as 4.9 wt% could be incorporated in the HA structure while retaining phase purity. This may be attributed to the stringent control and selection of the processing parameters and conditions to prevent the formation of carbonated HA as silicate (SiO_4^{4-}) and carbonate (CO_3^{2-}) ions are known to replace phosphate ions competitively [28, 36]. Hence, the magnetron co-sputtering method with annealing allows production of coatings with predictable properties.

8.4 *In Vitro* Study: Acellular Simulated Body Fluid

The rate at which a material is able to induce CaP precipitation on its surface from a solution of physiologically relevant ions is a measure of its level of bioactivity. A relatively simple, inexpensive way to assess the bioactivity of materials has been the use of acellular simulated body fluid (SBF). SBF with an ionic composition similar to human blood plasma was prepared in accordance with the formulation described by Kokubo et al. [37].

Thian et al. [38] performed an SBF study on the as-deposited and annealed SiHA thin coatings by immersing them in SBF solution maintained at 37°C and pH 7.35. These samples were then removed from the SBF solution at periodic intervals, rinsed with deionized water to remove any excess SBF, and allowed to air-dry. The solution was not renewed during the study. Uncoated Ti substrates and as-deposited HA thin films were used as controls.

After 1 day of immersion in SBF, random submicrometer-sized pits were observed on the surface of the as-deposited SiHA coating, increasing in number from ~2 to ~5 μm^{-2} by day 4. Newly formed circular patches, comprising freshly nucleated crystallites of diameter ~25 nm appeared on the surface by day 7. A homogeneous, porous layer was obtained after immersion for 14 days (Fig. 8.2a).

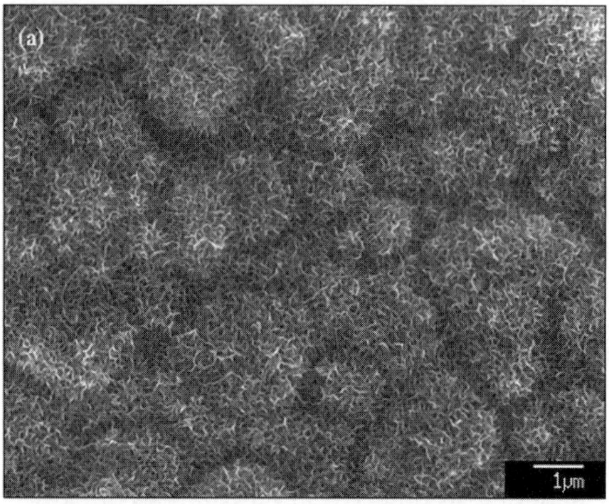

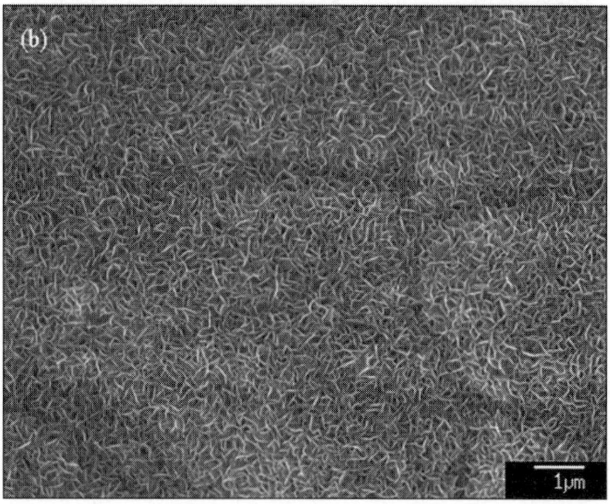

Fig. 8.2 Scanning electron microscopy images of the morphology of coating after immersion in simulated body fluid (SBF) for 14 days. **a** As-deposited silicon-substituted hydroxyapatite (SiHA). **b** Annealed SiHA. **c** Uncoated titanium (Ti). **d** As-deposited HA. From [38], with permission

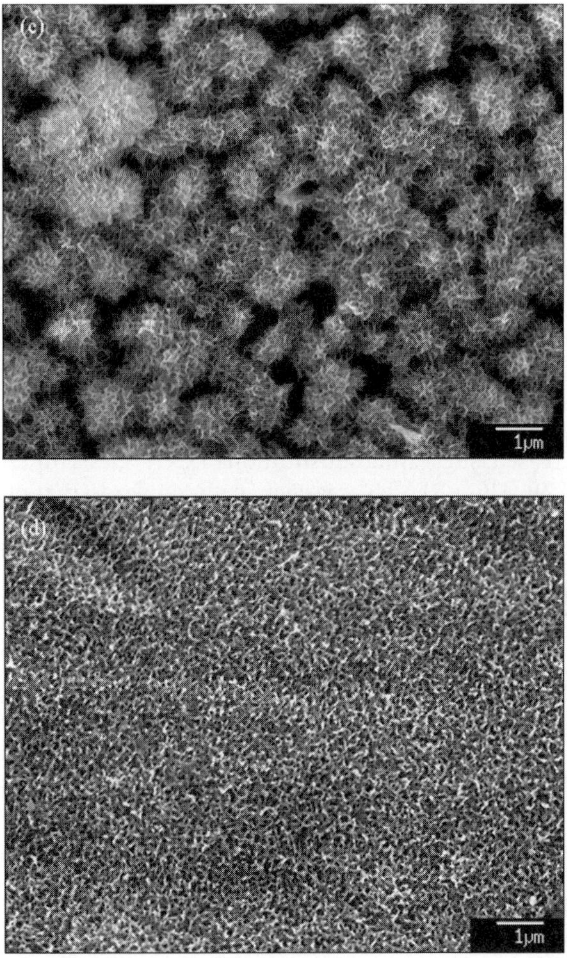

Fig. 8.2 (continued)

As for the annealed SiHA film, surface cracks on the coating appeared to be exacerbated after SBF immersion for 1 day, possibly due to preferential dissolution. As the immersion time reached day 4, freshly nucleated crystallites were observed on the surface, covering as much as ~85% of the coating surface with a newly formed layer. By day 7, the morphology of this layer was transformed into a homogeneous, porous structure consisting of short interconnecting micrometer rods covering the entire surface. After immersion in SBF for 14 days, a dense layer was achieved (Fig. 8.2b).

In contrast, a porous layer composed of loosely packed globules (Fig. 8.2c) and short interconnecting micrometer rods (Fig. 8.2d) formed on the surface of uncoated Ti and as-deposited HA after 14 days of immersion in SBF, respectively.

Energy dispersive x-ray spectroscopy (EDS) analysis confirmed that the dense layer formed on the annealed coating surface was rich in Ca and P. It was also possible to identify the incorporation of Na^+ and Mg^{2+} ions into the layer.

Detailed characterization of the newly formed layer in SBF for annealed SiHA film indicated that it was apatitic in nature, consisting of nano-sized crystallites characterized by broadening of the major HA XRD peak widths. With continued immersion, the intensity of the HA peak corresponding to lattice plane reflection (002) increased, indicating that the layer is preferentially aligned along the c-axis. It was further deduced that a broadening effect coupled with a reduction in the splitting of the P–O band between 1000 and 1100 cm^{-1} in the IR spectrum indicated formation of a new layer. The appearance of carbonate (C–O) bands at 867 and 1416 cm^{-1} confirmed the presence of a carbonate-containing HA (CHA) layer. In addition, the intensity of the O–H band at 3571 cm^{-1} decreased, suggesting substitution of CO_3^{2-} ions for OH^- ions in the HA structure [39]. This CHA layer is chemically similar to that of the inorganic mineral phase of bone, in which a coupled substitution of Na^+ and Mg^{2+} for Ca^{2+} ions is observed [40].

When comparing the as-deposited HA and SiHA coatings, results revealed that a newly precipitated dense layer was formed on SiHA by day 14; but this was not the case for HA, implying that SiHA was more bioactive than HA. During evaluation of the elemental changes in SBF solution upon immersion, a low level of Si^{4+} ions was detected in the SBF, and thereafter a decrease in the ionic concentration was noted. It is proposed that these Si^{4+} ions are attached to the coating surface as SiO_4^{4-} anions. As dissolution-precipitation is a surface-mediated process, the presence of these surface SiO_4^{4-} anions could have altered the surface properties of the material. This effect might be responsible for the higher bioactivity of SiHA s compared to that of HA. Zeta potential measurements have shown that the surface charge of SiHA was decreased by the presence of SiO_4^{4-} anions. This fact induced favorable sites for nucleation and crystallization of the apatite, which led to rapid apatite formation on SiHA [19, 41].

It can also be deduced from the immersion testing that the annealed coating underwent much earlier precipitation, compared to the as-deposited coating. However, in other reports in the literature, a reverse trend was observed where the rate of precipitation was much slower for the annealed coating, be it plasma-sprayed or magnetron-sputtered [42, 43].

In the case of as-deposited SiHA coating, this effect is attributed to the lack of crystallinity [42, 44]. Dissolution occurs during the initial stage when Ca^{2+} and P^{5+} ions are released into the SBF. It is proposed that these ions increased the degree of supersaturation of the SBF with respect to apatite, thereby facilitating the initial formation of CaP nuclei on the coating surface by consuming the Ca^{2+} and P^{5+} ions in the SBF. CaP crystallite growth then proceeded along with the continued formation of additional nuclei, thus promoting an apatite layer.

For the annealed SiHA film, the precipitation process proceeded at a much faster rate than the dissolution process, resulting in a decrease in the levels of Ca^{2+} and P^{5+} ions in SBF. It is suggested that this effect facilitated the formation of CaP nuclei on the coating surface before the formation of a crystalline apatite layer is completed. Although a mechanism by which bone-like apatite forms on bioactive ceramics has been proposed [45], enhancement of the kinetics of apatite nucleation can be related to the structural-scale factor, which explains why the annealed SiHA is more bioactive than as-deposited SiHA. It is proposed that the nanocrystalline structure creates an increased grain boundary area, providing an abundance of nucleation sites for the CaP crystallites to form because the process of crystallite formation commences at areas of low surface energy. Once formed, these crystallites grow spontaneously and are transformed into a carpet of bone-like apatite on the surface.

8.5 *In Vitro* Cell Culture

Cell culture has become increasing popular for the studying interactions at the bone–material interface. It is an accepted method for testing material safety, gaining a deeper understanding of the *in vivo* mechanisms of actions that determine the success or failure of skeletal implants and reducing the number of animals used for *in vivo* studies [46]. This section details the biological response of human osteoblast-like (HOB) cells to annealed SiHA thin films by investigating the effect of variation in Si substitution on the rate of biomineralization.

All samples were soaked in ethanol for 48 hours before sterilization with ultraviolet (UV) radiation for 30 minutes. HOB cells (Promocell, Heidelberg, Germany) of cell density 1×10^4 cells/test were then seeded onto the surfaces of these sterile samples before incubating at 37°C in a humidified atmosphere of 95% air and 5% carbon dioxide. Uncoated Ti substrates were used as test controls.

Thian et al. [47] conducted an alamarBlue™ assay test and found an increase in the growth of HOB cells with increased culture time on all samples, except samples containing 4.9 wt% Si (S3), which seemed to decline at day 14 (Fig. 8.3). When comparison was made between all SiHA films and the uncoated Ti substrate, significant differences were noted at days 4, 7, and 14, with SiHA coatings resulting in much higher HOB activity. When all the SiHA coatings were evaluated at each time point, S3 showed a statistically significant increase in cell growth compared to samples containing 0.8 wt% Si (S1). In addition, a significant increase was observed for samples containing 2.2 wt% Si (S2) when compared to S1 at days 4 and 7. On the whole, S2 exhibited the highest cell growth among all samples throughout the culture period.

The authors also performed immunofluorescence labeling of the actin filaments at day 1 to observe the cell–substrate interaction [47]. Although the

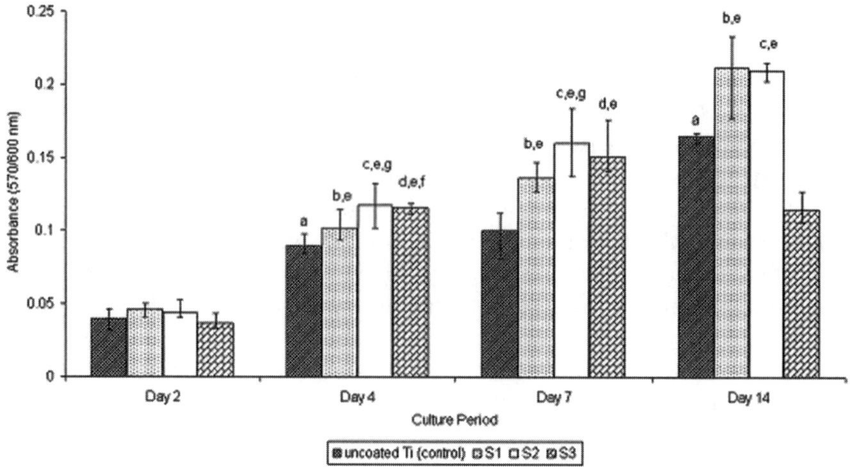

Fig. 8.3 Growth of human osteoblast (HOB) cells versus culturing time. [a]$P < 0.05$: growth activity was significantly higher on control between groups. [b]$P < 0.05$: growth activity was significantly higher at S1 between groups. [c]$P < 0.05$: growth activity was significantly higher at S2 between groups. [d]$P < 0.05$: growth activity was significantly higher at S3 between groups. [e]$P < 0.05$: growth activity was significantly higher on SiHA than the control within groups. [f]$P < 0.05$: growth activity was significantly higher at S3 than at S1 within groups. [g]$P < 0.05$: growth activity was significantly higher at S2 than at S1 within groups. From [47], with permission

cytoskeletons displayed a polygonal-like architecture on all surfaces, well developed actin filaments aligning along the long axis of the cells were apparent within HOBs on both S2 (Fig. 8.4a) and S3 samples but were less distinct and diffuse in HOBs in the S1 sample. HOBs cultured on uncoated Ti substrate seemed to be devoid of microfilaments in the cell membranes (Fig. 8.4b).

Basically, cells attached, spread, and grew on all samples, with filopodia extending from the cell edges. At day 2, a less confluent cell layer was obtained for the uncoated Ti substrate, synthesizing minute amounts of ECM (Fig. 8.5a). In addition, cell spreading was less pronounced and displayed underdeveloped lamellipodia. Well flattened cells were observed to cover all surfaces completely on SiHA films (Fig. 8.5b). Furthermore, dense ECM layers comprising of Ca and P (as determined by EDS spot analysis) were visible underneath the cell layers (Fig. 8.5c). At day 16, cells were seen adhering and spreading on top of each other for all samples, forming a multilayer of cells without any specific orientation (Fig. 8.5d). At day 42, there was little evidence of CaP mineral deposits on the uncoated Ti, whereas numerous randomly distributed, large mineral deposits of diameter > 1 μm were seen on all SiHA coatings, indicating signs of mineralization. Of all the samples, S3 appeared to show the highest level of mineralization.

The enhanced bioactivity exhibited by the coated Ti substrate (compared with uncoated Ti) was attributed to a combination of effects: (1) the presence of HA promoting cell attachment, proliferation, and differentiation; and (2) the incorporation of Si^{4+} ions into HA, which appeared to be an important factor for

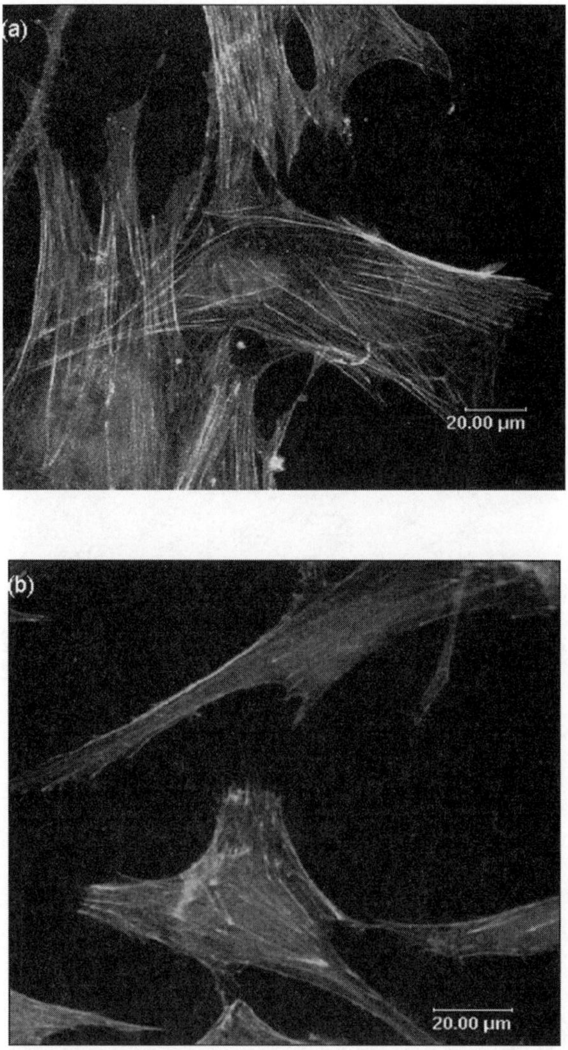

Fig. 8.4 Confocal fluorescence microscopy of nuclear DNA (stained blue) and actin cytoskeleton (stained green) in HOB at day 1 as revealed with double labeling using TOTO-3 and fluorescein isothiocyanate (FITC)-conjugated phalloidin S2 (**a**) or uncoated Ti (**b**). From [47], with permission

stimulating bone cell metabolism. It has been reported in several studies that Si inhibited the growth of HA crystals and that this effect was more significant as the Si level increased [32, 33]. As such, it might be expected that increased Si content would cause HA crystals to be more soluble, releasing more Ca^{2+}, P^{5+}, and Si^{4+} ions into the culture medium. This effect would then facilitate rapid development of a carbonated apatite layer on the coating surface. This phenomenon was observed here for coatings with high Si content (2.2 and 4.9 wt%).

The release of Si^{4+} ions has been shown to alter the surface properties of SiHA [41, 48], which in turn could have a positive effect on protein adsorption. It is proposed that the released Si^{4+} ions combine with oxygen ions, forming a $SiO_4{}^{4-}$ network structure on the surface that is capable of holding elements of the proteins together in an organized fashion, thereby contributing to the architecture of connective tissue [49]. It is possible that these proteins are adsorbed onto the bound $SiO_4{}^{4-}$ network, contributing to a higher protein concentration than would be found with either uncoated Ti substrates or HA films. In addition, Thian et al. found that

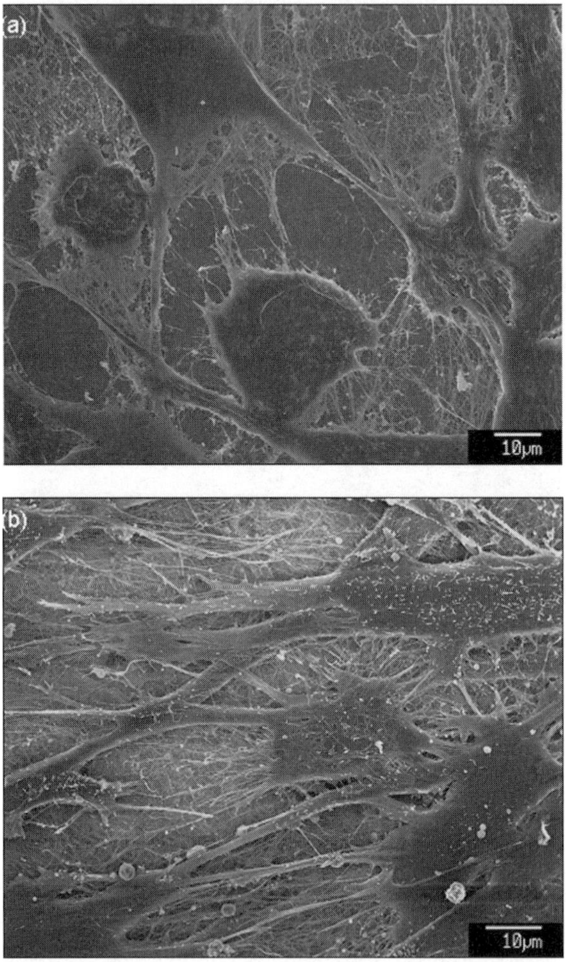

Fig. 8.5 Cell morphology at different time points. **a** Uncoated Ti at day 2. **b** S1 at day 2. **c** Extracellular matrix on S3 at day 2. **d** S1 at day 16. From Thian et al. [25, 47], with permission

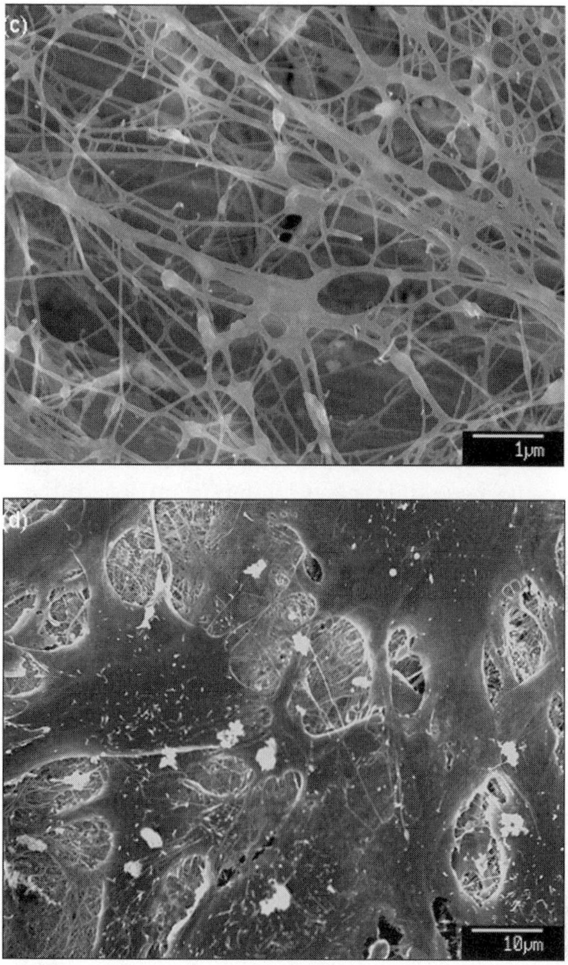

Fig. 8.5 (continued)

SiHA films showed a lower contact angle (29.54° ± 3.10° for 0.8 wt% Si) than the uncoated Ti film (67.87° ± 5.09°) or HA film (47.60° ± 2.52°). A low contact angle, and thus increased surface wettability, has been demonstrated to enhance protein adsorption and, consequently, cell attachment on biomaterial surfaces [50, 51]. Both of these effects influence the regulators of DNA synthesis in the HOBs that promote cell attachment via interaction with integrins. These interactions, in turn, trigger certain specific signals that regulate cellular functions, such as cell attachment, proliferation, and differentiation or even mobility and shape [52], which could have a stimulatory effect on the bone mineralization process.

This effect can be clearly seen from this study, where rapid cell growth, well organized cytoskeletal architecture, and enhanced biomineralization were achieved with increasing Si content. HOBs displayed more mature cytoskeleton organization on SiHA coatings than on the uncoated Ti, as actin is involved in the transport mechanism of RNA between the nucleus and cytoplasm. However, the precise mechanism by which Si affects cell activity requires further investigation.

It may also be deduced from this study that cell growth was retarded at the early stages of culture for coatings with high Si content. This could be due to the rapid dissolution of the coatings owing to their small HA crystallite size, thereby rendering the surface unfavorable for osteoblast attachment. At a later stage, when the surface had been modified by the growth of a newly formed carbonated apatite layer, many cells began to migrate, attach, proliferate, and differentiate on the surface.

All these findings suggest that Si controls the rate of dissolution of the coatings and, at the same time, plays an important role in the early stages of mineralization. As such, a balance between both factors is desirable. Of the three compositions studied, 2.2 wt% SiHA seems to be the preferred optimal composition and merits further investigation.

8.6 Conclusion

Novel SiHA thin coatings have been deposited on Ti substrates by magnetron co-sputtering. *In vitro* studies in SBF and HOB cells have shown that these coatings exhibit enhanced bioactivity and biomineralization over uncoated Ti samples and HA coatings. The rate at which dissolution-precipitation and biomineralization mechanisms proceed is directly related to the presence of Si in the HA structure. High Si levels result in the promotion of bone mineralization but also lead to rapid dissolution of the coating. The mechanical properties of these coatings and the behavior of this novel SiHA film *in vivo* require further investigation. Overall, the choice of coating depends on the desired application, but these SiHA thin films offer a good alternative to both plasma-sprayed coatings and HA thin films.

References

1. H. Aoki, in "Science and Medical Applications of Hydroxyapatite" (JAAS, Tokyo, 1991).
2. C. A. van Blitterswijk, S. C. Hesseling, J. J. Grote, H. K. Koerten and K. de Groot. *J. Biomed. Mater. Res.* **24** (1990) 433.
3. K. de Groot, in "Bioceramics of Calcium Phosphate" (Boca Raton, FL, USA: CRC Press Inc, 1983).
4. W. Bonfield. *Phil. Trans. R. Soc. A* **364** (2006) 227.
5. C. P. A. T. Klein, A. A. Driessen, K. de Groot and A. van den Hooff. *J. Biomed. Mater. Res.* **17** (1983) 769.

6. E. M. Carlisle. *Science* **167** (1970) 279.
7. E. M. Carlisle. *Science* **178** (1972) 619.
8. E. M. Carlisle. *Fed. Proc.* **32** (1973) 930.
9. E. M. Carlisle. *J. Nutr.* **110** (1980) 1046.
10. W. J. Landis, D. D. Lee, J. T. Brenna, S. Chandra and G. H. Morrison. *Calcif. Tissue Int.* **38** (1986) 52.
11. C. Ohtsuki, T. Kokubo and T. Yamamuro. *J. Non-Cryst. Solids* **143** (1992) 84.
12. A. Pazo, E. Saiz and A. P. Tomsia. *Acta Mater.* **46** (1998) 2551.
13. I. D. Xynos, M. V. Hukkanen, J. J. Batten, L. D. Buttery, L. L. Hench and J. M. Polak. *Calcif. Tissue Int.* **67** (2000) 321.
14. I. D. Xynos, A. J. Edgar, L. D. Buttery, L. L. Hench and J. M. Polak. *J. Biomed. Mater. Res.* **55** (2001) 151.
15. D. Arcos, D. C. Greenspan and M. Vallet-Regi. *J. Biomed. Mater. Res.* **65A** (2003) 344.
16. J. E. Gough, J. R. Jones and L. L. Hench. *Biomaterials* **25** (2004) 2039.
17. J. E. Gough, D. C. Clupper and L. L. Hench. *J. Biomed. Mater. Res.* **69A** (2004) 621.
18. I. R. Gibson, J. Huang, S. M. Best and W. Bonfield, in Proceedings of the 12th International Symposium on Ceramics in Medicine, Nara, 1999, edited by H. Ohgushi, G. W. Hasting and T. Yoshikawa (Trans Tech Publications, Switzerland, 2000) p.191.
19. F. Balas, J. Perez-Pariente and M. Vallet-Regi. *J. Biomed. Mater. Res.* **66A** (2003) 364.
20. N. Patel, S. M. Best, W. Bonfield, I. R. Gibson, K. A. Hing, E. Damien and P. A. Revell. *J. Mater. Sci. Mater. Med.* **13** (2002) 1199.
21. N. Patel, R. A. Brooks, M. T. Clarke, P. M. T. Lee, N. Rushton, I. R. Gibson, S. M. Best and W. Bonfield. *J. Mater. Sci. Mater. Med.* **16** (2005) 429.
22. A. E. Porter, N. Patel, J. N. Skepper, S. M. Best and W. Bonfield. *Biomaterials* **25** (2004) 3303.
23. A. E. Porter, S. M. Rea, M. Galtrey, S. M. Best and Z. H. Barber. *J. Mater. Sci.* **39** (2004) 1895.
24. E. S. Thian, J. Huang, S. M. Best, Z. H. Barber and W. Bonfield. *J. Mater. Sci. Mater. Med.* **16** (2005) 411.
25. E. S. Thian, J. Huang, M. E. Vickers, S. M. Best, Z. H. Barber and W. Bonfield. *J. Mater. Sci.* **41** (2006) 709.
26. N. Hijon, M. V. Cabanas, J. Pena and M. Vallet-Regi. *Acta Biomater.* **2** (2006) 567.
27. E. L. Solla, P. Gonzalez, J. Serra, S. Chiussi and B. Leon. Pulsed Laser Deposition of Silicon Substituted Hydroxyapatite Coatings from Synthetical and Biological Sources. E-MRS Spring Meeting, Strasbourg, France, May 28th – June 1st 2007.
28. I. R. Gibson, S. M. Best and W. Bonfield. *J. Biomed. Mater. Res.* **44** (1999) 422.
29. K. van Dijk, H. G. Schaeken, J. G. C. Wolke and J. A. Jansen. *Biomaterials* **17** (1996) 405.
30. W. J. Lo, D. M. Grant, M. D. Ball, B. S. Welsh, S. M. Howdle, E. N. Antonov, V. N. Bagratashvili and V. K. Popov. *J. Biomed. Mater. Res.* **50** (2000) 536.
31. Y. Yang, K. H. Kim, C. M. Agrawal and J. L. Ong. *Biomaterials* **24** (2003) 5131.
32. I. R. Gibson, S. M. Best and W. Bonfield. *J. Am. Ceram. Soc.* **85** (2002) 2771.
33. D. Arcos, J. Rodriguez-Carvajal and M. Vallet-Regi. *Chem. Mater.* **16** (2004) 2300.
34. M. Neo, T. Nakamura, C. Ohtsuki, T. Kokubo and T. Yamamuro. *J. Biomed. Mater. Res.* **27** (1993) 999.
35. S. R. Kim, J. H. Lee, Y. T. Kim, D. H. Riu, S. J. Jung, Y. J. Lee, S. C. Chang and Y. H. Kim. *Biomaterials* **24** (2003) 1389.
36. I. R. Gibson and W. Bonfield. *J. Biomed. Mater. Res.* **59** (2002) 697.
37. T. Kokubo, H. Kushitani, S. Sakka, T. Kitsugi and T. Yamamuro. *J. Biomed. Mater. Res.* **24** (1990) 721.
38. E. S. Thian, J. Huang, S. M. Best, Z. H. Barber and W. Bonfield. *J. Biomed. Mater. Res. (Appl. Biomater.)* **76B** (2006) 326.
39. I. Rehman and W. Bonfield. *J. Mater. Sci. Mater. Med.* **8** (1997) 1.
40. R. Z. LeGeros. *Prog. Crystal Growth Charact.* **4** (1981) 1.

41. C. M. Botelho, M. A. Lopes, I. R. Gibson, S. M. Best and J. D. Santos. *J. Mater. Sci. Mater. Med.* **13** (2002) 1123.
42. J. G. C. Wolke, K. van Dijk, H. G. Schaeken, K. de Groot and J. A. Jansen. *J. Biomed. Mater. Res.* **28** (1994) 1477.
43. L. Sun, C. C. Berndt, K. A. Khor, H. N. Cheang and K. A. Gross. *J. Biomed. Mater. Res.* **62** (2002) 228.
44. J. Weng, Q. Liu, J. G. C. Wolke, X. Zhang and K. de Groot. *Biomaterials* **18** (1997) 1027.
45. H. M. Kim, T. Himeno, M. Kawashita, T. Kokubo and T. Nakamura. *J. R. Soc. Interface* **1** (2004) 17.
46. M. Fini and R. Giardino. *J. Appl. Biomater. & Biomech.* **1** (2003) 155.
47. E. S. Thian, J. Huang, S. M. Best, Z. H. Barber, R. A. Brooks, N. Rushton and W. Bonfield. *Biomaterials* **27** (2006) 2692.
48. A. E. Porter, N. Patel, J. N. Skepper, S. M. Best and W. Bonfield. *Biomaterials* **24** (2003) 4609.
49. K. Schwarz. *Fed. Proc.* **33** (1974) 1748.
50. R. M. Shelton, A. C. Rasmussen and J. E. Davis. *Biomaterials* **9** (1988) 24.
51. J. G. Stelle, C. Mcfarland, B. A. Dalton, G. Johnson, M. D. M. Evans, C. R. Howlett and P. A. Underwood. *J. Biomater. Sci. Polym. Edn.* **5** (1993) 245.
52. B. G. Keselowsky, D. M. Collard and A. J. Garcia. *J. Biomed. Mater. Res.* **66A** (2003) 247.

Chapter 9
Electrochemically Assisted Deposition of Thin CaP Coatings

Dieter Scharnweber and Susanne Bierbaum

Abstract Calcium phosphate (CaP) coatings have long been known to have a positive influence on implant integration into bone. Several methods for the formation of such coatings are known; this chapter focuses on the process of electrochemically assisted deposition (ECAD). With this highly reproducible biomimetic method, CaP coatings are generated on electrically conductive substrates in aqueous solutions. The fact that the process can take place at ambient temperature and neutral pH allows the deposition of coatings containing inorganic and especially organic components. Following a general description of the method and its basic principle, the influence of the deposition conditions on the coating properties is discussed in detail regarding a number of parameters. Among them are electrolyte composition, temperature, electrochemical mode used, and the effect of organic or inorganic additives. Variations of the said parameters can affect the composition of the phases deposited, the total coating mass, the mechanical characteristics, and a number of other properties. In addition to the physicochemical stability of ECAD coatings, another important aspect is the biological efficiency and compatibility of the coatings. In this context, cell biological investigations, animal studies, and experience from clinical applications are reviewed. The final aspect addressed in the chapter focuses on the characterization of ECAD-derived coatings in relation to the regulatory pathway and the prospects for industrial applications.

9.1 Introduction

The main focus of this chapter is the electrochemically assisted deposition (ECAD) of calcium phosphate phases (CPPs), a process possible only with electrically conductive substrates in Ca and P containing electrolytes. Cathodic polarization of these substrates results in the formation of OH ions,

D. Scharnweber (✉)
Institute of Materials Science, Max Bergmann Center of Biomaterials, Technische Universität Dresden, Budapester Str. 27, 01069 Dresden, Germany
e-mail: Dieter.Scharnweber@tu-dresden.de

B. León, J.A. Jansen (eds.), *Thin Calcium Phosphate Coatings for Medical Implants*, DOI 10.1007/978-0-387-77718-4_9, © Springer Science+Business Media, LLC 2009

causing a local increase in pH at the substrate surface. As the solubility of CPP is pH-dependent, this rise in pH leads to an increase in the relative supersaturation σ of the electrolyte with respect to CPP, resulting in the formation of particulate CPP. The term electrochemically assisted reflects the fact that although electrochemical reactions play a major role in the overall process during the actual deposition of CPP there is no transfer of charge carriers in the sense of an electrochemical reaction comparable to metallic galvanic coatings.

In contrast, with the electrophoretic (EP) deposition process (discussed later in the chapter), macroscopic particles from CPP are already present in the electrolyte and are deposited on the substrate under the influence of an electric field. This division is reflected in Table 9.4 (at the end of the chapter), which attempts to give a complete overview of articles published on the ECAD process itself, the characterization of resultant coatings, and their use in animal experiments and clinical applications. Table 9.4 also contains some articles dealing with EP coatings, but the latter do not constitute a complete literature review.

9.1.1 Advantages of the ECAD Method

- The deposition of thin, not monolithic layers with a composition, crystal size, and chemical history close to that of bone mineral is possible.
- The thickness and chemical composition of coatings can be controlled down to the submicrometer level.
- The coatings have excellent homogeneity on structured and porous surfaces as well as on irregularly formed structures, as it is no line of sight process.
- Generation of coatings with a high specific surface area is possible.
- Compared to the biomimetic method of incubation in simulated body fluid (SBF), there is more defined, higher relative supersaturation at the interface, resulting in shorter processing times.
- Owing to possible physiological processing parameters (pH, temperature, aqueous solution), the deposition of CPP can be combined with the immobilization/incorporation of organic components such as proteins (peptides).
- There is no adverse effect of heat on the substrate material.
- It is a low energy process.
- It is a low cost process (with respect to production and waste management).

9.1.2 Disadvantages of the ECAD Method

- There is potentially low adhesive strength of the coatings (unlikely for rough surfaces common for implants in bone), which can be overcome by combination with anodic growth of oxide layers [1].
- An electrically conductive substrate or substrate top layer is necessary.

- For extreme electrochemical conditions (high current densities, long duration polarization) there is a risk of hydrogen embrittlement for metallic substrates.

9.2 ECAD: The Technique

9.2.1 *Basic Principles*

As already mentioned, the ECAD technique takes advantage of the pH-dependent solubility of CPP and is based on a local increase of the pH close to the substrate surface in an aqueous system. A prerequisite for deposition of CPP is therefore cathodic polarization of the substrate, which increases the pH on the surface. Considering the substrate as inert, in air-saturated solutions the two following overall reactions take place.

$$2H_2O + 2e^- \rightarrow H_2 + 2OH^- \tag{9.1}$$

$$O_2 + 4e^- + 2H_2O \rightarrow 4OH^- \tag{9.2}$$

In air-saturated aqueous solutions, the oxygen-limiting diffusion current is in the range of about 30 $\mu A/cm^2$ [2, 3]. At the typical ECAD current density of several milliamperes, the predominant electrochemical reaction is the formation of hydrogen according to Eq. 9.1. This is summarized in Fig. 9.1 together with the influence of the local pH on the dissociation of phosphate ions.

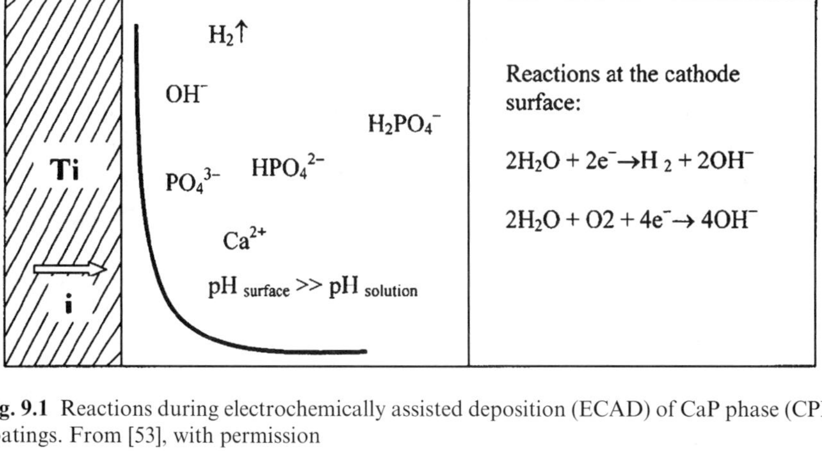

Fig. 9.1 Reactions during electrochemically assisted deposition (ECAD) of CaP phase (CPP) coatings. From [53], with permission

Nitrate-containing electrolytes constitute a special case, as the reduction of this ion as an additional cathodic process also contributes to the total current (discussed by Montero-Ocampo et al. [4]); but similar to the reduction of oxygen, the contribution is negligible because of the low (millimolar) nitrate concentrations.

Three methods can be used for polarization of the substrate.

- *Constant cell voltage.* A constant voltage between the working electrode (substrate) and the counter electrode is applied, similar to the galvanic deposition of metal coatings. With this technique, any variation of the cell geometry ultimately alters the electrochemical conditions (current density) because of a change in the ohmic relations of the whole system.
- *Constant potential of the working electrode (potentiostatic).* The potential of the working electrode is kept constant with respect to a reference electrode. In this constellation a third electrode (counter electrode) is needed to pass the necessary current. Typically, the overall current decreases with increasing deposition time, consequently decreasing the pH close to the substrate surface. As the substrate is increasingly covered with CPP, the surface area of the substrate available for the electrochemical process is reduced. As this second effect overcompensates the first one, the current density increases during the deposition process.
- *Constant current (galvanostatic).* The current in a system of two electrodes is held constant, keeping the turnover of the electrochemical reactions at the working and counter electrodes independent of time. Compared to the potentiostatic polarization, the galvanostatic regime results in a stronger increase of the current density over time for surface areas available for electrochemical reactions. This can be taken into consideration by decreasing the current density during deposition.

Independent of the polarization method, the increase in current density due to increasing coverage by CPP can be described by

$$i_{eff} = i_{total} \frac{1}{(1 - \theta)} \tag{9.3}$$

where i_{eff} is the current density with respect to the substrate surface available for electrochemistry (not coated by CPP); i_{total} is the current density with respect to the total substrate surface; θ is the fraction of the surface covered by CPP. Thus, irrespective of the electrochemical modus, no absolutely dense coatings can be obtained.

The first parameter influencing the CPP coating is the composition of the electrolyte. The absolute concentrations of Ca und PO_4 and their concentration ratio as well as the electrolyte pH and possible additives play major roles in this context.

A number of investigations were performed under defined atmospheres [5–9] to investigate the effect of CO_2, which may result in the deposition of carbonate-containing CPP. The effect of further additives on the composition of the coatings is discussed in Chapter 2.

Going through the literature, the main CaP phases produced by the ECAD process—depending on the electrochemical conditions and the electrolyte solution composition—are brushite (BR), amorphous CaP (ACP), octacalcium phosphate (OCP), and hydroxyapatite (HA) with different carbonate contents. The consumption of OH ions for these CPPs given in the brutto reaction equations below is a measure of the influence of pH on the formation of the respective CPP. As indicated by the indexes and factors x in the equations, the consumption is clearly a function of the pH of the used electrolyte. Furthermore, x depends on the concentration of the electrolyte, as it is related to the buffer capacity.

- Formation of brushite [$M_{BR} = 172\ \mathrm{g\ mol^{-1}}$]

$$Ca^{2+} + H_xPO_4^{(3-x)-} + (x-1)OH^- + (3-x)H_2O \rightarrow CaHPO_4 \cdot 2\ H_2O \quad (9.4)$$

- Formation of OCP [$M_{OCP} = 892\ \mathrm{g\ mol^{-1}}$]

$$Ca^{2+} + 6\ H_xPO_4^{(3-x)-} + (6x-2)OH^- \rightarrow Ca_8H_2(PO_4)_6 + (6x-2)H_2O \quad (9.5)$$

- Formation of ACP [$M_{ACP} = 310\ \mathrm{g\ mol^{-1}}$]

$$3Ca^{2+} + 2H_xPO_4^{(3-x)-} + 2xOH^- \rightarrow Ca_3(PO_4)_2 + 2x\,H_2O \quad (9.6)$$

- Formation of HA [$M_{HA} = 1004\ \mathrm{g\ mol^{-1}}$]

$$10Ca^{2+} + 6H_xPO_4^{(3-x)-} + (6x+2)OH^- \rightarrow Ca_{10}(PO_4)_6(OH)_2 + 6x\,H_2O \quad (9.7)$$

For pH 3 to 6 (common for most investigations in the literature), it follows from the acidic constants (pK_s) of phosphoric acid [10] that x is close to 2 in Eqs. 9.5 to 9.7. With this value, the OH/Ca consumption ratios for the formation of each CPP (Table 9.1) can be calculated from these equations.

The values for the charge balance given in the third column of Table 9.1 are based on the assumption that the Faraday effectivity for the formation of OH ions is 100% and that all the OH ions formed at the interface are participating in the formation of CPP. The OH/Ca ratio as well as the charge consumption

Table 9.1 OH/Ca ratios and charge balance relevant for the formation of CPP in the ECAD process

CPP	OH/Ca ratio	Charge balance (C/mg)
Brushite	1:1 = 1	0.561
OctaCaP	10:8 = 1.25	1.082
Amorphous CaP	4:3 = 1.33	1.245
Hydroxyapatite	14:10 = 1.40	1.346

clearly reflects the transition from the acidic CPP brushite to increasingly alkaline CPPs in the sequence OCP to ACP to HA.

However, it must be noted that the real charge efficiency of the ECAD process is far from being 100% and is highly dependent on the pH and composition of the electrolyte, electrochemical parameters, and the CPP to be deposited. In a study by Redepenning et al. [11], charge efficiencies varied between 5% and 50%. Moreover, it significantly decreased with processing time during the deposition process, reaching values as low as 3%. When working in systems with much lower electrolyte concentrations and higher pH [12], the current efficiency can decrease to well below 1%.

The deposited amount of CPP does not depend linearly on the deposition time. Ban and Maruno [13] and Montero-Ocampo et al. [4] demonstrated a square root relation between the deposited mass and the deposition time for potentiostatic conditions. This clearly indicates that the deposition is limited by diffusion processes.

The second parameter influencing the formation of CPP coatings is the process temperature. Ban and Maruno [13–15] demonstrated that rising temperature not only increased the deposited amount of CPP but also favored the formation of crystalline phases with larger crystal sizes. The temperature is thus important for the deposition of highly crystalline coatings, with the temperature range studied extending to $> 100^\circ C$ for hydrothermal ECAD processes [15] in aqueous solutions.

Another aspect where the process temperature is of special importance is the formation of coatings containing heat-sensitive organic components such as proteins. Changing the ambient pressure is a fourth possible parameter. Wang et al. [16] used low pressure conditions in the ECAD to avoid possible negative effects of hydrogen formation on the homogeneous coatings of CPP.

9.2.2 Influence of Processing Conditions on Coating Properties

9.2.2.1 Influence on Coating Composition

First applications of the ECAD process for deposition of CPP layers on metallic implants used relatively acidic solutions and produced coatings of brushite [17]. To improve osseointegration, the further developments aimed at creating a product closer to natural bone apatite and focused on two preparation methods.

One method is a two-step process beginning with ECAD of CPPs other than HA and then transforming them to the required phase. Several processes have been developed in this context, such as incubation in SBF [18] or in aqueous solutions of high pH [11, 19–22] or hydrothermal treatments [5, 7, 23, 24].

The second method is direct deposition of HA. This is achieved either by increasing the temperature [4, 6, 14, 25–30] during deposition, using electrolytes of higher pH (and consequently lower Ca and phosphate ion concentrations) [12, 13, 31], or combinations of these strategies. The advantage of raising the temperature without changing the electrolyte pH is that higher ionic concentrations in Ca and phosphate, and thus lower implant surface/electrolyte volume ratios, are possible. On the other hand, a process conducted at physiological temperatures allows for co-deposition of temperature-sensitive components such as proteins.

9.2.2.2 Influence on Coating Mass

As already discussed at the beginning of the chapter, the deposition rate of CPP is substantially determined by diffusion. Therefore, higher concentrations of calcium and phosphate ions in the electrolyte (which always have to correlate with lower pH values because of the limitations imposed by the solubility products of CPPs) together with higher current densities result in faster growth of layers and consequently in higher coating masses. This has been illustrated in a number of experiments.

Montero-Ocampo et al. [4], for instance, used conditions similar to those described by Shirkhanzadeh et al. [7–9, 32] and obtained layer masses of 650 to 2200 μg/cm^2 depending on the potential and the deposition time (20–60 minutes). For these layers, the thickness ranged from 2.7 to 7.0 μm. Kuo and Yen [3], using twofold higher concentrations at room temperature in the galvanostatic mode with –10 mA/cm^2, obtained layer masses between 500 and 2500 μg/cm^2 for deposition times ranging from 5 to 40 minutes.

For neutral electrolytes with low concentrations of Ca and phosphate ions (4 and 2 mM, respectively), Wang et al. [33] with a current density of –2 mA/cm^2 produced relatively thick coatings (40–50 μm), but with a polarization time of 10 hours. For deposition times of more technical relevance (60 minutes), their data are in agreement with those of Rössler et al. [1, 12, 34], who prepared layers $<$10 μm thick with ion concentrations lower by half. With a similar electrolyte and the same polarization time but under hydrothermal conditions, Ban and Maruno [15] produced coating masses between 1 and 4 mg/cm^2 for temperatures between 80° and 150°C, respectively, which indicates the strong influence of temperature on the deposition rate.

Thus, deposition of coatings from acidic electrolytes typically results in layer masses of 2 to 3 mg/cm^2 for 1 hour of deposition, which is comparable to layer masses deposited from neutral electrolytes under hydrothermal conditions. The use of neutral electrolytes at ambient temperatures, however, results in much lower layer masses (~0.1 mg/cm^2), which can be increased by longer deposition times (square root dependence between layer mass and time).

9.2.3 Influence of Electrochemical and Solution Parameters

This section is a more detailed discussion of the literature on the deposition of pure CPP coatings using the ECAD process. It covers both the formation conditions and the resulting phases. The formation of composite coatings is addressed in Chapter 2.

Although formation and morphology of the CPP generated during the ECAD process are determined by a variety of parameters (electrochemical conditions, electrolyte composition, temperature, deposition time). For ease of reading, not all of them are described in detail. For these, the reader is referred to Table 9.4 at the end of this chapter.

9.2.3.1 Processing with Constant Cell Voltage

The constant cell voltage method was used in only a small number of studies owing to the comparatively undefined conditions for cathodic polarization of the substrate. Most of the contributions studied the effect of cell voltage on the composition of the coatings with results that confirm the influence of pH on the formation of CPP, discussed in Chapter 2. Thus, Okamura et al. [35] reported that for cell voltages below 10 V coatings composed of brushite, monetite, and HA are produced, whereas higher voltages give rise to pure HA as determined by x-ray diffraction (XRD). Similar results were gained by Wang et al. [16] at 80 torr for a temperature range of 0° to 60°C in a comparatively acidic electrolyte of pH 3. For cell voltages up to 6 V they detected brushite with increasing crystal sizes, whereas for voltages > 7 V HA starts to appear, becoming the major phase at 10 V. With rising process temperature, the coating thickness increases, as does the HA/brushite ratio.

Haddow et al. [27] studied the influence of the carbonate content of the electrolyte on the phase composition of the coatings. HA was identified by XRD to be the only product deposited in a carbonate-free environment. A carbonate content of the electrolyte as created by atmospheric equilibrium only decreases the typical size of the crystallites by increasing the amount of carbonate-substituted HA of the b type (i.e., CO_3^{2-} substituting OH^- ions). With a further increase in the carbonate content, aragonite and calcite are also detected.

9.2.3.2 Potentiostatic Processing

The ground work in the use of potentiostatic conditions for the deposition of CPP has been laid by Shirkhanzadeh et al., who between 1991 and 1998 published at least nine articles in this field [7–9, 25, 32, 36–39]. Typically, their experiments were run with potentials between –1.4 and –1.6 V_{SCE} at 65°C in an electrolyte with 21 mM Ca and 12.5 mM PO_4 and pH 4.4. Their first experiments [25, 36], however, were performed with electrolyte solutions prepared by dissolution of CaP tribasic powder (20 g/L) in 1 M NaCl solution, resulting in coatings that formed interlocking networks of nonoriented plate-like crystals with the largest dimensions 2 to 5 μm, as shown Fig. 9.2a. With a deposition temperature of 25°C, the coating morphology did not change; the size of the crystals, however, increased to about 40 μm (Fig. 9.2b).

Using the deposition conditions mentioned above (21 mM Ca, 12.5 mM PO_4, pH 4.4, 65°C), a series of articles were published where (1) coatings were

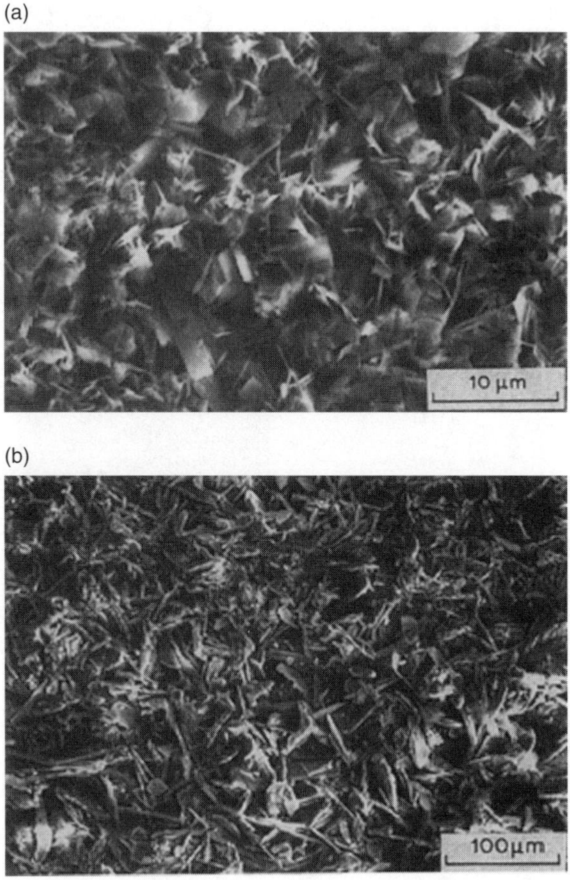

Fig. 9.2 Influence of temperature on the morphology of CPP coatings deposited from electrolytes prepared by dissolution of CaP tribasic powder (pH 4.4). **a** Deposition at 65°C. **b** Deposition at 25°C. From [25], with permission

investigated in detail by XRD and Fourier transform infrared (FTIR) spectroscopy [7]; (2) fluorinated CPPs were deposited by working with a F^- concentration of 1 mM [8, 9]; (3) coatings were loaded with Ag ions after the ECAD process [38]; (4) coatings were deposited on porous substrates of Co-Cr-MO (ASTM F-75) [8]; and (5) deposited coatings were loaded with vesicles from mussel adhesive protein [32]. As concluded from XRD investigations [7], the coatings consist of poorly crystalline, Ca-deficient HA with a crystal size of about 35 nm. Coatings prepared in fluoride-containing electrolytes had slightly different FTIR spectra, with a new peak at 3540 cm^{-1} and a shift of the OH librational band from 632 cm^{-1} to 735 cm^{-1} [8, 9], indicating the formation of fluoride-containing phases.

Benhayoune et al. [5] and Montero-Ocampo et al. [4] used conditions similar to those of Shirkhanzadeh [8] and prepared coatings under N_2 atmosphere. Working at –1.6 V_{SCE}, brushite was formed [5] and converted to HA under hydrothermal conditions similar to those used by Han et al. [24]. Montero-Ocampo et al. varied the substrate potential between –1.6 and

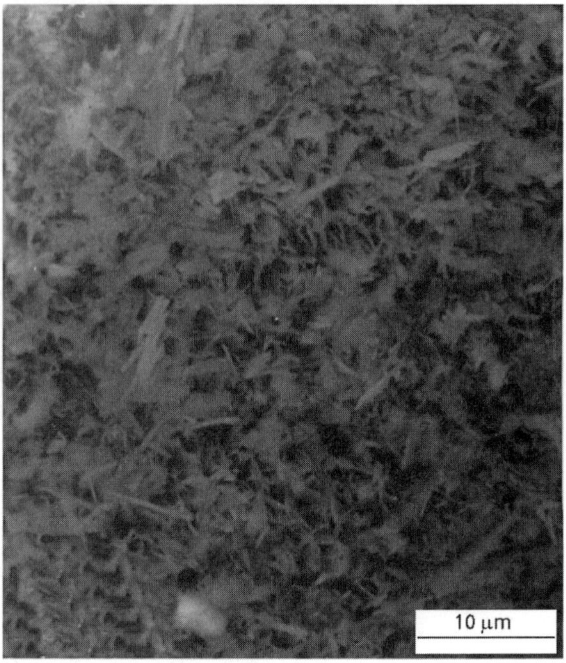

Fig. 9.3 CPP coating deposited at pH 4.2 with $-1.4\ V_{SCE}$ at 85°C for 120 minutes. From [37], with permission

$2.0\ V_{SCE}$; for -1.6 V, the coatings were given as $Ca_3(PO_4)_2 \cdot n\ H_2O$, called TCP; whereas for the more negative potential, hexagonal HA was detected as the main phase.

Holding the potential constant at $-1.4\ V_{SCE}$, Shirkhanzadeh [37] varied the Ca concentration between 20 and 0.61 mM (corresponding to pH values of the electrolytes between 4.2 and 6.0) with a constant Ca/PO_4 ratio of 1.67. Starting with relatively large plate-like crystals in the range of 4 to 6 μm at pH 4.2 (Fig. 9.3), the morphology of the coatings changed to fine crystals (not described closer either in shape or size) at pH 6.0 (Fig. 9.4). Coatings prepared at pH 4.2 exhibited apatitic characteristics in the XRD diffraction pattern; but because OCP-like structures could not be excluded, these coatings are likely to have had a composition different from that of HA. Coatings prepared at pH 6.0, however, gave clear evidence of HA layers according to both electron diffraction and XRD data.

Experiments with higher ionic strength electrolyte using potentiostatic polarization of $-2\ V_{SCE}$ at 22°C were performed by Ban and Maruno [40]. They used 37.8 mM NaCl, 2.4 to 4.0 mM Ca, and 1.0 to 2.5 mM PO_4 with resulting Ca/PO_4 ratios between 1.0 and 4.0. Furthermore, they added 50 mM trishydroxyaminomethane to avoid an increase in bulk pH and thus homogeneous nucleation within the electrolyte. The presence of trishydroxyaminomethane did not change the morphology or the Ca/P ratio of the coatings, but the amount of CPP deposited at low Ca/PO_4 ratios was increased by a factor of 10. Scanning electron microscopy (SEM) images show globular precipitates

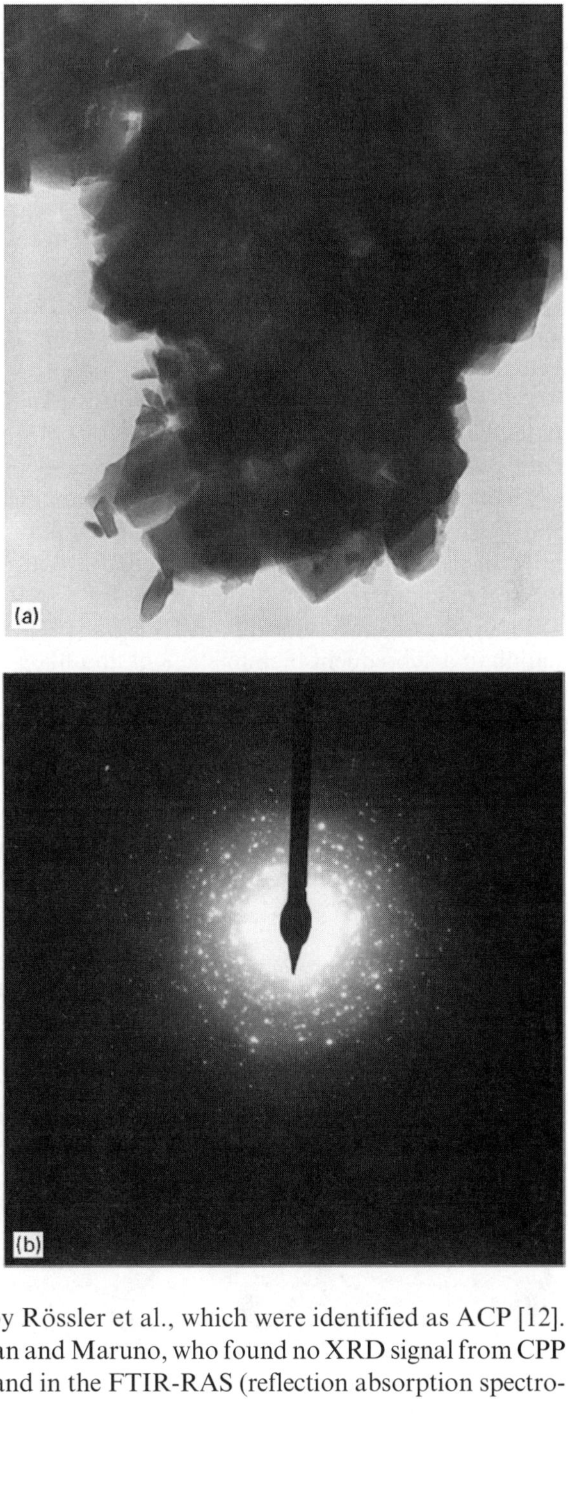

Fig. 9.4 Transmission electron microscopy (TEM) image (**a**) and electron diffraction pattern (**b**) of coating material deposited at pH 6.0 with $-1.4\ V_{SCE}$ at 85°C for 120 minutes. From [37], with permission

similar to those observed by Rössler et al., which were identified as ACP [12]. This is in agreement with Ban and Maruno, who found no XRD signal from CPP but a badly resolved PO_4 band in the FTIR-RAS (reflection absorption spectroscopy) spectra.

In the same basic electrolyte system with Ca and PO_4 concentrations constant at 2.5 and 1.0 mM, respectively, but with the inclusion of SBF instead of NaCl, Ban and Maruno [13] studied the influence of temperature and deposition time on the formation of CPP layers on titanium. Coatings produced at temperatures up to 37°C were amorphous, whereas higher temperatures led to the formation of HA with low crystallinity. Based on solution analysis after dissolution of the coatings (Ca + Mg)/PO_4 ratios between 1.0 and 1.7 were determined, with small ratios for low temperatures and short deposition times and vice versa.

An article published by Neumann et al. [41], which described applying conditions analogous to those used by Shirkhanzadeh [25, 42], may be considered the starting point of the BONIT® process. The deposit prepared on X5CrNi8.10 and Ti6Al4V substrates consists of separate 10 to 25 μm long, plate-like crystals. In their later articles [19, 43] the coatings (Fig. 9.5) are identified as single-phase brushite, but no exact deposition conditions are given.

Zhang et al. [10, 44] combined the ECAD method with the formation of CPP coatings by soaking in SBF following the Kokubo process [45–47] and compared the resultant coatings. Using an SBF solution with pH 6.0 as electrolyte and cathodic polarization at 1.625 V_{SCE} for 5 to 10 minutes at room temperature [10], they formed amorphous CPP films that greatly enhanced CPP formation in a subsequent biomimetic Kokubo-like process, resulting in coatings of OCP irrespective of the time of exposure to SBF. On porous titanium, both CPP coatings deposited from a NaCl-based electrolyte (pH 7.4, polarization at –1.425 V_{SCE}) and coatings prepared according to the Kokubo process (BD)

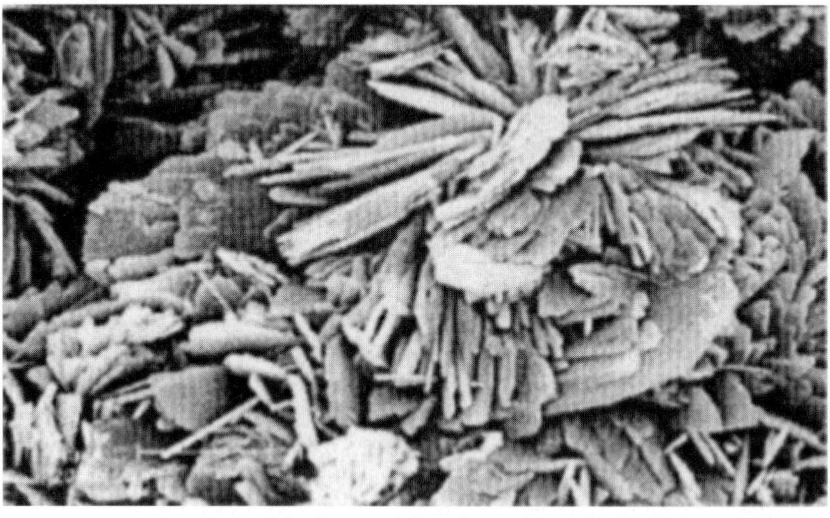

Fig. 9.5 Scanning electron microscopy (SEM) image of the initial coating deposited at room temperature. From [43], with permission

formed homogeneous, pure OCP layers. The BD coatings were comparatively uniform in thickness, whereas the ECAD coatings showed a thickness of only 5 to 10 μm in the pores of the substrate but about 20 μm on the outer surfaces, corroborating the diffusion control of the ECAD process.

9.2.3.3 Galvanostatic Processing

Because of the constant current used for galvanostatic processing, the amount of OH ions formed is also constant. As this gives the best control over the ECAD process and consequently the most reliable results, galvanostatic processing has been used for a number of detailed investigations on the structure and composition of CPP coatings. Among the parameters studied were the (1) current density, (2) pH, (3) polarization time, (4) electrolyte composition, and (5) temperature.

Redepenning and McIsaac [17], in 1990, were the first to use the ECAD method under galvanostatic conditions. Working at room temperature in saturated solutions of $Ca(H_2PO_4)_2$ at pH 3.5, they used current densities up to 10 mA/cm^2. Under all conditions, only plate-like brushite was detected, with the crystal size increasing with decreasing current density. The authors also performed the first experiments coating titanium mesh on stems of commercially available hip implants, demonstrating the potential of the ECAD process for generating a homogeneous coating on substrates with complex geometries (Fig. 9.6). Later, the same group [11], using current densities up to 50 mA/cm^2, showed that the current efficiency goes through a maximum for values between 3 and 8 mA/cm^2.

To transform the brushite prepared by ECAD into HA, the coatings were exposed to 0.1 M NaOH at different temperatures by Redepenning, whereas Shirkhanzadeh and Azadegan [48] used 1 mM $Ca(OH)_2$ solution at 70°C for 30 minutes. Kumar et al. [18] formed brushite coatings with an electrolyte similar to that described by Redepenning et al. [11], and for transformation they used different media including deionized water and various versions of Hank's balanced solution at room temperature. SEM images [11] show that the macroscopic morphology of brushite remains unchanged by the conversion except for a small degree of remodeling.

Monma et al. [28] used a similar electrolyte with $NaNO_3$ (1.65 M) instead of KCl and 24 mM fluoride. Working at elevated temperatures (mostly 80°C), they deposited apatite crystals with a morphology of ellipsoidal rods with a conical head. With increasing deposition time these changed first to hexagonal pyramidal rods, initially with pointed and later with flat ends, and then to hexagonal prismatic rods. As shown by TEM and electron diffraction studies, the apatite crystals are elongated in the [001] direction and surrounded with the (100) planes of the apatite structure.

Two groups performed detailed investigations on the influence of current density, deposition time [12, 14, 15, 34, 49–51], temperature [14, 15, 49], and electrolyte composition [12, 34, 50, 51] on the growth kinetics and composition

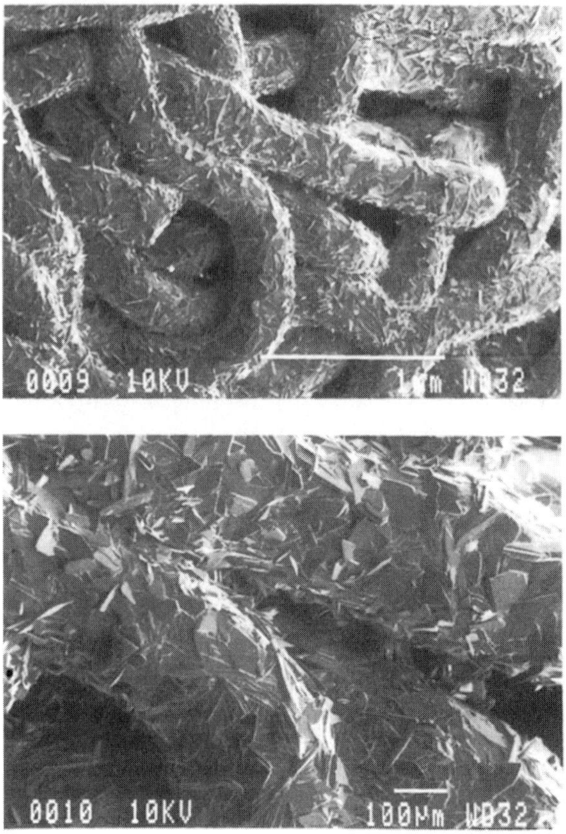

Fig. 9.6 Brushite coating prepared by Redepenning and McIsaac on titanium mesh. From [17], with permission

of ECAD-formed CPP layers. Whereas the electrolyte conditions used by both groups are rather similar (2.5 mM Ca/1.67 mM P/pH 7.2 or 1.67 mM Ca/1 mM P/pH 6.4) with a higher relative supersaturation for Bans electrolyte, different temperatures were used (Ban et al. 52°C; our group 36°C). These differences in the process temperature significantly influenced the deposited mass of CPP as a function of time and current density. Ban et al. [49] detected OCP coatings for a current density of 1.3 mA/cm^2, which changes to HA with increasing deposition time and process temperature. As shown in Figs. 9.7 and 9.8, the change from OCP to HA as a function of time (Fig. 9.7) is accompanied by significant changes in the morphology of the coatings (Fig. 9.8): from a fine, cauliflower-like appearance to much larger, plate-like crystals. For a current density of 12.9 mA/cm^2, the authors detected only HA irrespective of temperature or deposition time. The carbonate content of the deposited HA decreased from about 2.5% to 1.3% with temperatures increasing from 52° to 92°C.

Using the same electrolyte and hydrothermal conditions (80°–200°C), there was no major change in crystal morphology; temperature changed the needle-like

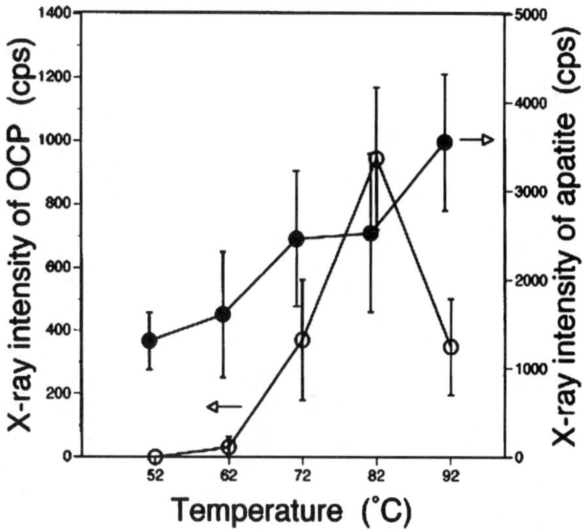

Fig. 9.7 Intensities of signals assigned to octa-CaP (*OCP*) and hydroxyapatite (HA) for coatings prepared for 1 hour at a current density of 1.3 mA/cm^2 as a function of the electrolyte temperature. From [14], with permission

hexagonal crystals only in longitudinal length [15]. However, the Ca/PO_4 ratio of the deposits increased from about 1.35 for 80°C to about 1.65 for 200°. From 80°C to 150°C, the deposited mass concomitantly increased by a factor of nearly five and decreased again slightly for higher temperatures. Although the authors failed to explain the change in the Ca/PO_4 ratio, the dependence of layer mass on the temperature is explained as a superposition of several effects such as the temperature-dependent solubility of HA and the change in pH due to increasing solubility of the electrolyte for H_2. Moreover, the lower pH in the growth region of the crystals is due to the longer distance from substrate surface and thus the source of OH ions. For this reason, it is of importance only for CPP formation on the outside of thicker layers.

In contrast to Ban's findings given above, in the investigations of Rössler et al. [12] and Sewing at al. [34] the initial phase of the deposition process of the CPP coatings does not depend on the current density but always starts with the formation of a CPP base layer (investigated range 0.5–10.0 mA/cm^2). For a current density of 1 mA/cm^2, small islands formed after 5 seconds with diameters < 15 nm. After 15 seconds, the surface was completely covered with a thickness of about 6 nm (Fig. 9.9).

Because no favored sites of nucleation were observed for diverse surface structures, roughness, or the α- and β-phase in the case of the titanium alloy Ti6Al4V, nucleation does not appear to be site-specific and probably occurs close to the substrate surface in homogeneous solutions. Analysis of the electrolyte showed that further growth of the nuclei occurs only after they are deposited on the substrate surface. Nuclei that do not reach the surface dissolve again.

With increasing deposition time (10 minutes), spherical deposits with typical diameters of 100 to 200 nm are formed atop this base layer (Fig. 9.10). In TEM

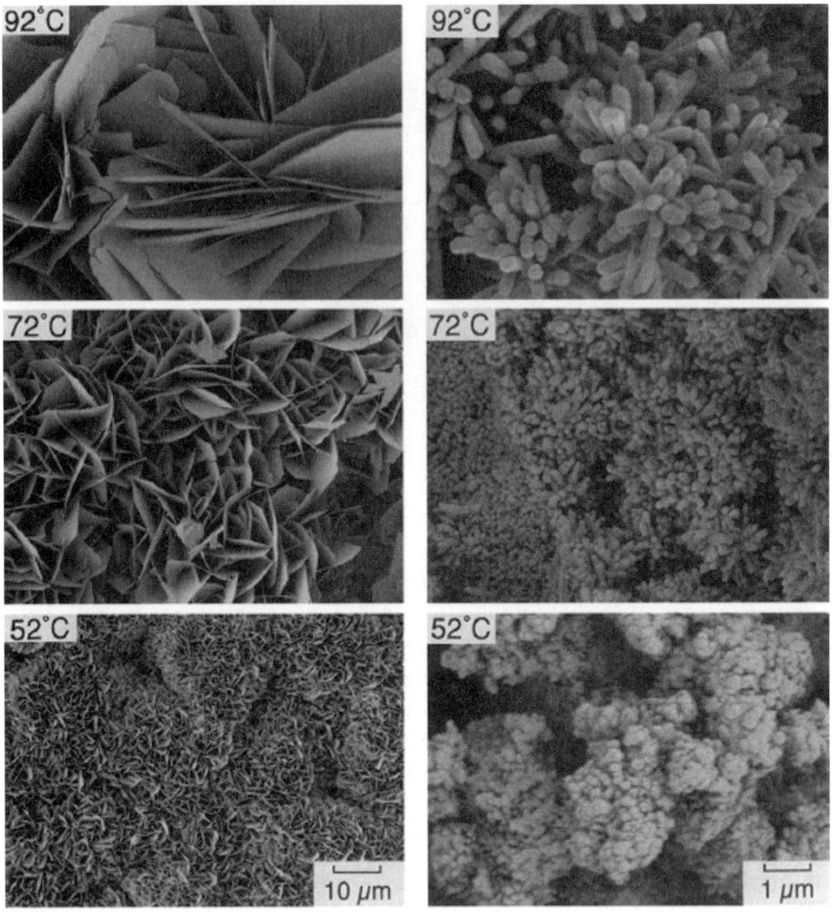

Fig. 9.8 Field emission (FE)-SEM micrographs of deposits prepared for 1 hour with current densities of 1.3 mA/cm^2 (*left*) and 12.9 mA/cm^2 (*right*) at electrolyte temperatures of 52°, 72°, and 92°C. From [14], with permission

diffraction studies and FTIR investigations (Fig. 9.10), these globuli were identified as amorphous CaP ACP ($Ca_3(PO_4)_2 \cdot n\, H_2O$) with a clustered spherical substructure in the globules. Continuous irradiation by the TEM electron beam causes thermal fluctuations in these substructures and finally results in rupture of the globules and the onset of crystallization (Fig. 9.11b), both indicating a high water content in the spheres.

The above formula for amorphous CaP is supported by chemical analysis of CPP layers generated for various current densities and deposition times where, irrespective of the applied current density, the Ca/PO_4 ratio for short deposition times was 1.5. With a further increase in deposition time, the first crystalline phases start to appear. Formation of the nanocrystalline HA seems to start

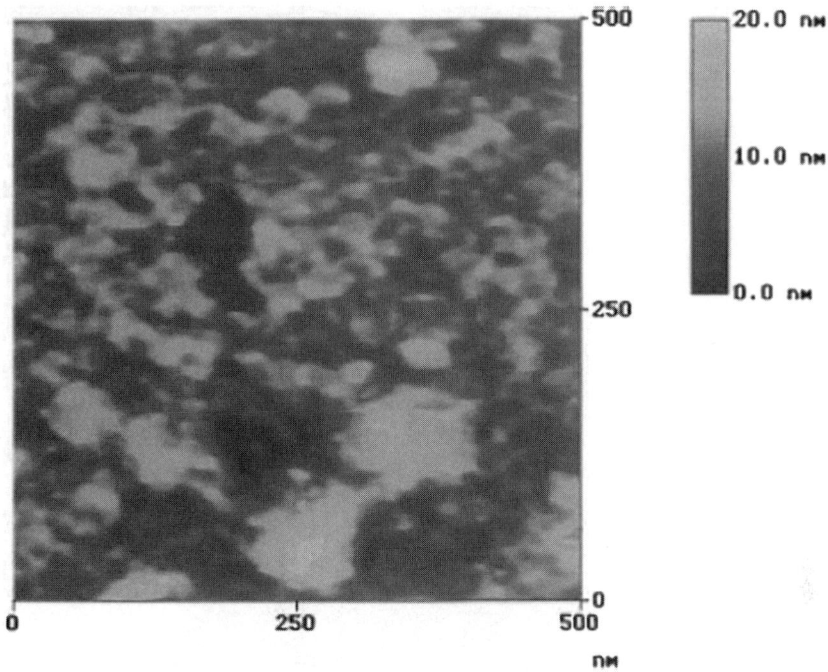

Fig. 9.9 Atomic force microscopy (AFM) image of a titanium surface after cathodic polarization at –1 mA/cm^2 for 15 seconds. It shows complete coverage with amorphous CaP (ACP) at the substrate surface with a thickness of about 6 nm (including the thicker islands). From [12], with permission

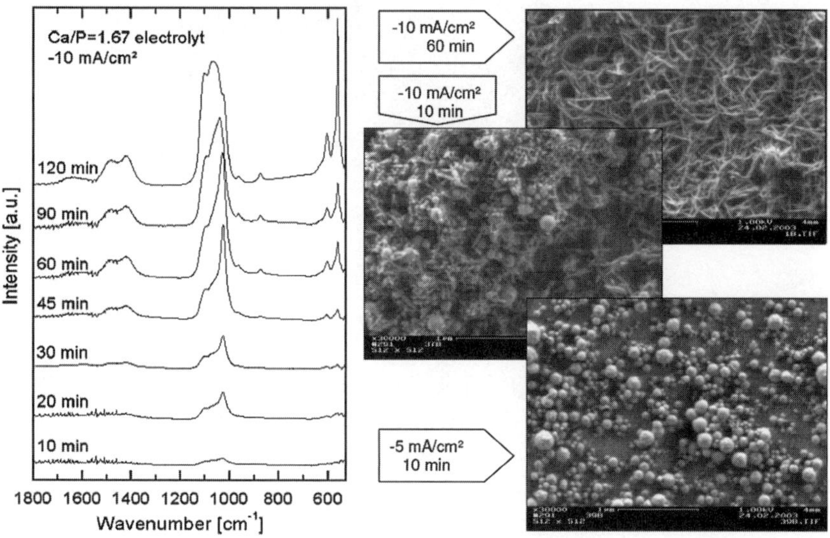

Fig. 9.10 Coating morphology (*right*) and respective Fourier transform infrared (FTIR) spectra (*left*) for various current densities and deposition times. From [34], with permission

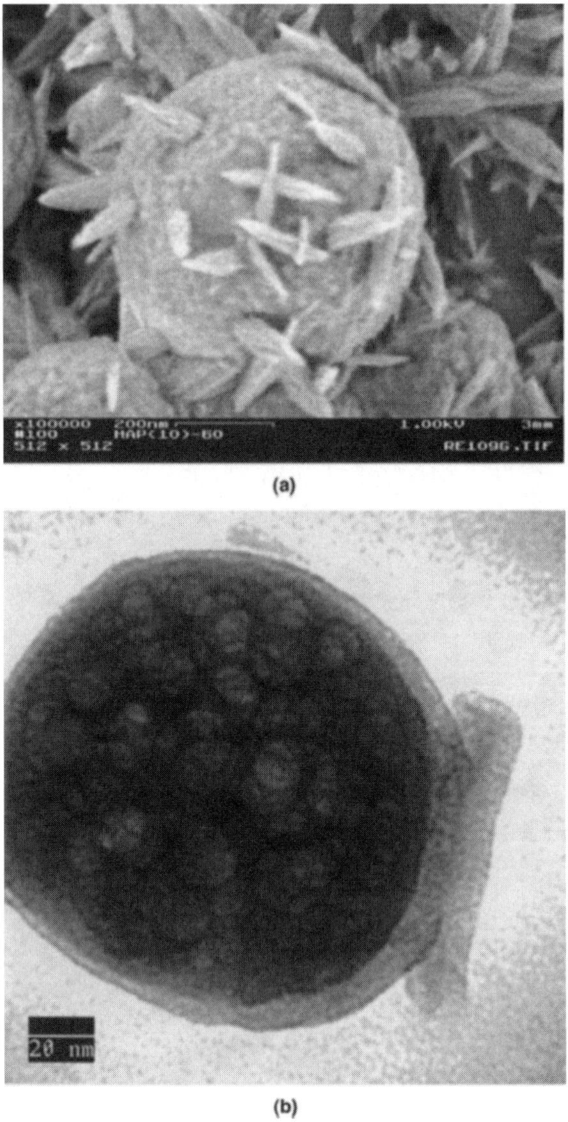

Fig. 9.11 Amorphous CaP (ACP) sphere with starting crystallization into HA on titanium for –10 mA/cm^2 and 15 minutes deposition time. **a** SEM image. **b** TEM micrograph. From [12], with permission

directly on the surfaces of ACP spheres as well as on the initially formed CPP layer (Fig. 9.11a), which probably also consists of ACP. Following the suggestions of Johnsson and Nancollas [52], the formation of HA from ACP can thus be described by the following Eq. 9.8 as a transformation into a crystalline product accompanied by dehydration.

$$3Ca_3(PO_4)_2 \cdot nH_2O + Ca^{2+} + 2OH^- \rightarrow Ca_{10}(PO_4)_6(OH)_2 + 3nH_2O \quad (9.8)$$

With continuing polarization the substrate surface is finally completely covered with needle-like HA crystals with typical dimensions of < 500 nm length and < 60 nm diameter (Fig. 9.10).

The FTIR spectra and SEM images in Fig. 9.10 reflect the changes in the deposited CPP coatings as a function of deposition time and applied current density. The phase diagrams given in Fig. 9.12 describe the main components of the deposited coatings as a function of the deposition time and current density. Figure 9.12b shows further the influence of a parameter not discussed until

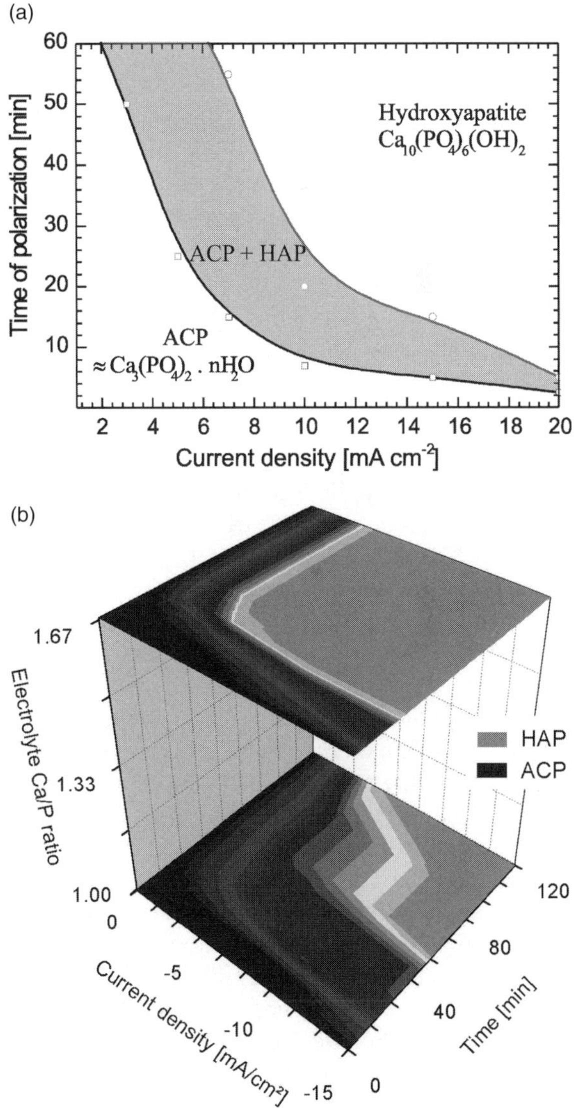

Fig. 9.12 Phase diagrams of the composition of ECAD CPP layers as identified by SEM and FTIR as a function of current density and deposition time. **a** For 1.67 mM Ca and 1 mM PO_4. *ACP*, amorphous CaP; *HAP*, hydroxyapatite. From [12], with permission. **b** For 1 mM PO_4 and Ca/PO_4 ratios between 1.00 and 1.67. From [34], with permission

now – the effect of the Ca/PO_4 ratio on the onset of HA crystal formation starting from an ACP coating. It seems to delay the transformation process of ACP to HA, resulting in a much larger parameter field where ACP and HA coexist (the range of different levels of gray between the black ACP area and the light gray HAP area in the lower plane of Fig. 9.12b).

LeGeros' group described a pulsed galvanostatic method with currents between 4 and 14 mA/cm^2 to improve the adhesion behavior of CPP coatings on different substrates (Ti6Al4V and Co-Cr alloy) [53–56]. Working mostly at 60°C with on/off times between 5 and 40 seconds and typically of equal duration, depending on the current density coatings from OCP [53], HA and fluoride-substituted apatite [54] were deposited. The crystal size of the CPP decreased with current density and pulse time.

Using conditions similar to those described by Ban et al. (2.5 mM Ca, 1.5 mM PO_4, 80°C), Lu et al. [6] studied the influence of the gas atmosphere on the deposition of CPP around pH 4.5. Coating morphology changed from submicrometer needles of HA for an N_2 atmosphere to plate-like OCP crystals, some micrometers in size, in a pure CO_2 atmosphere, with no changes detected as a function of the deposition time (30–60 minutes). Based on this result, Lu et al. were able to produce layered coatings from OCP and HA by changing the atmosphere during deposition. Working under air, deposition starts with HA for $t < 30$ minutes, which transforms to OCP for longer deposition times.

9.2.3.4 Summary

Application of the ECAD process for the deposition of CPP on metallic biomaterials accounts for nearly 70 publications since 1990, cited in ISI Web of Science® and/or PubMed (Fig. 9.13). Whereas experiments performed under potentiostatic conditions dominated during the early years, the galvanostatic processing has been preferred in later publications because of its advantages and applicability for industrial purposes.

Electrolytes with relatively high Ca and phosphate concentrations and thus comparatively low pH values (3.54.5) yielded deposition of brushite. As HA is the main inorganic component of bone, methods for the transformation of brushite to HA were developed, among them soaking in NaOH solutions or hydrothermal processes, sometimes followed by thermal processing to improve adhesion of the coatings. Later studies investigated the influence of process temperature, electrochemical conditions, and composition as well as the pH of the electrolyte in great detail, finally allowing direct deposition of HA coatings, although mostly at temperatures above body temperature.

With detailed data on the temporal development of the phase composition of coatings, the direct deposition of brushite, OCP, ACP, and apatites of different composition (carbonate, fluoride) is now well established. Especially for apatites, stable processing conditions are available for the deposition of nanocrystalline layers with highly specific surface areas. These coatings can be

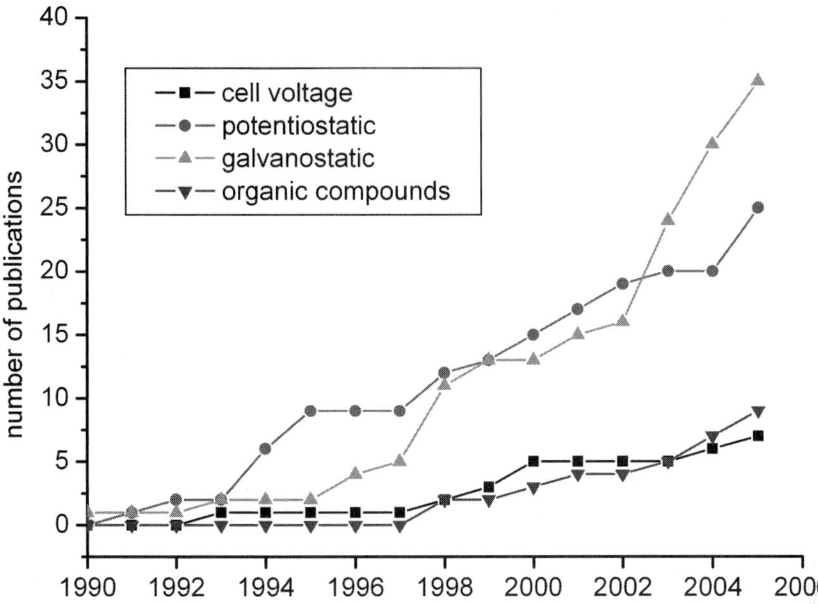

Fig. 9.13 Publications on the use of the ECAD process for coating metallic biomaterials with CPP. Publications performing co-deposition with organic components are also counted in the respective method

applied to substrates with structured surfaces on the submicrometer level with hardly any change in the surface morphology.

9.2.4 Formation of Composite Coatings

Composite coatings can be produced based on the ECAD process in two ways. The first method is to start with the deposition of pure CPP and then expose the coating to solutions of the second component. Depending on the stability of the coating, the second component is then either incorporated into (partial) dissolution/redeposition of the coating or adsorbed to the stable CPP. Usually the latter, especially, results in fast, uncontrolled release.

The second way to form composite coatings is co-deposition already in the ECAD process with the advantage of a single process step and incorporation of the second component. However, greater care has to be taken with the ECAD conditions if temperature- or pH-sensitive organic components such as proteins are used.

Although only a few articles have been published on composite coatings including inorganic components [20, 38, 57, 58], an increasing number of publications deal with the formation of coatings containing organic components, with the main focus on proteins [1, 32, 35, 59] and chitosan [22, 60].

9.2.4.1 Composite Coatings with Inorganic Additives

The doping of CPP coatings with silver ions by exposure to silver nitrate solutions has been investigated by Shirkanzadeh et al. [38, 58]. The release kinetics of the ions that are assumed to replace Ca ions in the coatings show about 50% elution after 1 day in SBF at 37°C and another 15% after 7 days. Under these conditions, the silver content of the coatings favors transformation into carbonate-containing HA, something discussed as a possible enhancement of bone-bonding properties.

A process similar to the co-deposition of cermets has been applied by Dasarathy et al. [57] to prepare coatings from HA and cobalt on titanium substrates aiming to form strongly adhesive coatings. The adhesion strength of the layers, as determined by a Sebastian five bond tester, was 10.7 ± 5.4 MPa, which was significantly lower than for pure cobalt coatings (50.6 ± 5.5 MPa) prepared under similar conditions. The HA coverage as determined from SEM image analysis was approximately >50% for all grain sizes, with a high variance in the order of ± 20%. Smaller particles gave lower values but more homogeneous coatings with better adhesion.

Zhang et al. [20] formed similar composite coatings from cobalt and CPP by the potentiostatic deposition of cobalt following the galvanostatic ECAD process. Quite homogeneous coating (at the micrometer level) with Co contents of 12 to 33 wt% were obtained. Bonding strength values were 6.7 ± 24.4 to 20.4 ± 3.1 MPa, which is twofold higher than the highest values found by Dasarathy et al. [57].

9.2.4.2 Composite Coatings with Organic Additives

Shirkhanzadeh and Liu [39] investigated the adsorption of L-lysine to CPP layers prepared by ECAD at 85°C under condition similar to those used for the integration of silver [38, 58]. FTIR detected no phases other than HA, indicating that lysine adsorption did not affect the CPP coating. The lysine spectra changed, however, which is interpreted as hydrogen bonding between C=O groups of the lysine and polar OH groups in the hydration layer of the HA. Although desorption behavior of the amino acid has not been investigated, adsorption was shown to reach an equilibrium after about 5 minutes.

Shirkhanzadeh [61] prepared CPP coatings on acupuncture needles with the goal of immobilizing α-D-glucopyranosyl-α-D-glucopyranoside (trehalose), as this component stabilizes protein structures. Depending on the electrolyte conditions, the composition of the coatings changed: Decreasing Ca concentrations gave rise to more resolved and intense FTIR bands corresponding to HA, whereas higher Ca concentrations resulted in mixtures of OCP and HA.

Hurteaux et al. [62] allowed that alginate from a 3 wt% solution adsorbs to preformed CPP coatings. In scanning transmission electron microscopy (STEM) investigations, the authors found three layers: CPP coating, alginate layer, and a homogeneous interface of about 2 μm thickness. Applications of such layered structures as drug delivery system for bioactive molecules were envisaged by the authors.

First attempts to use the ECAD process to form composite coatings containing collagen, the organic main component of bone, can be traced back to a study by Okamura et al. [35]. Working in electrolytes of low pH (2.1–3.3), they added unspecified collagens. From ESR investigations after irradiation with x-rays, they conclude that hydrogen bonds exist between H^+ in HPO_4^{2-} groups of the defective apatite and carbonyl groups of collagen. This is taken as an indication that HA–collagen compound layers formed.

In more detailed experiments, Rössler et al. [1] adsorbed fibrils from collagen type I on a HA layer prepared by the ECAD process and then mineralized this collagen again using ECAD at 36°C with HA. Because of the short polarization time, the collagen structures remained visible in SEM investigations (Fig. 9.14). The characteristic banding pattern of collagen fibrils (63–67 nm) remained visible, but no periodic correlation of HA crystals with the banding pattern was found. FTIR spectra of the HA–collagen coating can be interpreted as a superposition of pure HA and collagen, but a broadening and shift to lower wave numbers for the amide-I band in the mineralized coating corresponds well with the broad amide-I band of bone, indicating an interaction between the two components of this coating analogous to the situation *in vivo*.

Contrary to the two-step method chosen above, Fan et al. [59] added acid-soluble collagen type I to the deposition electrolyte and performed ECAD at 30°C, intending to combine fibrillogenesis of collagen with deposition of CPP. Typical layer morphologies for variable deposition times are shown in Fig. 9.15. Starting with a thin basic layer after 5 minutes (Fig. 9.15a), a three-dimensional porous network of mineralized collagen fibers formed. Crystal clusters 300–500 nm in size seem to nucleate on the collagen fibers and increase in number with the deposition duration and ion concentration of the electrolyte.

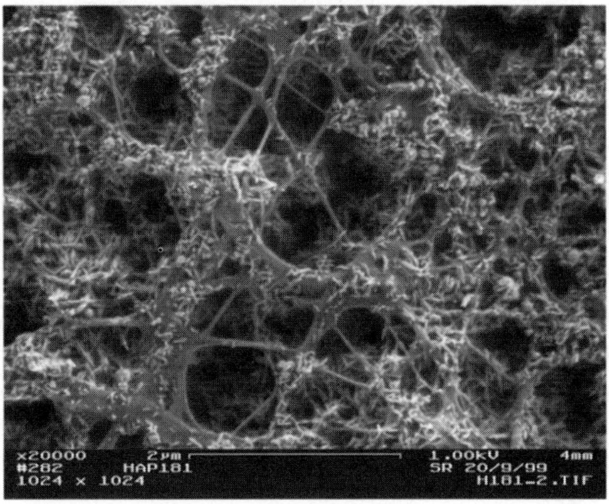

Fig. 9.14 Mineralized fibrillar collagen type I derived by ECAD formation of HA onto collagen adsorbed to a preformed HA base coating. From [1], with permission

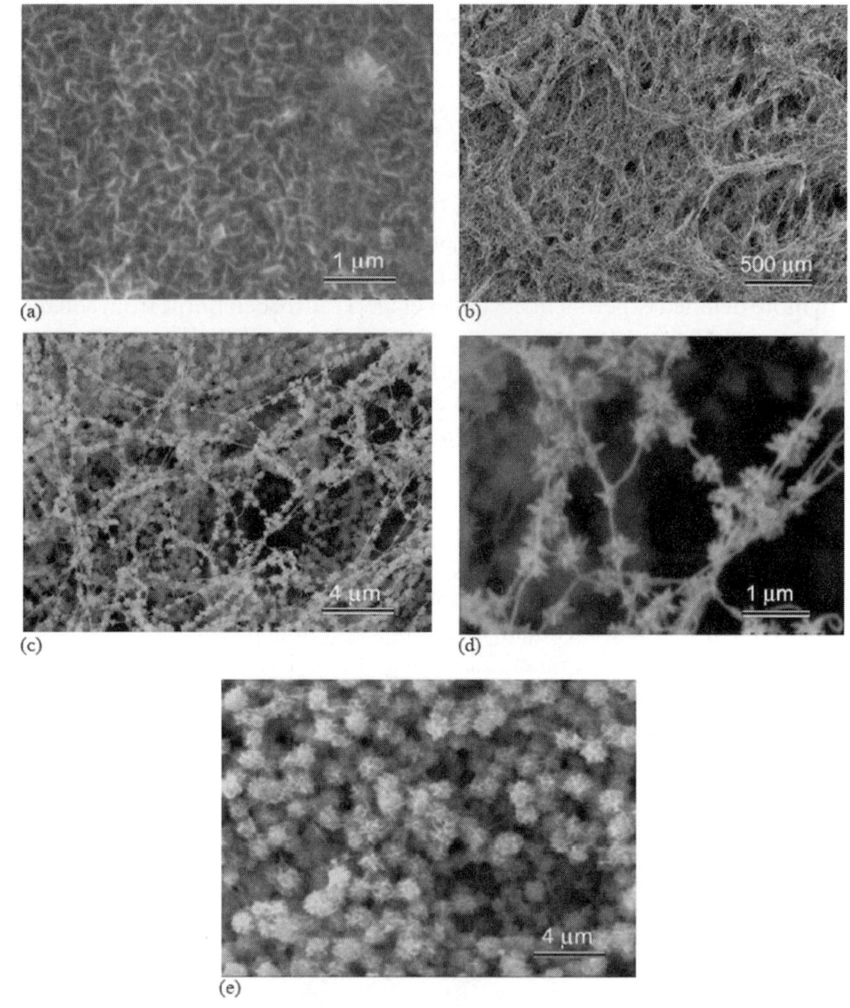

Fig. 9.15 SEM images of collagen–OCP composite coatings. (**a**) Thin initial CPP basic layer formed within 5 minutes. (**b**) Uniform coating formed within 30 minutes at low magnification. (**c, d**) Crystal clusters associated with collagen fibrils after 30 minutes with higher magnification. (**e**) Highly mineralized composite after 60 minutes of polarization. From [59], with permission

The final CPP deposit consists of flake-like crystals identified as OCP. No banding of the collagen fibres could be shown, indicating that the self-assembly of tropocollagen to supramolecular structures under the chosen conditions does not result in the formation of fibrils with native substructure.

Similar to Fan, Cheng et al. [63] performed the ECAD process in the presence of a protein. The aim in this case was the inclusion of potential therapeutic agents into CPP layers for sustained release. Bovine serum albumin

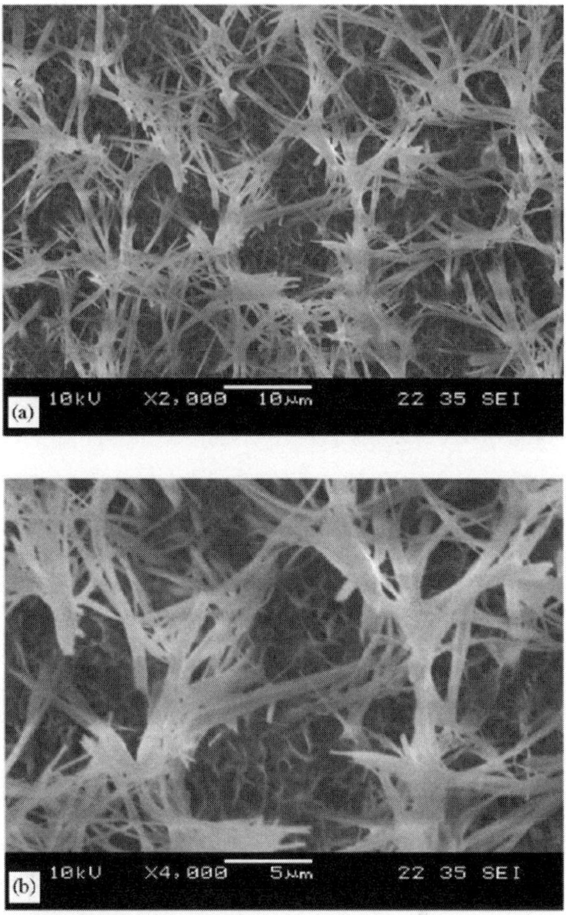

Fig. 9.16 SEM images of coating containing bovine serum albumin (BSA) prepared as described in the text. From [63], with permission

(BSA) was used as a model protein and co-deposited with brushite on pre-formed HA layers. These layers were prepared by ECAD from an electrolyte similar to a process described elsewhere [3, 64, 65]. Coatings prepared by this method with an overall process time of 3 days are shown in Fig. 9.16. Of the protein added, at least 85% was stably incorporated into the layers, resulting in a surprisingly high protein content of 500 µg/cm^2 in layers with a total mass of 3.3 mg/cm^2. By comparison, adsorption of BSA resulted in only ~7 µg BSA/cm^2, which was quickly desorbed within about 2 hours.

Redepenning et al. [22] and Wang et al. [30] described co-deposition of CPP with chitosan. Chitosan–brushite composite coatings obtained under conditions similar to former experiments of the Redepenning group [11, 17] were converted to chitosan–HA coatings by immersion in 0.1 M NaOH. Thermogravimetric analysis of these coatings gave chitosan contents between 1.2 and 16 wt%.

Wang et al. [30] performed detailed experiments in electrolytes based on various simulated physiological solutions in galvanostatic mode with additions of chitosan (0–0.2 g/L). In the SEM images, CPP and chitosan are clearly visible as different phases for all deposition times. XRD and FTIR results indicate that carbonated HA is formed first, with OCP appearing after 3 hours of deposition, with the maximum after 6 hours. After 12 hours, carbonated HA is the main component of the coatings, with minor amounts of OCP. Neither XRD nor FTIR results give clear evidence of chitosan in the coatings, which was determined by thermogravimetry to be in the range of 2% to 5% (depending on the chitosan concentration in the deposition electrolyte and the current density used).

With the main focus on adhesion between the CPP coating and the substrate, Hu et al. [29] performed the ECAD process in electrolytes containing 0.0125 vol% of vinyl acetate. The co-deposition was confirmed by XPS analysis and was assumed to proceed via polymerization, which is induced by hydrogen radicals formed on the cathode surface. Interestingly, the authors found well defined HA crystals as early as 30 seconds (Fig. 9.17), contrary to Rössler et al.

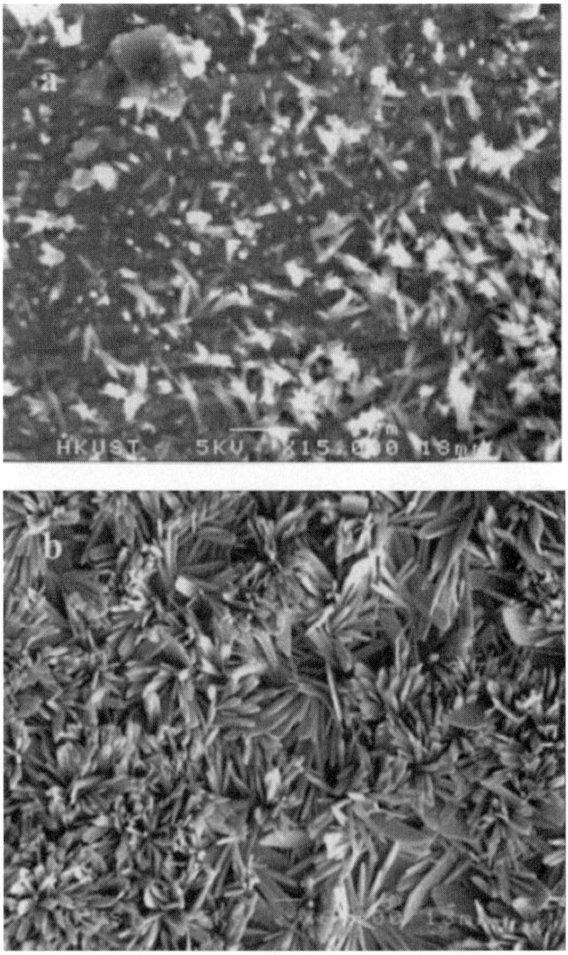

Fig. 9.17 SEM images of HA coating obtained in the presence of vinyl acetate for deposition times of 30 seconds (**a**) and > 30 minutes (**b**). From [29], with permission

[12] and Sewing at al. [34], who in similar electrolytes found only ACP after short times. However, these differences may possibly be explained by the different temperatures used, with 80°C in this work compared to 37°C in the latter two studies [12, 34].

9.2.4.3 Summary

The first experiments concerning the deposition of collagen and its mineralization were published after ECAD allowed deposition of HA at body temperature in 1998. The aim was to obtain a coating more bone-like than pure HA and with a better biological effect. As was shown in Chapter 7, these coatings have been successfully tested in cell culture and animal experiments.

For components conformationally more unstable than collagen (i.e., growth factors), BSA has been used as a model. It must be kept in mind, though, that the ECAD process significantly increases pH at the substrate surface, which may adversely affect the conformation and thus the biological activity of unstable proteins. An alternative may be the deposition of CPP coatings with highly specific surface areas followed by the adsorption of the proteins or peptides. This method has the additional advantage that adsorptive binding can be performed from small volumes, an aspect of interest when using expensive organic compounds such as growth factors.

Apart from proteins, the co-deposition of CPP with chitosan has recently been a point of interest in some publications.

In the future, a further increase in the combination of CPP with organic components can be expected, ranging from comparatively simple components such as chlorhexidine or antibiotics to complex structures such as specifically designed artificial extracellular matrices. These structures can be composed of structural proteins, glycosaminoglycans, proteoglycans, or their derivatives, with the aim of improving osteoconductivity and even osteoinductivity of implant surfaces. Such coatings might offer improved healing chances for patients with systemic diseases such as osteoporosis and diabetes.

9.2.5 Basic Principles of the Electrophoretic Deposition Process

In contrast to the ECAD process, the electrophoretic deposition process (EPD) utilizes a CPP suspension already present in the electrolyte. An overview of the theoretical background and fundamental aspects of the method is given by Zhitomirsky [66]. As the (predominantly positively) charged particles have to be moved to the substrate surface by means of an electrical field, the "current efficiency" is much higher for the EPD process than for ECAD. Because the deposition rate is proportional to the strength of the electric field, fields in the range of ~10 V/cm are applied [67–70]. To avoid gas evolution at the electrodes, nonaqueous solutions are used for suspension of the CPP particles. Isopropanol [67, 70, 71] is the most common choice, but a combination of ethanol with hexadecyltrimethylammonium bromide (CTAB) has also been used as the conducting electrolyte [69]. Typical processing times to deposit layers with coating weights in the range of about 10 mg/cm^2 are < 1 minute [67, 68], although experiments have been performed for up to 5 minutes [69, 71]. Because of the nature of the deposition process, the initial adherence of the coatings is poor. For this reason, the deposition is followed in all cases by thermal treatment (mostly in vacuum), typically at 800° to 1200°C for at least 1 hour [67, 69, 71].

Owing to the nature of the method, the lowest possible layer thickness is determined by the average diameter of particles suspended in the electrolyte. Because particle diameters generally are in the micrometer range, coatings produced by EPD commonly have a thickness of 10 to 1000 μm.

9.3 Physicochemical Properties of Thin Coatings

Concerning the brushite that was the first phase produced by the ECAD process, the question arose in the medical field if a coating consisting of brushite (not HA) could improve the bony integration of implants. The current status in this regard is that a brushite coating is commercially available as BONIT® for a number of implant surfaces in various applications.

An important difference between coatings prepared by ECAD and those resulting from plasma spraying lies in their morphology. Wheres plasma-sprayed coatings are rather monolithic, coatings from ECAD form a more or less dense aggregation of CPP crystals. Thus, the specific surface area of the coatings, which equals the contact area with the biological system, is different. A potential advantageous effect of large surface areas is the ability to adsorb larger amounts of proteins, as discussed for CPP-based bone substitute materials with highly specific surface areas [72, 73]; however, owing to the low coating mass, there are no methods for directly measuring specific surfaces. Rough calculations for HA coatings prepared according to Rössler et al. [12] gave specific surfaces areas of about 45 m^2/g. These coatings have the morphology of nanocrystalline HA crystals, as shown in Fig. 9.10 and in higher magnification in Fig. 9.21b (see later). Such HA films are highly homogeneous; and for layer masses as small as 100 μg/cm^2, they increase the total surface area by a factor of 40 compared to the geometrical surface. These values are in good agreement with those of a commercial HA sold by Merck (for SEM image see Fig. 9.18), which gave BET data of 51.5 m^2/g. This high total surface area might be one reason for the favorable biological behavior of such coatings [74].

Coating composition can be determined in various ways. Especially predominant in the reviewed literature is EDX analysis as well as ICP-OES analysis, which is performed after dissolution of the layers. Although a number of studies relied on EDX results, according to our own investigations and some more critical articles [59], analysis after dissolution of layers is needed to obtain an accurate Ca/PO_4 ratio of the coatings.

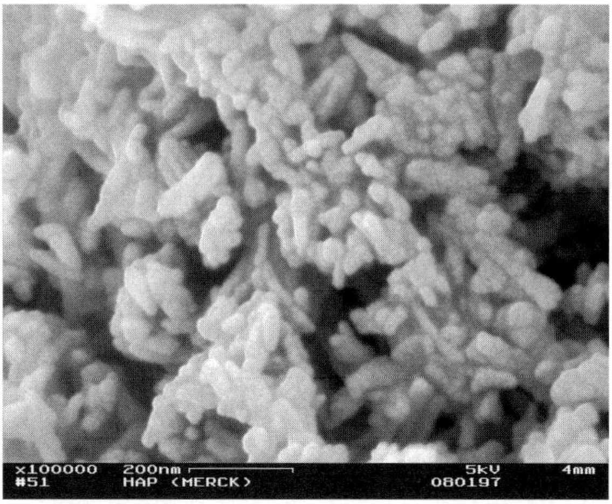

Fig. 9.18 SEM image of a commercial HA powder produced by precipitation from aqueous solution. (Merck KGaA, Darmstadt, Germany)

As described by Sewing et al. [34]. The $CaPO_4$ ratio of 1.67, which is indicative of a pure HA coating, was exceeded by the CPP layers described by Sewing et al. [34], whereas a number of other authors [42] found ratios of CPP layers much closer to that of HA. The comparatively high Ca content of their layers is explained by Sewing et al. as a result of the morphological development of the coatings. Because the local current density in the pores strongly increases with increasing surface coverage, the migration of both Ca and phosphate ions is enhanced, and the local pH increases. This, in turn, gives rise to the deposition of amorphous $Ca(OH)_2$. This phosphate-free compound explains Ca/PO_4 ratios that are higher than for HA, which is the CPP with the highest Ca/PO_4 ratio that can be produced by ECAD. Transformation of amorphous $Ca(OH)_2$ to carbonate upon exposure to air was discussed without giving details.

9.4 Mechanical Properties of Thin Coatings

To increase the adhesion strength of CPP layers, Rössler et al. [1] increased the thickness of the initial air-formed passive layer of titanium oxide (typically 3–5 nm) by combining the cathodically assisted deposition with subsequent anodic polarization (Fig. 9.19). Because anodic thickening leads to decreased pH close to the oxide surface due to hydrolysis of titanium ions, the anodic polarization (in galvanostatic mode with $+10$ mA/cm^2) was performed in 0.133 M phosphate buffer of pH 12. As the increase in oxide thickness is about 2 nm/V [75–78], an end potential of 40 V_{SCE} results in a final oxide thickness of about 80 nm. The estimated incorporation depth of the CPP into the oxide layer is about 50% of oxide thickness and thus roughly 40 nm [75, 79]. After dissolution of the HA layer in Soerensen's glycine buffer of pH 3.0, the SEM image given in Fig. 9.20 clearly shows a number of irregularly formed

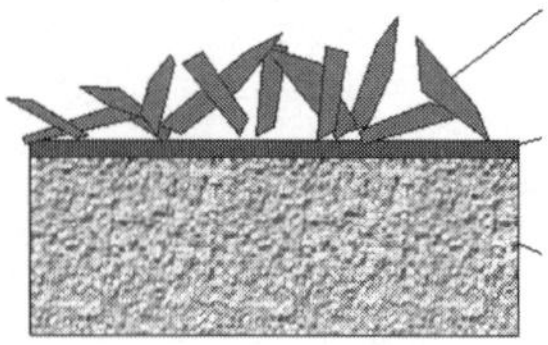

(a)

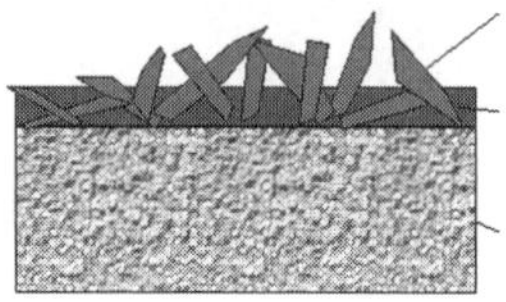

(b)

Fig. 9.19 Principle of the partial incorporation of HA into anodically thickened oxide layers on titanium materials. (**a**) Deposition of HA onto the air-formed passive layer. (**b**) Anodic thickening of the oxide layer

holes in the anodic oxide layer that associate with some remaining HA crystals. This morphology is not observed for similar oxide layers on HA free surfaces and can only be explained as imprints of HA crystals that were partially embedded in the thickening oxide layer formed during anodic polarization. This shows that it is possible to create a compound layer of titanium oxide and HA at the interface. However, no data about the adhesion strength was given.

Kumar et al. [18] studied the influence of the deposition time on bonding strengths of brushite coatings deposited from $Ca(H_2PO_4)_2$ electrolytes. As tested by the Sebastian five pull test, the bonding strength decreased for higher coating thickness, starting with 1350 psi for 10 seconds and reaching about

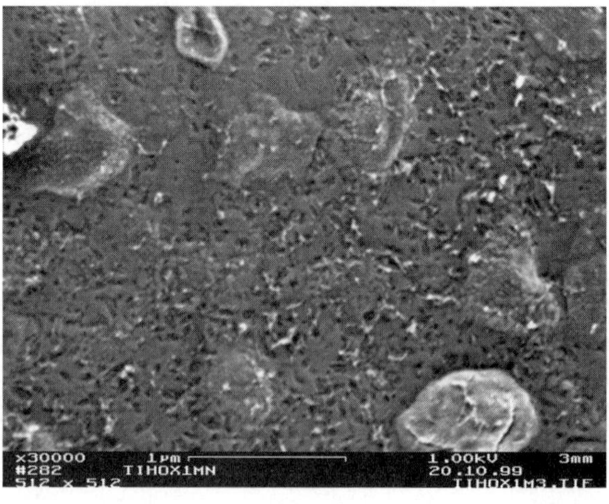

Fig. 9.20 SEM image of a surface state according to Fig. 9.19b after 300 seconds of layer degradation in Sörensen's glycine buffer pH 3.0. HA deposition and anodic oxide formation were done as described by Rössler et al. [1] and in the text. From [91], with permission

60 psi at 60 seconds. The titanium samples used were gound with 320 SiC grit paper followed by grit blasting with the same type of SiC.

Friction load curves for coatings from HA (determined from poorly resolved XRD spectra) were measured by Kuo and Yen [3] in scratch tests. For loads > 23 N, the entire coating was scraped off. From a friction of 2.85 N – corresponding to a load of 30 N – and for about 86 μm width of the scratch, the authors calculated a shear stress of about 105 MPa, which is higher than the adhesion strength of plasma-sprayed coatings (50–60 MPa).

The composite layers from HA and vinyl acetate formed by Hu et al. [29] could not be removed by the simple Scotch™ tape test, unlike their pure HA layers. In scratch and shear tests with polished substrate surfaces, the vinyl acetate containing coatings gave an adhesive strength of 3 MPa compared to only 0.5 MPa for the pure HA coating.

Lin et al. [53] performed tensile strength measurements (according to ASTM specifications for CPP coatings) with OCP coatings deposited by a pulse galvanostatic method. For Ti6Al4V with three surface morphologies (grit-blasted with apatitic abrasive, arc-deposited Ti, and chemically textured) and Co-Cr beads on a Co-Cr alloy, values ranged between 32 and 52 MPa, with the grit-blasted surface being significantly better than the others. Without details given, this surprising result is attributed to differences in the surface roughness introduced by the different treatments.

Composite layers from CPP and chitosan have been characterized regarding their adhesive strength with an automatic scratch tester by Wang et al. [30]. For chitosan contents in the coatings of 0 to 6 wt%, no significant differences were detected in the critical load forces for the first crack (~6 N) or complete delamination (11–14 N). In another study by these authors [33], the same method was used to compare coatings from OCP, carbonate apatite prepared biomimetically (soaked in simulated body fluids supersaturated with respect to CPP), and carbonate apatite prepared by the ECAD process. Significant differences of about 2 N were detected only for the critical load forces for the first crack with the OCP coating. The carbonate apatite prepared by ECAD gave the highest forces (close to 6 N) and differed at the $P < 0.05$ level from the biomimetically prepared apatite coating (close to 5 N). Values for complete delamination were in the range of 10 to 11 N for all three coatings.

Fan et al. [59] investigated the mechanical integrity of their CPP–collagen composite layers with a nanoindentation machine and determined elastic moduli and scratch test critical load values (defined as the normal load that causes the coating to fail or detach from the substrate), which are given in Table 9.2. The moduli of all coating types are low and indicate the porous structure of the coatings. When the collageneous network is not fully covered by CPP, both the modulus and the critical load for scratch failure are lower than for the pure OCP coating. Both values, however, can be greatly increased by a higher degree of mineralization.

Further experimental work on the adhesion strength of (modified) ECAD coatings is discussed in Chapter 2.4.1.

Table 9.2 Elastic modulus and scratch test critical load of various coatings

Coating	E (GPa)	Scratch critical load (mN)
OCP	0.92 ± 0.37	40.0 ± 14.7
Collagen/OCP, 30 min, 4.5 mM Ca	0.45 ± 0.14	33.6 ± 11.2
Collagen/OCP, 60 min, 12 mM Ca	1.46 ± 0.77	256.6 ± 37.6

From [59], with permission

9.5 Similarities and Differences Between Plasma-Sprayed HA and Thin CaP Coating

As already discussed at the beginning of the chapter, significant advantages of the ECAD process consist in the ability to prepare thin (< 10 μm) but nevertheless homogeneous coatings of a defined phase composition. Another advantage mentioned is the high surface area of ECAD coatings compared to the monolithic morphology of plasma-sprayed coatings, as illustrated in Fig. 9.21. The reader should note the different magnification in the images of this figure, illustrating the different length scales of the typical morphological features of the two coatings. Consequences for the dissolution behavior are discussed in the following section.

The composition of plasma-sprayed layers differs from that of ECAD coatings. Because of the thermal processing, including the typical high cooling rate, plasma-sprayed layers contain amorphous components such as oxyapatite and TCP. Consequently, degradation behavior is inhomogeneous and is associated with the danger of the release of particulate CPP, which may cause inflammatory reactions [80–82].

9.6 Physicochemical Stability *In Vitro* and *In Vivo*

Similar to that described by Wang et al. [33] and Lin et al. [53] but with a higher temporal resolution, the degradation behavior of CPP coatings on c.p. (commercially pure) titanium (in Sörensen's glycine buffer, pH 3.0, 37°C) has been investigated in our group by analysis of orthophosphate. With plasma-sprayed HA layers on sand-blasted surfaces as a reference (Fig. 9.21a), ECAD coatings generated under two conditions were investigated.

- Galvanostatic cathodic polarization with –10 mA/cm^2 for 60 minutes (according to Rössler et al. [12])
- Galvanostatic anodic polarization with + 10 mA/cm^2 up to a potential of 60 V_{SCE} in 0.5 M phosphate buffer pH 12.0 (similar to that described by Rössler et al. [1]), subsequently followed by galvanostatic cathodic polarization with –10 mA/cm^2 for 60 minutes (according to Rössler et al. [12])

Fig. 9.21 SEM images of a plasma-sprayed coating (**a**) and an HA coating prepared by the ECAD process (**b**)

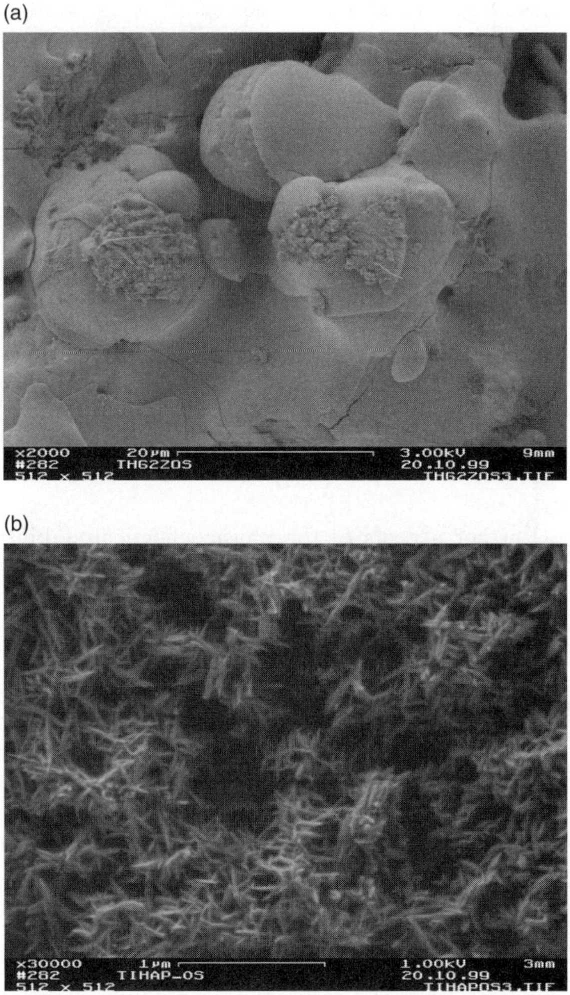

The investigations show that dissolution of the ECAD layers is completed at 60 to 120 seconds at the most, in contrast to plasma-sprayed HA layers, which took more than 100 minutes. Although the initial dissolution rate of the layers is comparable despite the different morphologies and specific surface areas (ECAD 1.5 µg cm^{-2} s^{-1} for 10 seconds, plasma-sprayed 1.6 µg cm^{-2} s^{-1} for 2 minutes), the degradation rate for plasma-sprayed layers then decreases to approximately 0.5 µg cm^{-2} s^{-1}.

The SEM images of the plasma-sprayed layers (Fig. 9.22) show an increase of the total surface area with increasing degradation time, a phenomenon caused by selective dissolution. The dissolution kinetic of the layers is mainly determined by the phase composition, which results from the thermal history of the plasma-spray process.

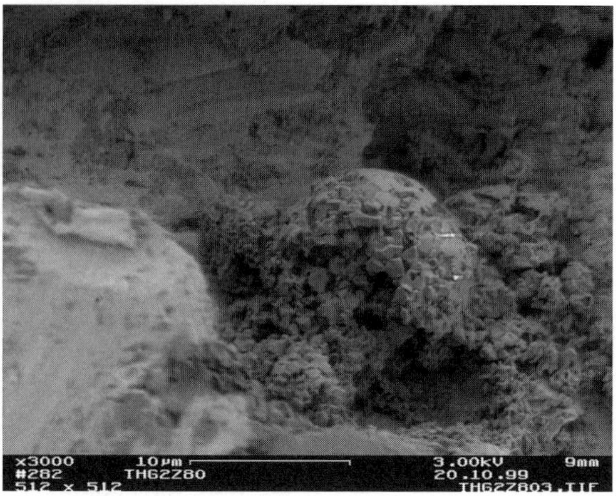

Fig. 9.22 SEM image of a plasma-sprayed coating after 180 minutes of degradation in Sörensen's glycine buffer pH 3.0

Further aspects of the physicochemical stability of ECAD coatings were discussed in the description of the method earlier in the chapter and in the following points on biological efficiency.

9.7 Biological Efficiency of the Thin CaP Coating

9.7.1 Cell Culture Investigations Using ECAD-CPP Coating

Rössler et al. [1] performed cell culture studies for a number of coatings, some of them based on ECAD CPP on Ti6Al4V. HaCaT human keratinocytes and MC3T3-E1 mouse osteoblasts were used as model systems for the gingival region and bone contact, respectively, and cell adhesion was determined 1 hour after seeding (animal experiments with these coatings are described later in the chapter).

As shown in Fig. 9.23, all coatings and additional functionalizations with adhesion peptides (RGD and TWYKIAFQRNRK as part of the laminin sequence) increase cell adhesion to different extents. The best results for HaCaT cells were obtained for collagen coatings and surfaces functionalized with the laminin sequence. MC3T3-E1 cells as a model for bone response gave the best adhesion on mineralized collagen and RGD-functionalized surfaces, with the positive effect of the adhesion peptide more pronounced on the pure HA coating.

Coatings consisting of brushite (BONIT®), monetite, and HA—obtained from BONIT® coatings through heat (parameters not given) and chemical treatment (0.5 M NaOH at 37°C), respectively—were compared by Becker et al. [19] using the MG-63 osteosarcoma cell line. A collagen type I coating (preparation not specified) served as a positive control. Cell morphology

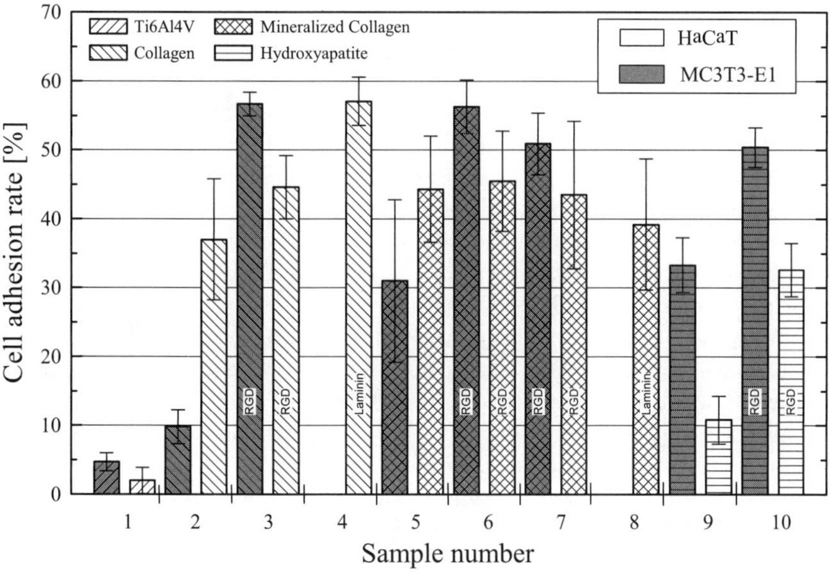

Fig. 9.23 Cell adhesion of MC3T3-E1 and HaCaT cells on various coatings. *1*, Ti6Al4V (reference); *2-4*, collagen; *5-8*, mineralized collagen; *9*, *10*, hydroxyapatite. Adhesion peptides were bound to collagen (*3*, *4*, *6*, *8*) or to hydroxyapatite (*7*, *10*). From [1], with permission

investigated after 48 hours of culture by phalloidine-TRITC staining of the cytoskeleton showed no differences between any of the tested surfaces. As stated by the authors, proliferation after 7 days of culture was high on the BONIT® and HA coatings compared to the collagen coating, with no numbers given. After the same time, the numbers of proliferative cells (in S and G_2/M phases) determined by FACScan was 14% for monetite, 22% for brushite, 25% for the collagen reference coating, and 38% for a composite HA–brushite coating.

In a preliminary study, Hu et al. [29] investigated the proliferation of SAOS-2 (ATCC HTB-85) cells on coatings of HA and vinyl acetate simultaneously deposited by ECAD. After 4 days of culture, the cell number was 6-fold higher on the HA-vinyl acetate coatings than on the HA coatings, and 12-fold higher than on the controls (cell culture polystyrene).

A more detailed investigation of ECAD coatings using primary human osteoblasts isolated from the femoral head of patients undergoing total hip replacement was performed by da Silva et al. [65]. Cells were cultured for up to 14 days on surfaces of CP titanium with the surface states (1) as-machined; (2) Al_2O_3-blasted ; (3) Ti-plasma sprayed; and (4) HA-coated, with the HA crystals showing a plate-like morphology with dimensions of 1 to 5 μm. After 3 days, cell proliferation was highest on the HA-coated samples (significant versus as-machined and Al_2O_3-blasted at $P < 0.01$), and lowest on the

Al_2O_3-blasted surfaces. Alkaline phosphatase (ALP), a marker for osteoblast differentiation, increased from day 3 to day 14 two- to threefold for all surface states, although there was no statistical significance. The number of filopodia as a measure of cell adhesion was highest for HA surfaces (day 3), to which fact not only surface chemistry but also surface roughness at the submicron scale might contribute.

Wang et al. [30, 33] described the behavior of bone marrow stromal cells derived from goat iliac crest on various CPP coatings with and without chitosan. Cell adhesion, determined after 1 and 3 days by the DNA content, was significantly higher—about 9-fold (for 1 day) and about 20-fold (3 days)—for chitosan-containing surfaces. The cells showed a more polygonal shape and were connected with each other through cytoplasmatic processes compared to cells on pure CPP coatings. Comparing coatings from OCP, carbonate apatite biomimetically prepared and a coating of carbonate apatite prepared by the ECAD process [33], the highest cell adhesion was found for the biomimetic carbonate apatite, followed by the OCP coating (~7-fold less at day 1 and ~20-fold less at day 3) and the ECAD coating (~18-fold less at day 1 and ~65-fold less at day 3).

The behavior of monocytes on a number of surfaces, among them HA and HA–collagen coatings according to Rössler et al. [1, 12], was investigated by Warmuth et al. [83]. With no statistically significant differences, only tendencies for the various surfaces are discussed with respect to cell metabolism, expression of interleukin-6 (IL-6) and the ratio IL-1β/IL-1ra, i.e. between the interleukin and its receptor agonist. A ranking of the coatings with respect to the inflammatory potential is deduced to be in this order: collagen III < collagen I < collagen I–fibronectin < HA < HA–collagen.

9.7.2 Animal Experimental Investigations

Due to the comparative newness of the process (first papers were published in 1990 [17, 67]) only a few CPP coatings based on the ECAD process are as yet on the market for biomedical applications, and for those in clinical trials only preliminary results are available. Hence, this chapter focuses on a number of animal experiments as well as on results from the commercially available coatings.

Coatings consisting of brushite and brushite converted to HA by immersion in 0.1 M NaOH for 18 to 24 hours at 95° to 100°C were the object of an experiment in a rabbit model conducted by Redepenning et al. [11]. Cylindrical samples (diameter 4 mm, length 9 mm) were press-fitted into holes in femoral shafts. After 6 weeks, pushout tests and histological analyses were performed. Bone ingrowth for the HA coating was found to be significantly increased compared to that of the uncoated reference samples ($P < 0.018$) and the brushite coated ones ($P < 0.035$). The results of the pushout tests supported these findings but with no statistical significance.

Ban et al. [26] investigated the effect of HA coatings prepared by the ECAD method in galvanostatic mode (current density 160 mA/cm^2, electrolyte pH 7.2, 62°C for 20 minutes) on the bonding strength to bone in the femurs of Japanese white rabbits. Healing times were 3, 6, and 9 weeks. Two types of substrate were used: sand-blasted pure titanium and the same substrate precoated with a mix of glass and HA powder in different ratios, then fired at 800° to 900°C after drying at 70° to 100°C. The samples (11–12 mm length, 2 mm diameter) were placed in transverse holes through the lateral cortex of the femur prepared by a drill (2.3 mm diameter). Bone bonding strengths were investigated by a pullout method analysed according to Weibull [84]. This analysis gives both a value for the homogeneity of the specimens and the bonding situation in the interface (Weibull's modulus m) and allows the prediction of fracture probabilities at various stress levels. After 3 and 6 weeks of healing time, higher values for the bone bonding strength σ, Weibull's modulus m, and the strength at a predicted failure level of 5% ($\sigma_{0.05}$) were determined for both substrate materials (titanium and HA glass precoating) when coated by the ECAD process (Table 9.3). From the start, the values of m for the ECAD-coated samples were higher than for the uncoated ones and increased from week 3 to week 6, whereas the values for uncoated samples began to increase only after 9 weeks. As the levels for σ and $\sigma_{0.05}$ were also higher for the ECAD samples, it clearly indicates earlier fixation of the bone–implant surface. This is supported by field emission (FE)-SEM and micro-FTIR data indicating enhanced formation of new bone on the ECAD coating at week 3. The underlying substrate material also showed an effect in the test: The HA glass precoating resulted in higher values for

Table 9.3 Summary of pullout testing and Weibull's analysis

Implantation time	Group	No. of samples	m	$\sigma_{0.05}$ (MPa)	σ (MPa)
Titanium					
3 Weeks	– ECAD	10	1.4	0.6	4.5 (2.7)[a]
	– ECAD	10	1.8	1.8	8.5 (4.2)
6 Weeks	– ECAD	8	1.4	1.5	9.9 (5.4)
	+ ECAD	8	2.5	4.2	12.4 (4.1)
9 Weeks	– ECAD	8	4.3	10.0	18.5 (3.6)
	+ ECAD	8	3.8	9.3	18.8 (4.3)
Titanium + HA glass precoating					
3 Weeks	– ECAD	10	2.1	2.5	9.0 (3.8)
	+ ECAD	10	2.5	4.7	13.2 (5.0)
6 Weeks	– ECAD	8	2.0	3.5	13.8 (6.1)
	+ ECAD	8	3.1	7.6	17.8 (4.8)
9 Weeks	– ECAD	8	4.0	13.3	25.7 (5.4)
	+ ECAD	8	4.0	14.0	27.0 (6.3)

From [26], with permission

m, Weibull modulus; $\sigma_{0.05}$, strength predicted at the 5% level of failure; σ, pull-out bonding strength

[a]Numbers in parentheses are SDs

bonding strength (σ and $\sigma_{0.05}$) and Weibull's modulus for all healing times. A major reason for this effect could be the surface roughness, which SEM images show to be higher for the precoated surfaces.

The BONIT® coating (brushite of 15–20 µm thickness, deposited at room temperature) on conventional tooth implants has been tested by Szmukler-Moncler et al. [85] in a pilot study in pig maxilla. Three months after premolar extraction, eight implants were placed in each hemi-maxilla and were left to heal in a submerged fashion for 6 weeks. Titanium (plasma sprayed) surfaces were used as reference implants. Bone appositions for test and control groups were 73.0% ± 6.2% and 49.8% ± 16.4%, respectively, with $P = 0.009$. In the histological examinations no macrophages or multinuclear giant cells were detected, and minute particles of remaining BONIT® were found in only a small number of cases, indicating a resorption rate of > 99%.

Schliephake et al. [74] used the mandible of beagle dogs as a model in which to investigate five surface preparations on Ti6Al4V implants with square cross sections: (1) polished; (2) fibrillar collagen type I partially integrated into an anodic oxide layer; (3, 4) collagen type I mineralized with HA by the ECAD process according to Rössler et al. [1] with a thickness of 500 nm (3) or 2 to 3 µm (4); and (5) HA coating produced by the ECAD process according to Rössler et al. [12]. Implants with an oblique diameter of 4.6 mm (length 13 mm) were inserted by press-fit into trephine burr holes of 4.6 mm. The model was chosen because it allowed analysis of both bone formation in the periimplant space and assessment of osteoconductive properties of the surface modifications in the defect zones. Healing periods were 1 and 3 months, respectively, during which time sequential fluorochrome labeling of bone formation was performed. Before sectioning the explants for histological evaluation of bone/implant contact and bone apposition in the defect zones, quantitative micro-computed tomography was performed, using different setups and radiation sources [86].

After 1 month, a significantly higher percentage of mean bone–implant contact was found in the HA-coated implants (group 5) compared to the polished ones (group 1) and those with the collagen coating (group 2). No differences were detected for groups 3 and 4 for this time period. After 3 months, no more differences could be detected among the five groups.

In contrast, bone apposition next to the implants after 3 month was found to be significantly higher for the 2- to 3-µm collagen–HA coating (group 4) compared to the 500 nm coating (group 3) and the polished surfaces. No other differences could be detected. Results after 1 month of healing showed the same tendency but were not statistically significant.

The authors conclude, in agreement with Ban et al. [26], that HA coatings produced by the ECAD process clearly tended to increase bone–implant contact at an early stage, and the additional inclusion of collagen may be beneficial when used as a sequential HA–collagen coating of sufficient thickness.

McAfee et al. [87] used the BONIT® coating deposited on intervertebral disc prostheses without a reference surface in a baboon model. Seven mature animals underwent L5-L6 total disc replacement through an anterior transperitoneal approach. Six months after surgery, the range of motion of the animals that had undergone surgery was compared to that of the nonoperative control subjects (axial compression, flexion-extension, lateral bending). No statistically significant differences ($P > 0.05$) could be detected. Histopathological analysis showed excellent ingrowth without evidence of fibrous tissue or synovium. The total endplate area showed a mean ingrowth (per volume) of 47.9% ± 9.12% and a total ingrowth range of 35.5% to 58.8%, which was more favorable than for cementless total joint components in the appendicular skeleton (range 10%–30%). However, the authors attributed this not to the coating itself but to the fact that ligamentosis causes sustained compression across the metal–bone interface for the total disc replacement prosthesis.

9.7.3 Experience from Clinical Applications

An application with human volunteers was reported by Shirkhanzadeh [61] concerning the mechanical properties of porous CPP coatings with and without trehalose, a disaccharide. Stainless steel acupuncture needles of 200 μm diameter with said coatings were inserted into forearms to an average depth of approximately 100 to 300 μm for a short time (< 30 seconds). Subsequent SEM analysis showed largely intact CPP layers with no sign of cracking or physical fragmentation as a result of the insertion into skin.

Clinical experience for coatings prepared by the ECAD process is available only for BONIT®-based surfaces that were characterized with respect to their cell biological behavior by Becker et al. [19]. Since 1995, the BONIT® coating has been in use on corundum-blasted surfaces of hip stems. A follow-up study from 2002 [88] with 826 cementless stems (1433 patients), with no differentiation between coated and uncoated stems, gave an overall loosening rate of 1.4%, which was low compared to the loosening rate of 9.2% for 6 years and plasma-spray-coated stems. This rate, established at 12 weeks of postoperative follow-up, did not increase for the next 10 years. Heterotopic ossification was observed in 7.16% of the follow-up group, and infections occurred at a rate of 1.11%.

In a study covering 200 cementless, mobile-bearing STAR total ankle replacements implanted between 1993 and 2000, Wood and Deakin [89] stated that BONIT®-coated implants seem to be associated with the radiological appearance of the interface of the implant, which can be interpreted as a positive bone response to the coating.

Birkenhauer et al. [90] reported on the BONIT® coatings on conical, self-cutting femoral neck prostheses inserted cementless. Within 3 months they implanted 38 prostheses in 34 patients with a preoperative Harris hip score (HHS) of 51 ($n = 38$). After 1 year, the HHS_1 was 94 ($n = 23$). During that time no prosthesis-specific complications were discovered, and the rehabilitation time showed a tendency to be shorter than after stem arthroplasty. Radiological follow-up investigations after 3 months showed the development of increasing trabecular reinforcement of the femoral neck and pertrochanteric regions.

9.7.4 Summary

CaP coatings prepared by the ECAD process have shown positive effects in cell experiments with cell lines as well as different primary cells, especially with respect to adhesion, proliferation, and cell morphology. These effects could be further improved by combinations of pure CPP coatings with cell adhesion peptide sequences, chitosan, or vinyl acetate. Experiments with monocytes indicated a relatively high inflammatory potential of the coatings; however, nothing comparable was ever reported from animal experiments or clinical studies.

In animal experiments, bone ingrowth (partially investigated in defect models) was significantly improved by HA coatings especially during the early healing phase compared with both uncoated and brushite-coated surfaces. Additionally, bone bonding strength was shown to be significantly improved in a number of experiments. No adverse effects of ECAD coatings related to delamination have been reported. This is in accordance with the reports on clinical studies including ECAD coatings: Without exception, positive effects of the coatings are documented.

ECAD coatings can be summarized as providing a positive effect, especially on early bone response, accelerating healing behavior without adverse effects (e.g., increased overall loosening rates and/or inflammatory effects due to emission of particulate CPP). This might be important not only for a faster recovery and thus an improved quality of life for healthy patients but also for patients with systemic diseases detrimental to bone healing.

9.8 Characterization of Thin CaP Coating in Relation to the Regulatory Pathway

Hydroxyapatite and a number of other CPPs of various preparations have already been admitted as class III products or devices for a number of biomedical applications. For coatings with brushite, octaCaP, amorphous CaP, and a number of apatites, the ECAD process is already in use for biomedical devices that are approved for both the European and US markets. Thus, the admission of new types of thin CaP coatings prepared by the ECAD process can be based on well established procedures.

For details concerning the characterization of ECAD coatings in relation to the regulatory pathway, the reader is referred to the *CaP (Ca-P) Coating Draft Guidance for Preparation of FDA Submissions for Orthopedic and Endosseous Implants* (February 21, 1997 version), which provides help for preparing submissions for CPP coated implant devices, such as premarket notifications [510(k)], Investigational Device Exemption (IDE) applications, Premarket Approval (PMA) applications, reclassification petitions, and master files. The document provides a list of standards, methods, and publications that may be used for characterizing ECAD coatings with respect to the following.

- Sterilization process
- Elemental analysis including the Ca/PO_4 ratio
- X-ray diffraction (but infrared spectrometry should also be applied)
- Solubility
- Coating thickness
- Surface roughness
- Tensile strength
- Shear strength
- Fatigue testing
- Animal and clinical studies

Furthermore, parameters are given in the *ASTM Draft Specification for CaP Coatings for Implantable Materials* (F4.2.3.5) that have to be met by legally marketed devices.

9.9 Critical Assessment on the Prospects of Future Industrial Applications (Advantages and Difficulties)

When discussing the applicability of laboratory processes for industrial applications, points of interest are good controllability combined with a reasonable process time (preferably in the range of 10 minutes or less), the possibility of performing the process in parallel for up to several hundred (potential) products, low energetic effort, and low amounts of inexpensive and harmless waste. Under these aspects the ECAD process (the advantages of which are given at the beginning of the chapter) is destined to be used for coatings of metallic implants for bone contact with thin layers of CPP.

Nevertheless, when going from the laboratory to the industrial scale, a few issuses have to be considered. First, the potentiostatic method of polarization cannot be used for simultaneous deposition of coatings on a large number of substrates. Thus, only galvanostatic polarization or the less defined method using constant cell voltage can be applied. Second, cathodic polarization is performed in a system with a low ohmic resistance that is mainly determined by the resistance of the electrolyte. Thus, in addition to the geometry of the counter electrode, the general geometry of the deposition bath is important for the homogeneity of the coating. Another point to be considered is the ratio between the surface to be coated and the electrolyte volume in use. A rough calculation for the deposition of HA coatings with a mass of 100 $\mu g/cm^2$ from the electrolyte in Rössler et al. [12] gives the result that 20 ml of electrolyte are needed to coat 1 cm^2 of surface, with the assumption that the change in electrolyte concentration is less than 5%. For the deposition of brushite coatings with a typical mass of 1000 $\mu g/cm^2$, more acidic electrolytes of much higher concentrations can be used, and thus electrolyte volume/substrate surface ratios of close to 1:1 can be achieved.

One possibility for a new product using the ECAD process is corundum-blasted and acid-etched implant surfaces as substrate, as are increasingly applied especially for dental implants. Thin coatings would preserve the sub-micrometer morphology of such surfaces and further improve the healing behavior, perhaps with a view to dental implants for patients with poor bone quality. Additionally, coatings containing organic components to improve the biological reaction to the implant are not only a topic of high interest in the scientific literature but are on their way to clinical studies and will hopefully arrive on the market in the near future.

Table 9.4 List of articles published on electrochemically assisted deposition of CPP

		Specificity of the particular system										Physicochemical characterization techniques used							Testing		
		Method					Products														
Year	Author	CV	PS	GS	EP	Other	Bru/mon	OCP	A	Other	Organic	FTIR/Raman	SEM/TEM	XRD	EDX	AFM	AES/XPS	Other	Mechanical	Invitro	Invivo
1990	Ducheyne [67]				x				x	x		x	x	x						x	
1990	Redepenning [17]			x			x						x	x				x			
1991	Shirkhanzadeh [25]		x						x?				x	x	x						
1992	Shirkhanzadeh [36]		x						x?				x	x	x			x			
1993	Shirkhanzadeh [42]	x							x?			x	x	x				x			
1993	Shirkhanzadeh [48]			x					x?			x	x	x							
1994	Ban [40]		x							x		x	x	x	x						
1994	Shirkhanzadeh [9]		x						x			x	x	x							
1994	Shirkhanzadeh [39]		x						x?		x	x									
1994	Shirkhanzadeh [7]		x						x			x	x	x							
1995	Ban [13]		x						x	x		x	x	x				x			
1995	Shirkhanzadeh [8]		x						x			x	x	x							
1995	Shirkhanzadeh [38]		x						x	x		x						x			
1996	Dasarathy [57]			x					x	x		x	x						x		
1996	Redepenning [11]			x			x		x					x				x			

Table 9.4 (continued)

		Specificity of the particular system										Physicochemical characterization techniques used							Testing		
		Method					Products														
Year	Author	CV	PS	GS	EP	Other	Bru/mon	OCP	A	Other	Organic	FTIR/Raman	SEM/TEM	XRD	EDX	AFM	AES/XPS	Other	Mechanical	Invitro	Invivo
1997	Ban [26]			x					x?			x	x								x
1997	Gottlander [70]				x				x	x								x			x
1997	Radin [92]				x				x	x	x										
1997	Zhitomirsky [93]				x				x				x	x				x			
1998	Ban [15]			x					x			x	x	x	x			x			
1998	Ban [14]			x				x	x			x	x	x							
1998	Born [50]			x					x	x	x	x	x								
1998	Chen [64]		x				x		x?				x	x							
1998	Neumann [41]		x				x				x									x	
1998	Radin [94]				x				x	x		x	x	x				x		x	
1998	Shirkhanzadeh [37]		x				x		x?			x	x	x							
1998	Shirkhanzadeh [32]		x					x	x?			x	x							x	
1998	Shirkhanzadeh [58]			x				x	x	x		x	x							x	
1998	Worch [51]			x					x	x	x		x								
1998	Zhang [20]			x			x	x?	x	x	x	x	x	x			x	x	x		
1999	Haddow [27]	x							x	x		x	x	x							
1999	Han [24]		x				x		x			x	x	x	x						
1999	Kumar [18]			x			x		x				x	x	x		x		x	x	
1999	Monma [28]			x					x			x	x	x	x			x		x	
1999	Wei [95]				x				x				x	x					x		
2000	Huang [23]	x					x		x			x	x	x							
2000	Manso [96]		x			x			x			x	x	x	x	x					
2000	Okamura [35]	x					x		x		x			x				x			
2000	Oliveira [97]		x				x?		x			x	x	x							
2001	Smukler-Moncler [85]	x?					x						x					x			x
2001	Da Silva [21]		x				x		x			x	x	x							
2001	Manso [98]		x			x			x			x	x	x	x						
2001	Nie [99]				x		x		x			x	x	x	x						
2001	Roessler [1]			x		x			x		x	x	x			x				x	
2001	Wei [100]				x				x				x						x		
2002	Becker [43]	x?					x		x				x	x	x					x	
2002	Benhayoune [5]		x				x		x			x	x		x						
2002	De Sena [101]				x				x			x	x	x					x		
2002	Kuo [3]		x			x	x		x				x	x	x			x	x		
2003	Aksakal [69]				x				x				x								

Table 9.4 (continued)

		Specificity of the particular system										Physicochemical characterization techniques used							Testing		
		Method					Products														
Year	Author	CV	PS	GS	EP	Other	Bru/mon	OCP	A	Other	Organic	FTIR/Raman	SEM/TEM	XRD	EDX	AFM	AES/XPS	Other	Mechanical	Invitro	Invivo
2003	Da Silva [65]		x						x?				x						x	x	
2003	Hu [29]			x					x?		x		x	x			x		x	x	
2003	Lin [53]			x				x				x	x	x				x	x	x	
2003	Ma [102]				x				x	x			x					x	x		
2003	McAfee [87]	x?					x		x?												x
2003	Redepenning [22]			x			x		x		x		x	x	x			x			
2003	Roessler [12]			x					x	x		x	x	x		x					
2003	Schliephake [74]			x		x			x		x		x								x
2003	Wood [89]	x?					x		x?												x
2004	Almeida [103]				x				x				x		x						x
2004	Becker [19]	x?					x		x			x	x	x				x		x	
2004	Birkenhauer [90]	x?					x		x?												x
2004	Cheng [63]			x			x	x?	x		x	x	x	x				x			
2004	Sewing [34]			x					x	x		x	x					x			
2004	Shibata [31]	x?							x?			x	x	x	x		x				
2004	Wang [30]			x				x	x		x		x	x				x	x	x	
2004	Wang [33]			x					x			x	x	x				x	x	x	
2005	Eliaz [71]				x				x				x	x	x					x	
2005	Fan [59]		x					x			x	x	x		x			x	x	x	
2005	Hurteaux [62]			x						x	x		x	x	x			x			
2005	LeGeros [54]			x				x	x			x	x	x							
2005	Lu [6]			x				x	x			x	x	x	x						
2005	Montero-Ocampo [4]		x						x	x		x	x	x				x			
2005	Pang [60]				x				x		x		x	x				x		x	
2005	Skirkhanzadeh [61]		x					x	x		x	x	x							x	x
2005	Wang [16]	x					x		x		x		x	x	x						
2005	Wei [104]				x				x				x	x							
2005	Yildirim [105]				x				x				x	x				x			x
2005	Zhang [10]		x					x		x			x				x	x		x	
2005	Zhang [44]		x					x				x	x	x			x				
2005	Warmuth. [83]			x																x	

CV, polarization with constant cell voltage; PS, potentiostatic polarization; GS, galvanostatic polarization; EP, electrophoretic deposition; bru/mon, deposition of brushite and/or monetite; OCP, deposition of octa-CaP; A, deposition of apatitic phases; organic, preparation of organic components containing coatings; (?), incomplete information and/or uncertainty of results

References

1. S. Roessler, R. Born, D. Scharnweber, H. Worch, A. Sewing, M. Dard, J Mater Sci Mater Med 12 (2001) 871.
2. F. Song, D. Kirk, J. Graydon, D. Cormack, J Electrochem Soc 149 (2002) B479.
3. M. Kuo, S. Yen, Mater Sci Eng C 20 (2002) 153.
4. C. Montero-Ocampo, D. Villegas, L. Veleva, J Electrochem Soc 152 (2005) C692.
5. H. Benhayoune, P. Laquerriere, E. Jallot, A. Perchet, L. Kilian, G. Balossier, J. L. Bubendorff, G. D. Sockalingum, J Mater Sci Mater Med 13 (2002) 1057.
6. X. Lu, Z. Zhao, Y. Leng, J Cryst Growth 284 (2005) 506.
7. M. Shirkhanzadeh, NanoStruct Mater 4 (1994) 677.
8. M. Shirkhanzadeh, J Mater Sci Mater Med 6 (1995) 90.
9. M. Shirkhanzadeh, M. Azadegan, V. Stack, S. Schreyer, Mater Lett 18 (1994) 211.
10. Q. Zhang, Y. Leng, Biomaterials 26 (2005) 3853.
11. J. Redepenning, T. Schlessinger, S. Burnham, L. Lippiello, J. Miyano, J Biomed Mater Res 30 (1996) 287.
12. S. Rossler, A. Sewing, M. Stolzel, R. Born, D. Scharnweber, M. Dard, H. Worch, J Biomed Mater Res A 64 (2003) 655.
13. S. Ban, S. Maruno, Biomaterials 16 (1995) 977.
14. S. Ban, S. Maruno, Biomaterials 19 (1998) 1245.
15. S. Ban, S. Maruno, J Biomed Mater Res 42 (1998) 387.
16. S. Wang, W. Shih, W. Li, M. Hon, M. Wang, J European Ceramic Soc 25 (2005) 3287.
17. J. Redepenning, J. Mcisaac, Chem Mater 2 (1990) 625.
18. M. Kumar, H. Dasarathy, C. Riley, J Biomed Mater Res 45 (1999) 302.
19. P. Becker, H. G. Neumann, B. Nebe, F. Luthen, J. Rychly, J Mater Sci Mater Med 15 (2004) 437.
20. J. Zhang, C. Lin, Z. Feng, Z. Tian, J Mater Sci Lett 17 (1998) 1077.
21. M. Da Silva, J. Lima, G. Soares, C. Elias, M. De Andrade, S. Best, I. Gibson, Surf Coat Technol 137 (2001) 270.
22. J. Redepenning, G. Venkataraman, J. Chen, N. Stafford, J Biomed Mater Res A 66A (2003) 411.
23. L. Huang, K. Xu, J. Lu, J Mater Sci Mater Med 11 (2000) 667.
24. Y. Han, K. Xu, J. Lu, J Mater Sci Mater Med 10 (1999) 243.
25. M. Shirkhanzadeh, J Mater Sci Lett 10 (1991) 1415.
26. S. Ban, S. Maruno, N. Arimoto, A. Harada, J. Hasegawa, J Biomed Mater Res 36 (1997) 9.
27. D. B. Haddow, M. S. Thompson, S. R. Berry, J. T. Czernuszka, J Mater Sci Mater Med 10 (1999) 219.
28. H. Monma, O. Nemoto, S. Takahashi, H. Kobayashi, J Electroceram 4 (1999) 135.
29. H. Hu, C. Lin, P. P. Lui, Y. Leng, J Biomed Mater Res A 65 (2003) 24.
30. J. Wang, J. De Boer, K. De Groot, J Dent Res 83 (2004) 296.
31. Y. Shibata, H. Takashima, H. Yamamoto, T. Miyazaki, Int J Oral Maxillofac Implants 19 (2004) 177.
32. M. Shirkhanzadeh, J Mater Sci Mater Med 9 (1998) 503.
33. J. Wang, P. Layrolle, M. Stigter, K. De Groot, Biomaterials 25 (2004) 583.
34. A. Sewing, M. Lakatos, D. Scharnweber, S. Roessler, R. Born, M. Dard, H. Worch, Key Eng Mater 254–256 (2004) 419.
35. H. Okamura, M. Yasuda, M. Ohta, Electrochemistry 68 (2000) 486.
36. M. Shirkhanzadeh, Mater Lett 14 (1992) 27.
37. M. Shirkhanzadeh, J Mater Sci Mater Med 9 (1998) 67.
38. M. Shirkhanzadeh, M. Azadegan, G. Liu, Mater Lett 24 (1995) 7.
39. M. Shirkhanzadeh, G. Liu, Mater Lett 21 (1994) 115.
40. S. Ban, S. Maruno, Jpn J Appl Phys 33 (1994) L1545.

41. H. Neumann, U. Beck, M. Drawe, J. Steinbach, Surf Coat Technol 98 (1998) 1157.
42. M. Shirkhanzadeh, J Mater Sci Lett 12 (1993) 16.
43. P. Becker, P. Zeggel, F. Luthen, B. Nebe, J. Rychly, H. Neumann, Key Eng Mater 218–220 (2002) 653.
44. Q. Zhang, Y. Leng, R. Xin, Biomaterials 26 (2005) 2857.
45. M. Kawashita, M. Nakao, M. Minoda, H. M. Kim, T. Beppu, T. Miyamoto, T. Kokubo, T. Nakamura, Biomaterials 24 (2003) 2477.
46. M. Tanahashi, T. Kokubo, T. Matsuda, J Biomed Mater Res 31 (1996) 243.
47. M. Tanahashi, T. Yao, T. Kokubo, M. Minoda, T. Miyamoto, T. Nakamura, T. Yamamuro, J Appl Biomater 5 (1994) 339.
48. M. Shirkhanzadeh, M. Azadegan, Mater Lett 15 (1993) 392.
49. S. Ban, S. Maruno, A. Harada, M. Hattori, K. Narita, J. Hasegawa, Dent. Mater. J. 15 (1996) 31.
50. R. Born, D. Scharnweber, S. Rossler, M. Stolzel, M. Thieme, C. Wolf, H. Worch, Fresenius J Anal Chem 361 (1998) 697.
51. H. Worch, D. Scharnweber, Zeitschrift für Metallkunde 89 (1998) 153.
52. M. Johnsson, G. Nancollas, Crit Rev Oral Biol Med 3 (1992) 61.
53. S. Lin, R. Z. Legeros, J. P. Legeros, J Biomed Mater Res A 66 (2003) 819.
54. J. Legeros, S. Lin, D. Mijares, F. Dimaano, R. Legeros, Key Eng Mater 284–286 (2005) 247.
55. J. Legeros, S. Lin, R. Legeros, J Dent Res 79 (2000) 560.
56. R. Legeros, J. Legeros, C. Bautista, J Dent Res 74 (1995) 405.
57. H. Dasarathy, C. Riley, H. D. Coble, W. R. Lacefield, G. Maybee, J Biomed Mater Res 31 (1996) 81.
58. M. Shirkhanzadeh, M. Azadegan, J Mater Sci Mater Med 9 (1998) 385.
59. Y. Fan, K. Duan, R. Wang, Biomaterials 26 (2005) 1623.
60. X. Pang, I. Zhitomirsky, Mater Chem Phys 94 (2005) 245.
61. M. Shirkhanzadeh, J Mater Sci Mater Med 16 (2005) 37.
62. R. Hurteaux, H. Benhayoune, F. Edwards-Levy, S. Bouthors, G. Balossier, D. Laurent-Maquin, J Mater Sci Mater Med 16 (2005) 9.
63. X. Cheng, M. Filiaggi, S. G. Roscoe, Biomaterials 25 (2004) 5395.
64. J. S. Chen, H. Y. Juang, M. H. Hon, J Mater Sci Mater Med 9 (1998) 297.
65. M. Da Silva, G. Soares, C. Elias, S. Best, I. Gibson, L. Disilvio, M. Dalby, J Mater Sci Mater Med 14 (2003) 511.
66. I. Zhitomirsky, Adv Colloid Interface Sci 97 (2002) 279.
67. P. Ducheyne, S. Radin, M. Heughebaert, J. C. Heughebaert, Biomaterials 11 (1990) 244.
68. P. Ducheyne, W. Vanraemdonck, J. Heughebaert, M. Heughebaert, Biomaterials 7 (1986) 97.
69. B. Aksakal, O. S. Yildirim, A. Okur, J Int Med Res 31 (2003) 418.
70. M. Gottlander, C. B. Johansson, A. Wennerberg, T. Albrektsson, S. Radin, P. Ducheyne, Biomaterials 18 (1997) 551.
71. N. Eliaz, T. Sridhar, U. Mudali, B. Raj, Surf Eng 21 (2005) 238.
72. P. Habibovic, H. Yuan, C. M. van der Valk, G. Meijer, C. A. van Blitterswijk, K. De Groot, Biomaterials 26 (2005) 3565.
73. H. Yuan, Z. Yang, Y. Li, X. Zhang, J. D. De Bruijn, K. De Groot, J Mater Sci Mater Med 9 (1998) 723.
74. H. Schliephake, D. Scharnweber, M. Dard, S. Robetaler, A. Sewing, C. Huttmann, J Biomed Mater Res A 64 (2003) 225.
75. N. Khalil, J. Leach, Electrochimica Acta 31 (1986) 1279.
76. D. Blackwood, R. Greef, L. Peter, Electrochimica Acta 34 (1989) 875.
77. T. Hurlen, S. Hornkjol, Electrochimica Acta 36 (1991) 189.
78. M. Pankuch, R. Bell, C. Melendres, Electrochimica Acta 38 (1993) 2777.

79. D. Scharnweber, R. Beutner, S. Rossler, H. Worch, J Mater Sci Mater Med 13 (2002) 1215.
80. M. Ogiso, J Long Term Eff Med Implants 8 (1998) 193.
81. L. Sun, C. C. Berndt, K. A. Gross, A. Kucuk, J Biomed Mater Res 58 (2001) 570.
82. R. J. Talib, M. R. Toff, Med J Malaysia 59 Suppl B (2004) 153.
83. S. Warmuth, M. Kosmann, J. Aigner, E. Wintermantel, D. Scharnweber, H. Worch, Materialprüfung 47 (2005) 107.
84. W. Weibull, J Appl Mech – Transactions of the ASME 18 (1951) 293.
85. S. Szmukler-Moncler, D. Perrin, V. Ahossi, P. Pointaire, Key Eng Mater 192–195 (2001) 395.
86. R. Bernhardt, D. Scharnweber, B. Muller, P. Thurner, H. Schliephake, P. Wyss, F. Beckmann, J. Goebbels, H. Worch, Eur Cell Mater 7 (2004) 42.
87. P. Mcafee, B. Cunningham, C. Orbegoso, J. SEFTER, A. Dmitriev, I. Fedder, Spine 28 (2003) 332.
88. J. Mockwitz, V. Dathe, Orthopädische Praxis 38 (2002) 260.
89. P. L. Wood, S. Deakin, J Bone Joint Surg Br 85 (2003) 334.
90. B. Birkenhauer, H. Kistmacher, J. Ries, Orthopäde 33 (2004) 1259.
91. D. Scharnweber, Biomaterialien 8 (2007) 8.
92. S. Radin, J. T. Campbell, P. Ducheyne, J. M. Cuckler, Biomaterials 18 (1997) 777.
93. I. Zhitomirsky, L. Gal-Or, J Mater Sci Mater Med 8 (1997) 213.
94. S. Radin, P. Ducheyne, P. Berthold, S. Decker, J Biomed Mater Res 39 (1998) 234.
95. M. Wei, A. Ruys, M. Swain, S. Kim, B. Milthorpe, C. Sorrell, J Mater Sci Mater Med 10 (1999) 401.
96. M. Manso, C. Jimenez, C. Morant, P. Herrero, J. Martinez-Duart, Biomaterials 21 (2000) 1755.
97. J. Oliveira, L. Sena, M. Da Silva, G. Soares, A. Rossi, Key Eng Mater 192–195 (2000) 271.
98. M. Manso, C. Jimenez, C. Morant, P. Herrero, J. Martinez-Duart, Surf Interface Anal 31 (2001) 1104.
99. X. Nie, A. Leyland, A. Matthews, J. C. Jiang, E. I. Meletis, J Biomed Mater Res 57 (2001) 612.
100. M. Wei, A. Ruys, B. Milthorpe, C. Sorrell, J. Evans, J Sol-Gel Sci Techn 21 (2001) 39.
101. L. De Sena, M. De Andrade, A. Rossi, G. Soares, J Biomed Mater Res 60 (2002) 1.
102. J. Ma, C. Liang, L. Kong, C. Wang, J Mater Sci Mater Med 14 (2003) 797.
103. C. Almeida, L. Sena, A. Rossi, M. Pinto, C. Muller, G. Soares, Key Eng Mater 254–256 (2004) 729.
104. M. Wei, A. Ruys, B. Milthorpe, C. Sorrell, J Mater Sci Mater Med 16 (2005) 319.
105. O. S. Yildirim, B. Aksakal, H. Celik, Y. Vangolu, A. Okur, Med Eng Phys 27 (2005) 221.

Chapter 10
Electrosprayed Calcium Phosphate Coating for Biomedical Purposes

Sander C.G. Leeuwenburgh, Joop G.C. Wolke, Marijke C. Siebers, Joop Schoonman and John A. Jansen

Abstract The suitability of the electrostatic spray deposition (ESD) technique was studied for biomedical purposes—i.e., deposition of calcium phosphate (CaP) coatings onto titanium substrates. Using ESD, which is a simple, inexpensive deposition method for inorganic and organic coatings, it was possible to obtain thin CaP layers with an extremely wide range of chemical and morphological characteristics. Various CaP phases and phase mixtures were deposited, and a broad diversity of coating morphologies was produced by varying deposition parameters related to the ESD-apparatus and/or the precursor solutions. Electrosprayed CaP coatings were shown to be biocompatible with soft tissue, and the osteoconductive nature of electrosprayed CaP coatings was also proven *in vivo*. Particular interest was given to a unique, reticular coating morphology consisting of a porous network of variable pore size. This specific coating morphology offers the possibility of varying the specific surface area of electrosprayed CaP coatings to a large extent. Consequently, the degradation rate of CaP coatings and the incorporation and subsequent release of biological agents (e.g., growth factors) can be influenced by chemical as well as physical coating properties using the ESD technique. In that way, control over the biological activity of drug-releasing CaP coatings can be improved significantly compared to conventional coating techniques, which lack this chemical and morphological variability.

10.1 Introduction to Electrostatic Spray Deposition

The synthesis technique called electrostatic spray deposition (ESD) was developed at the Laboratory for Inorganic Chemistry, Delft University of Technology, during the early 1990s [1] to be able to fabricate porous, thin ceramic films with a controlled morphology for solid electrolytes and lithium battery

J.A. Jansen(✉)
Department of Periodontology and Biomaterials, Radboud University Nijmegen Medical Center, Philips van Leijdenlaan 25, 6525 EX Nijmegen, The Netherlands
e-mail: j.jansen@dent.umcn.nl

B. León, J.A. Jansen (eds.), *Thin Calcium Phosphate Coatings for Medical Implants*, DOI 10.1007/978-0-387-77718-4_10, © Springer Science+Business Media, LLC 2009

electrode materials. Briefly, the basic principle of ESD is generation of an aerosol composed of organic solvents containing inorganic precursors under the influence of high voltage. An aerosol is defined as dispersion of solid or liquid particles in a gas. This is accomplished by pumping this liquid through a nozzle. Usually, a spherical droplet is then formed at the tip of the nozzle; but if high voltage is applied between the nozzle and substrate, this droplet transforms into a conical shape and fans out to form a spray of highly charged droplets. The generated spray droplets are attracted by the grounded and heated substrate as a result of the applied potential difference. Consequently, the droplets impinge on the heated substrate, where they lose their charge. After complete solvent evaporation, a thin layer is left on the substrate surface. Figure 10.1 shows such an experimental setup.

This coating technique has several advantages over conventional deposition techniques such as plasma-spraying.

- It is a simple, inexpensive setup.
- There is a wide choice of sprayable precursor solutions (dissolved salts, suspensions, sols) and coatable substrates.
- There is extensive control over surface properties. In view of the relation between the physicochemical characteristics of biomaterials' surfaces and their biological performance *in vitro* and *in vivo*, the flexibility of the ESD technique regarding deposition of coatings with a wide variety of surface chemical and morphological properties offers a specific advantage over many deposition techniques that lack this freedom.

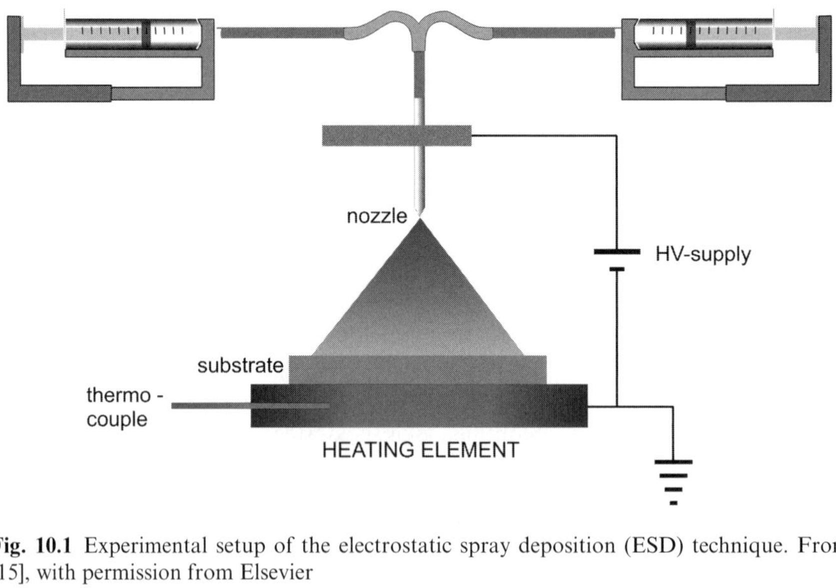

Fig. 10.1 Experimental setup of the electrostatic spray deposition (ESD) technique. From [15], with permission from Elsevier

- There is control over coating thickness. In contrast to plasma spraying, the thickness of electrosprayed thin films can be controlled easily from several nanometers to more than 30 μm.
- There is high deposition efficiency compared to conventional spraying processes without an applied electrical field. The trajectory of electrosprayed droplets is well defined owing to the external electric field, which can be modified by means of additional external electrodes to conform the electrical field to the desired shape. Moreover, droplet coagulation cannot occur because droplets are equally charged, yielding homogeneous, controllable sprays.

10.2 Electrospraying

10.2.1 Conventional Spraying

A large number of spraying techniques have been developed for various technical applications. In most cases, bulk liquid is atomized by means of mechanical energy, which disintegrates the liquid body into small droplets [2]. This mechanical energy can be added to the liquid by applying high pressure (ultrasonic) vibration and kinetic acceleration, among other methods. The mechanism of atomization is mainly based on a high relative velocity difference between the liquid and surrounding gas medium, as a result of which the liquid jet disintegrates into droplets.

10.2.2 Electrospraying

Compared to uncharged sprays, charged droplets and sprays offer the possibility of controlling the droplets' transport, evaporation, and lifetime by applying external electrical fields. The droplet trajectory can be directed toward the desired location by tailoring the external electrical field, which enhances deposition efficiency significantly [3]. Sprays can be charged by means of various droplet-charging mechanisms. Charging by induction is based on ionic bombardment of the droplets by ionized molecules after spray generation by means of mechanical forces (e.g., ultrasonic, pressure) [4]. In contrast, by applying a high voltage directly to the spray-generating nozzle, the processes of spray generation and charging of the droplets are no longer separated. In this case, the liquid is disintegrated by the disrupting influence of the applied electrical potential only. In the literature, this phenomenon is referred to as electrohydrodynamic or electrostatic atomization [5]. The purely electrostatic spraying method is used most frequently to produce charged droplets, but hybrid electrosprays are applied also. These sprays are generated by means of combined electrostatic and mechanical forces (e.g., for producing charged fuel sprays [6]) using conventional pressure nozzles in combination with external electrical fields.

Electrostatic atomizers make use of electrical forces to overcome the surface tension of the liquid. The electrical field acting on the droplet surface induces liquid acceleration and droplet breakup. Rayleigh [7] was the first to describe the instabilities of an electrically charged droplet when the outward electrostatic forces are balancing the surface tension forces, resulting in emission of a narrow liquid jet. Electrospraying in a capillary plate configuration is based on this effect. The liquid flows through the capillary outlet, where the high electrical field accelerates the liquid, resulting in jets that break up into droplets. Depending on the strength of the electrical stresses at the liquid surface relative to the surface tension stress and the kinetic energy of the flowing liquid, various electrospraying modes have been developed that were reviewed by Cloupeau and Prunet-Foch [8], Grace and Marijnissen [9], and Jaworek and Krupa [10].

10.3 Physicochemical Properties of Electrosprayed CaP Coatings

Generally, the phenomenon of bioactivity of calcium phosphate (CaP) bioceramics is determined by chemical factors (e.g., crystal and molecular structure of the material) and physical factors (e.g., surface roughness and porosity) [11–13]. In this respect, one of the main advantages of the ESD technique is the possibility of depositing CaP coatings with a wide range of physicochemical properties [14, 15].

10.3.1 Chemical Properties of Electrosprayed Coatings

To tailor the chemical characteristics of electrosprayed CaP coatings, several processing parameters can be varied using ESD. Regarding the composition of the precursor solutions, parameters such as the relative and absolute precursor solute concentrations, the solution acidity (in terms of addition of nitric acid), and the type of precursor salt were investigated. Concerning the influence of apparatus-related deposition parameters on coating properties, factors such as the nozzle-to-substrate distance, precursor liquid flow rate, deposition temperature, and the aforementioned nozzle geometry were studied.

10.3.1.1 Influence of Precursor Solution Parameters on Chemical Properties

The composition of the precursor solutions determined to a large extent the chemical properties of the deposited coatings. As an example of this influence, Fig. 10.2 shows x-ray diffraction (XRD) images (Fig. 10.2a) and corresponding Fourier transform infrared (FTIR) spectra (Fig. 10.2b) of coatings deposited using various solution acidities (between 0 and 2.0 vol% of extra nitric acid).

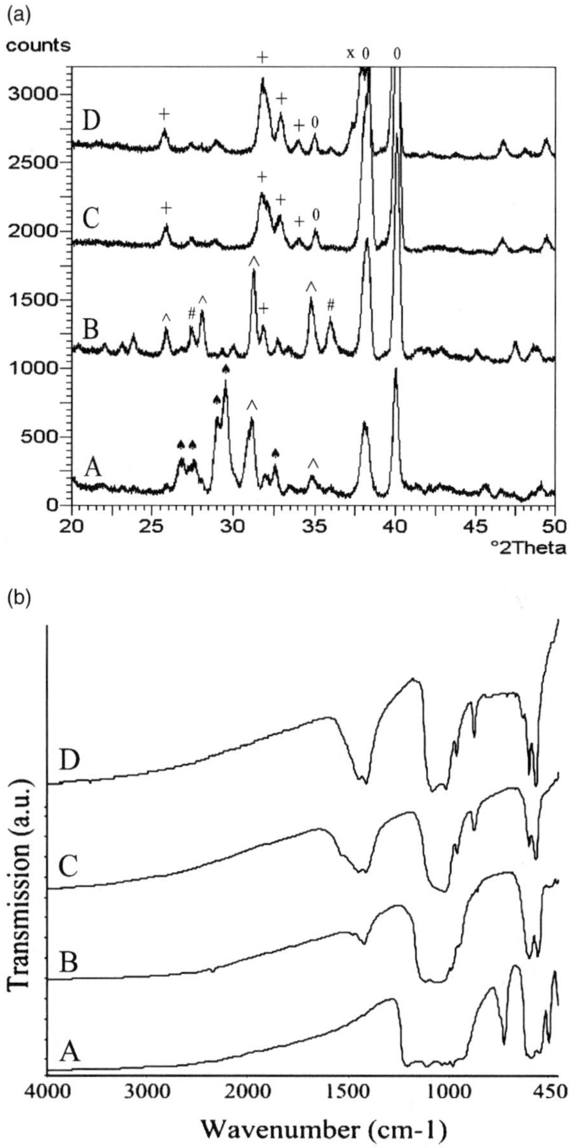

Fig. 10.2 X-ray diffraction (XRD) patterns (**a**) and Fourier transform infrared (FTIR) spectra (**b**) of electrosprayed calcium phosphate (CaP) coating, prepared using various amounts of HNO_3 added to the precursor solution. *A*, 2% HNO_3 addition. *B*, 1% HNO_3 addition. *C*, 0.1% HNO_3 addition. *D*, no HNO_3 addition. All coatings were heat-treated at 650°C. ♠ = β-pyrophosphate; ∧ = whitlockite; + = carbonate apatite; # = rutile; x = calcium oxide; 0 = Ti. From [14], with permission from Elsevier

All as-deposited coatings were amorphous. After heat treatment at 650°C, various CaP crystal phases were obtained, depending on the acidity of the precursor solutions. Using the most acidic precursor solution (2% HNO_3), β-pyrophosphate was the main crystal phase [Joint Committee on Powder Diffraction Standards (JCPDS) file no. 9-346]. However, diffraction peaks at 31.2° and 34.8° 2θ were assigned to whitlockite, corresponding to JCPDS file no. 13-404. Using less acidic precursor solutions (1% HNO_3), whitlockite was deposited with main reflections at 31.3° and 34.8° 2θ. A small peak at 31.8° 2θ could be related to minor contamination of apatitic nature. The XRD pattern of the coating, deposited using a slightly acidic solution (0.1% HNO_3) corresponded to a poorly crystalline apatite phase. Without any addition of HNO_3, the crystal phase was also apatitic, but a shoulder at 37.5° 2θ was assigned to calcium oxide as an impurity phase.

The FTIR spectrum, corresponding to the most acidic deposition with 2% HNO_3, resembled the FTIR spectrum of β-pyrophosphate, characterized by broad, feature-rich absorption bands of 900 to 1250 cm^{-1} (ν_3) and 450 to 650 cm^{-1} (ν_4). Small carbonate absorption peaks at 1482 and 1424 cm^{-1} were found in the IR spectrum of coatings deposited with 1% of HNO_3. The ν_3 phosphate absorption band was less broad and feature-rich, and it resembled the IR spectrum of precipitated, Mg-containing whitlockite [16]. Using 0.1% HNO_3, intense CO_3 absorption peaks at 878 (ν_2), 1415, 1453, and 1533 (ν_3) cm^{-1} indicated a considerable increase in carbonate incorporation. These ν_3 peaks indicated that carbonate anions were substituted for both phosphate (B type) and hydroxyl (A type) groups in a crystalline apatite lattice. The broad, featureless phosphate ν_3 band at 1050 cm^{-1} instead of a collection of sharply defined ν_3 absorptions was characteristic for poorly crystalline carbonate apatite. Absorption peaks at 960 (ν_1), 600, and 563 cm^{-1} (v_4) were assigned to phosphate groups. Without any HNO_3, intense carbonate absorptions peaks at 874, 1414, and 1454 cm^{-1} corresponded to high carbonate content (B type). Furthermore, small absorptions at 3570 and 630 cm^{-1} were assigned to OH^- stretch and libration absorption modes. Energy dispersive spectrometry (EDS) revealed that Ca/P ratios of the deposited coatings were strongly dependent on the amount of HNO_3 added to the precursor solutions. Without any HNO_3, a high Ca/P ratio (3.4) was measured, whereas this value decreased to 1.1 for coatings deposited using precursor solutions supplemented with nitric acid 2.0 vol%.

The influence of other precursor solution parameters on chemical properties of ESD-derived CaP coatings was described previously, to which article the reader is referred for specific details [14]. On the basis of these results, however, a chemical mechanism of coating formation was proposed. Briefly, deposition of the various crystal phases was suggested to be the result of the following acid-base reaction between basic CO_3^{2-} groups (originating from solvent decomposition reactions) and acidic HPO_4^{2-} groups from an intermediate monetite ($CaHPO_4$) phase of the CaP precipitate.

$$2\ HPO_4^{2-} + CO_3^{2-} \rightarrow 2\ PO_4^{3-} + CO_2 + H_2O$$

Evidence for the relevance of this intermediate monetite phase was threefold. First, it was observed by means of precipitation experiments that the monetite phase was formed upon precipitation of calcium and phosphate precursor solutes in the organic solvent butyl carbitol (at various absolute and/or relative concentrations) [14]. This observation was confirmed by the fact that the interior of all spraying nozzles was covered with a thin layer of monetite after several tens of hours of operation, as observed by FTIR spectroscopy [16]. Third, monetite coatings were deposited using highly concentrated—and consequently rapidly precipitating-precursor solutions [14]. Moreover, from the literature it is known that monetite reacts in hot carbonate solutions, yielding an apatite phase, often with simultaneous formation of calcite [17].

It was concluded that carbonate ions play an essential role in controlling the chemical properties of the deposited ESD coatings. The amount of carbonate incorporation determined the crystal and molecular structure of the deposited coatings. At low concentrations, carbonate acts as a base that eliminates protons from acidic, hydrogenated phosphate groups. With increasing carbonate content, carbonate is incorporated into apatitic CaP phases. At a higher carbonate wt% (typically more than 10 wt% CO_3), an extra calcite phase is formed as a result of a reaction between excessive Ca^{2+} cations and CO_3^{2-} anions.

10.3.1.2 Influence of Physical, Apparatus-Related Parameters on Chemical Properties

The chemical properties of ESD coatings appeared to be dependent also on apparatus-related parameters such as the deposition temperature, liquid flow rate, spraying nozzle geometry, and the distance between the spraying nozzle and the substrate surface. As an example of this influence, Fig. 10.3 shows the FTIR spectra of as-deposited coatings synthesized at different deposition temperatures. The minimum deposition temperature for the formation of CaP coatings by means of ESD was 300°C (at lower temperatures it was impossible to obtain solid, ceramic coatings). Thus, it was concluded that formation of CaP coatings was not just the result of solvent evaporation, as the boiling point of the solvent butyl carbitol ($C_8H_{18}O_3$) of 231°C was significantly lower than 300°C. This indicated that a chemical reaction was needed for coating formation. Remnants of the organic solvent were still present at 300°C, as indicated by several absorption peaks [18], such as intense CH stretch absorptions (2850–2940 cm^{-1}), a CH bending band at 1460 cm^{-1}, a symmetrical CH bending band of the CH_3 group at 1376 cm^{-1}, and a CH_2 rocking absorption at 722 cm^{-1}. Moreover, an absorption peak at 1713 cm^{-1} was assigned to C=O. At a deposition temperature of 350°C, the organic remnants and C=O groups were absent and two broad ν_3 carbonate absorptions were observed at 1487 cm^{-1} and 1425 cm^{-1}. Also, a small ν_2 carbonate peak at 870 cm^{-1} was found. These vibrations correspond to carbonate groups engaged in an amorphous CaP environment [19]. Moreover, absorption peaks at 782, 1323, and 1646 cm^{-1} corresponded to the presence of hydrated calcium oxalate [20]. At a deposition temperature of 450°C, the oxalate absorption peaks were hardly visible anymore, although the

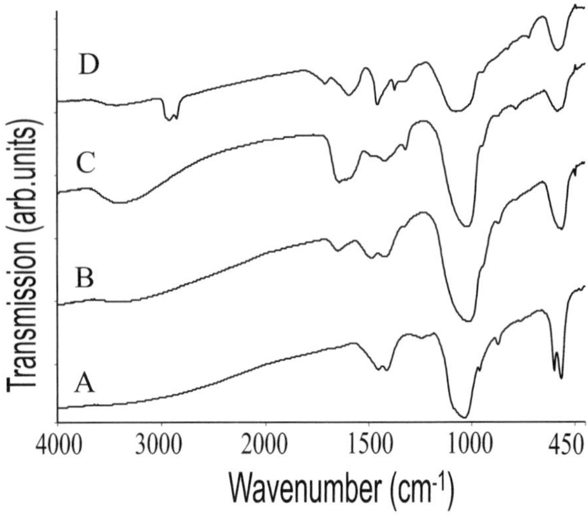

Fig. 10.3 FTIR spectra of as-deposited, electrosprayed CaP coatings prepared at different deposition temperatures. *A*, 600°C. *B*, 450°C. *C*, 350°C. *D*, 300°C. From [22], with permission from Wiley

carbonate bands at 1488, 1425, and 870 cm^{-1} were still present. It was concluded that carbonate ions were formed via intermediate oxalate groups as the result of thermal decomposition of the organic solvent butyl carbitol. From the literature it is known that oxalate decomposes to carbonate at around 425°C according to the following reaction [21]:

$$C_2O_4^{2-} \rightarrow CO_3^{2-} + CO$$

Phosphate absorptions between 1250 and 900 cm^{-1} (ν_3) and between 650 and 500 cm^{-1} (ν_4) remained broad and unresolved up to deposition temperatures of 550°C, but at 600°C these two absorption bands split into sharper bands at 1087, 1032 (ν_3), 962 (ν_1), 602, and 567 cm^{-1} (ν_4). Furthermore, sharp carbonate bands (ν_3) at 1455 and 1416 cm^{-1} revealed that carbonate was mainly substituting for phosphate anions (type B substitutions) in a crystalline CaP environment. The crystalline apatitic structure of these coatings was confirmed ny means of XRD analysis, as the main reflection lines were located at 25.8°, 31.9°, and 32.9° 2θ, which correspond to (002), (211), and (300) reflections of the apatite structure [16]. This indicated that the as-deposited coatings remained amorphous up to deposition temperatures of 600°C, which was the minimum temperature for crystallization of these B-type carbonate apatite coatings. Generally, all coatings transformed into crystalline carbonate apatite (CA) after additional heat treatment at 650°C, irrespective of their initial deposition temperature, indicating that the deposition temperature did not influence the final chemical structure of the heat-treated coatings.

The influence of other apparatus-related deposition parameters on chemical characteristics of electrosprayed CaP coatings was described previously, to which article the reader is referred for specific details [22].

10.3.2 Morphological Properties of Electrosprayed Coatings

10.3.2.1 Influence of Physical, Apparatus-Related Parameters on Morphological Properties

The topography of bioceramic surfaces (in terms of physical factors such as surface roughness, porosity, and specific surface) is suggested to have a strong influence on biological such processes as the adsorption of proteins, cell adhesion and spreading, and consequently the overall tissue response *in vivo* [23]. From this point of view, the versatility of the ESD technique regarding deposition of CaP coatings with a variable surface morphology is particularly interesting [15]. As an example of this strong relation between processing conditions and the resulting morphological properties, Fig. 10.4 shows the influence of the deposition temperature on CaP coating morphology. The influence of other apparatus-related deposition parameters on morphological properties of electrosprayed CaP coatings has been described elsewhere [15].

Various formation mechanisms have been suggested to explain the characteristic surface morphologies obtained using ESD [24–26]. However, these models are merely based on observations using scanning electron microscopy (SEM), and in some cases the models are contradictory [24, 26]. Therefore, a

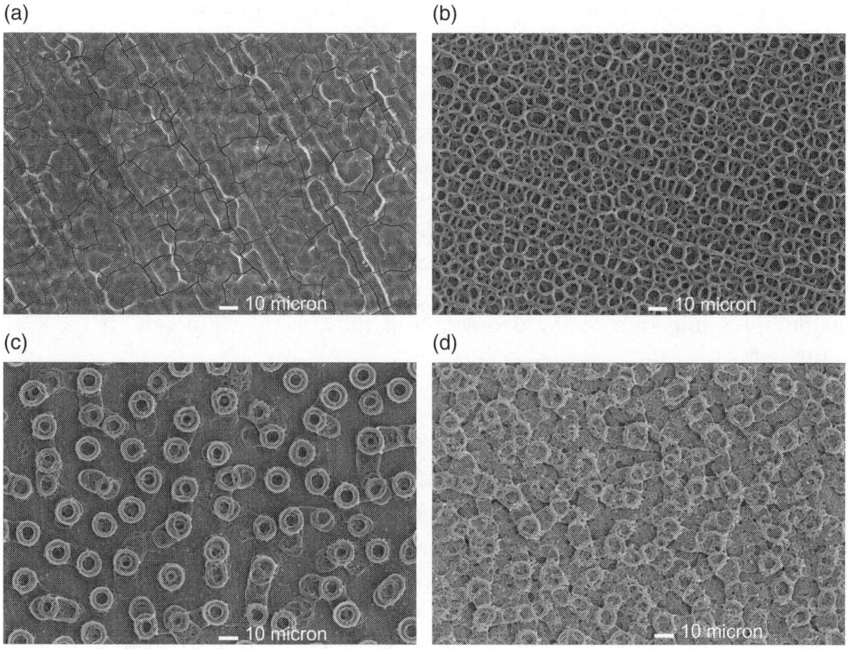

Fig. 10.4 Scanning electron microscopy (SEM) images of electrosprayed CaP coatings, deposited at various deposition temperatures. **a** 325°C. **b** 350°C. **c** 375°C. **d** 400°C. From [15], with permission from Elsevier

Phase Doppler Anemometer (PDA) was used to characterize the electrosprays in terms of droplet sizes and velocities in situ during formation of CaP coatings at high deposition temperatures. Mapping of droplet sizes and velocities was carried out in the axial direction along the central spray axis and in the radial direction from the center to the edge of the spray at a plane 5 mm above the substrate. Morphological features of ESD-derived coatings were correlated with the corresponding droplet characteristics of the electrosprays.

The results showed that droplet sizes and velocities do not depend on substrate heating or the nozzle-to-substrate distance using the solvent butyl carbitol with a high boiling point of 231°C. The resulting surface morphologies, however, varied considerably, ranging from porous morphologies with coalesced droplets to morphologies resembling separated doughnuts on top of submicron-porous or grainy underlayers. This indicates that ESD is a surface-controlled process using solvents with high boiling points without significant solvent evaporation during droplet flight. This means that conventional models on spray and droplet drying-including phenomena such as solvent evaporation, droplet shrinkage, and crust formation during droplet flight [27]-cannot be applied to ESD using the current setup. Droplet-derived features (e.g., micron-sized doughnut shapes) were formed after droplet spreading over the substrate surface, as the diameter of these features (typically about 12 μm) was generally a few microns larger than the corresponding droplet diameters before landing on the substrate (~7–8 μm). Chen et al. [24] suggested that solvent evaporation rates were higher at the edges of spreading droplets, which was confirmed by a mathematical model developed by Ajaev [28] for the spreading of liquid droplets on a uniformly heated plate. He confirmed that the evaporative mass flux strongly increases with decreasing thickness of the liquid film. As a result, heterogeneous concentration profiles of precursor solutes were formed for spreading droplets until CaP precipitation was initiated at the edges of the droplets after reaching critical supersaturation. Consequently, circular CaP doughnut shaped droplets were formed during droplet spreading and were deposited on the substrate as either isolated rings or coalesced pores, depending on the spreading rate of the droplets and the precipitation rate of the CaP solute.

10.3.2.2 Influence of Chemical, Precursor Solution Parameters on Morphological Properties

The chemical composition of the precursor solutions and the mixing characteristics of the calcium and phosphate precursor components strongly influenced initial electrospray droplet sizes, the precipitation kinetics of the CaP solute, and the corresponding coating morphologies, as shown in Fig. 10.5 for precursor solutions with different acidities. Droplet-derived structures, such as micron-sized doughnuts or pores, were completely absent in the surface morphology of coatings deposited using acidic precursor solutions (1 vol% HNO_3). PDA measurements revealed that the corresponding droplets were much

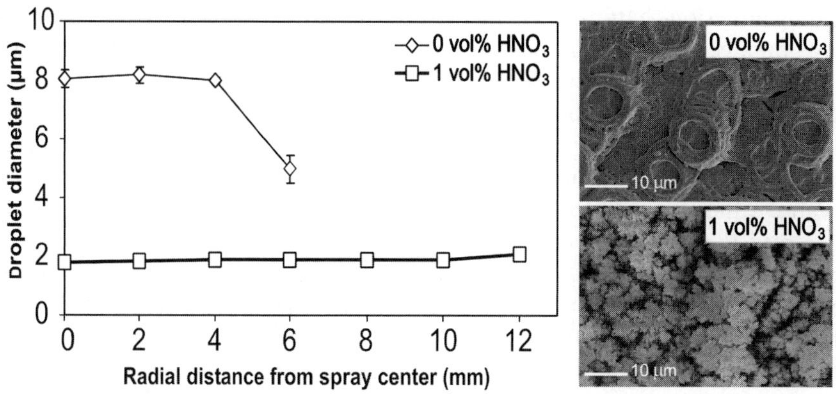

Fig. 10.5 Radial mapping of mean droplet diameters for precursor solutions with various acidities-0 vol% and 1 vol% extra nitric acid (HNO_3)-at a plane 5 mm above the substrate. Corresponding SEM images are depicted

smaller for these acidic precursor concentrations (droplets of about 3.0–3.5 µm) compared to the average droplet size of 8 µm for the precursor concentration without adding extra nitric acid. These observations are in agreement with the electrospraying theory [29, 30], which predicts that electrosprayed droplets decrease in size with increasing conductivity of the precursor solutions. Grainy surface morphologies for acidic precursor solutions were formed by particle formation from homogeneous solute precipitation in small droplets, whereas coatings consisting of droplet-derived structures were deposited by heterogeneous precipitation at the edge of large droplets during spreading over the substrate surface.

10.3.3 Conclusion

The ESD technique was shown to be appropriate for depositing CaP coatings with a large variety of morphological and chemical properties onto titanium substrates. This makes this technique especially suitable for investigating the fundamental relations between CaP coating characteristics and their biological performance *in vitro* and *in vivo*.

10.4 Mechanical Properties of Porous, Electrosprayed CaP Coatings

Calcium phosphate coatings must adhere satisfactorily to the underlying substrate to maintain their bioactive functionality after surgical installation. Generally, tensile adhesion testing according to standards such as ASTM C633 is the most common procedure for determining quantitative values for CaP coating adhesion to the underlying metallic substrates [31, 32]. In a preliminary study on mechanical properties of electrosprayed CaP coatings, we measured a tensile adhesion strength of 36 ± 5 MPa for reticular, 2 μm thick, as-deposited ESD coatings (mean of three coated substrates) according to this test method. However, it be noted that reliable data can be obtained only for coating thicknesses > 0.38 mm using ASTM C633 [33]. This limitation is imposed because adhesive epoxy bonding agents are used in the test, and they tend to penetrate the porosities of the coatings. Moreover, coatings do experience combined shear, bending, tensile, and compressive stresses *in vivo*. Thus, measurement of tensile adhesion strength can be regarded as an oversimplification of the *in vivo* situation [34]. Therefore, other approaches are needed to evaluate the mechanical properties of porous ESD coatings under various stress conditions.

In this study, the mechanical properties of reticular, electrosprayed CaP coatings have been characterized using a range of analytical techniques. First, the fatigue behavior of ESD coatings was investigated using a three-point bending test method in simulated body fluid (SBF) under cyclic loading conditions to simulate the discontinuous forces that act on an implant. Second, scratch testing was performed to obtain insight into the coating deformation mechanism under shear stress. Finally, the adhesion of ESD coatings to the surface of dental implants was evaluated by implanting cylindrical and conical commercially pure Ti implants into an osseous environment (femoral condyle of goat cadavers), followed by electron microscopic and chemical microanalysis of the explants to determine coating maintenance.

Electrosprayed CaP coatings were either left untreated or subjected to additional heat treatments at 500°C or 700°C for 2 hours at controlled heating and cooling rates of 100°C per hour. Untreated coatings were designated amorphous calcium phosphate (ACP), whereas heat-treated coatings were designated carbonate apatite (CA) heat-treated at 500°C or carbonated hydroxyapatite (CHA) heat-treated at 700°C. Briefly, the major structural difference between CA (heat-treated at 500°C) and CHA (heat-treated at 700°C) coatings was the presence of OH^- groups in the apatitic lattice of CHA coatings after heat treatment at 700°C; CA coatings did not display OH^- absorption and had a higher carbonate content. Consequently, CHA coatings were slightly more crystalline than CA coatings. More details on the chemical structure of these coatings can be found elsewhere [35].

10.4.1 Fatigue Testing

The fatigue behavior of ESD-derived CaP coatings (coating thickness about 1.5–2.0 μm) was investigated using a cyclic, three-point bending test method (ASTM E855) in SBF [36, 37]. XRD, FTIR, and SEM analyses revealed that amorphous ESD coatings gradually dissolved upon static immersion in SBF, and coating dissolution was slightly accelerated owing to cyclic loading. On the contrary, crystalline ESD coatings did not show any significant alterations in coating structure or morphology after cyclic loading in SBF. Clemens et al. [36] and Wolke et al. [37] also observed that crystallization of both plasma-sprayed and sputtered CaP coatings increased their resistance to crack formation and fatigue failure. The highly porous and compliant structure of the tested ESD coatings was expected to ensure relatively high bending flexibility, low amounts of internal stresses, and therefore a low tendency toward crack formation and coating degradation as a result of cyclic loading.

10.4.2 Scratch Testing

Scratch tests were performed on CaP-coated Ti disks (coating thickness ~2.0–2.5 μm) using a Universal Surface Tester (UST) (Innowep, Würzburg, Germany). This apparatus enabled separate measurement of plastic and elastic deformation by scanning three times over exactly the same track [38, 39]. The first and third scans were performed in the profilometer mode at a minimum vertical force of 1.0 mN, whereas the actual scratch was imposed on the coating surface during the second scan, in which the force was increased along the scratch path. The difference in recorded height profile between the third and second scans equals the reversible elastic deformation, whereas the difference between the first and third scan corresponds to permanent plastic deformation. Two styluses were used to produce scratches on the test specimens: A steel ball stylus with a tip radius of 0.40 mm was used to determine the influence of a blunt type of indenter on the mechanical integrity of the coatings, and a scratch diamond was employed to examine the localized deformation induced by a sharp stylus.

Scratch testing using a blunt ball stylus revealed a ductile failure mode of reticular CaP coatings. This ductile failure mode was described by Bull [40] as a failure mechanism characterized by small areas of uncovered substrate that are confined within the scratch track, whereas brittle failure is more extensive and often extends beyond the limits of the scratch track. Bull stated that there is a requirement for ductile failure for the best scratch adhesion, as critical loads L_c for ductile failure are much higher than those observed for brittle materials. Indeed, using a blunt ball stylus with a tip radius in the same size range as a conventional Rockwell C stylus (0.4 mm for the ball stylus vs. a tip diameter of 0.2 mm for Rockwell C), the maximum apparatus load of 100 mN was by far not enough to delaminate the coating. Still, the reticular surface structure of these ESD coatings appeared to be fragile. Wang et al. [41] reported the same effect for fragile octacalcium phosphate (OCP) coatings with flake-like morphologies, which displayed lower L_c values for initial deformation compared to denser CA coatings. The L_c values for total delamination were comparable to those for the CA coatings. These findings emphasize that caution should always be taken when determining critical load values L_c as a quantitative measurement for coating adhesion, as adhesion and mechanical strength (cohesion) of coatings are strictly separate phenomena. Without unambiguous definition of a well defined failure event (e.g., total coating delamination) by means of SEM, which illustrates the particular failure mode, determination of L_c values is a rather arbitrary method of quantifying coating adhesion. Scratch testing is a good comparative test for obtaining qualitative information on the major failure modes [41, 42]. Nevertheless, the scratch testing method is less suitable for acquiring absolute values of critical loads (L_c) owing to its dependence on numerous experimental parameters related to the testing system and the specific coating–substrate system [41–43]. As a consequence, it is hardly possible to compare rough, dense, plasma-sprayed coatings with flat, reticular electrosprayed coatings in a quantitative way using the scratch test because of the enormous differences in terms of roughness, thickness, morphology, crystallinity, and homogeneity, among other parameters. For example, plasma-sprayed coatings have a much higher average surface roughness (typically $>4.0\ \mu m$) and coating thickness (typically $\sim 50\ \mu m$). Scratch testing of electrosprayed coatings on top of roughened Ti substrates (R_a of about 1.0–1.5 μm) was impossible using the ball stylus because this coating was scratched only at the roughness peaks and remained intact at the roughness valleys.

Figure 10.6 show low- and high-magnification SEM images of 0.50 mm scratches on various reticular ESD coatings that were produced by means of a scratch diamond (final load 100 mN). Ductile failure modes were also dominant for ESD coatings using this sharp stylus, with the exception of amorphous ACP coatings, which displayed spallation of small coating fragments around the very

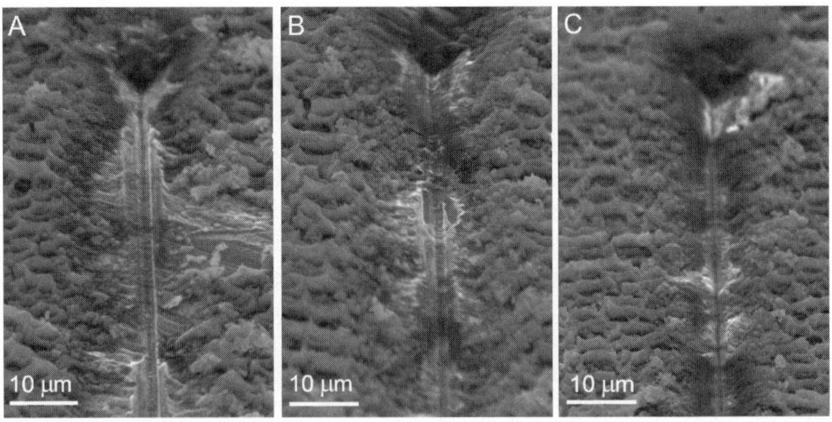

Fig. 10.6 SEM images of 0.50 mm scratches produced on various electrosprayed coatings by means of a sharp scratch diamond under a stepwise increasing load (final load 100 mN). **a** Tilted (60°) scratch endpoint on amorphous calcium phosphate (ACP) coating. **b** Tilted (60°) scratch endpoint on carbonate apatite (CA) coating. **c** Tilted (60°) scratch endpoint on carbonated hydroxyapatite (CHA) coating

end of the maximum apparatus load at 100 mN (Fig. 10.6b). Spallation is the result of total delamination (adhesive failure) due to a compressive stress field around the moving stylus [44] and typically occurs for poorly adhering coatings [40]. After heat treatment of as-deposited ESD coatings, the resistance to plastic deformation by the highly destructive scratch diamond stylus was enhanced most effectively for CHA coatings. Delamination did not occur for either type of heat-treated coating; instead, only simple ploughing through the coating material was observed. Scratches made on CHA coatings were considerably narrower than on ACP and CA coatings (10 μm for CHA vs. 20 μm for ACP and CA coatings, and delamination was never observed on CHA coatings (Fig. 10.6d). Chemical microanalysis of the deepest part of the scratches by the EDS technique revealed that the titanium (Ti) substrate was still partly covered with the CHA coating, as significant Ca and P peaks were still detected. Quantification of the ploughing depths using the profilometer mode of the UST apparatus revealed that all ESD coatings were plastically deformed initially at equal levels of about 0.4 to 0.5 μm under a vertical load of 5 mN. However, at the highest final load of 100 mN, ACP coatings were penetrated more than 2.0 μm by the scratch diamond, whereas CA coatings revealed a lower ploughing depth of about 1.5 μm. CHA coatings were resistant to plastic deformation even more than ACP and CA coatings, as reflected by low ploughing depths for CHA coatings of about 0.7 μm. To obtain more evidence for this latter observation, some of the earlier scratched ACP coatings were heat-treated at 700°C and subsequently scratched again on previously unscratched areas. Observed plastic scratch deformations decreased toward exactly the same values as found earlier for the CHA coatings that were not scratched prior to heat treatment.

Consequently, reticular electrosprayed CaP coatings can be described as ductile coatings with a good interfacial adhesion to the Ti substrate but with poor mechanical strength of the rather fragile superficial pore walls. Additional heat treatment at 700°C is necessary to restrict ploughing deformation into ESD-prepared CaP coatings.

10.4.3 Explantation of Dental Screw Implants

A study by Manders et al. [45] has proven the osteoconductive capacity of porous, electrosprayed CaP coatings. The mechanical behavior of these coatings, when applied to dental implants screws, was not previously addressed. Manders et al. showed that dental implants with complex surface geometries can be homogeneously coated with reticular CaP coatings using ESD, although local differences in nozzle-to-substrate distances, surface temperature, and/or the electrical field (in terms of preferential landing effects [46]) were supposed to hamper controlled deposition of these surface morphologies onto curved substrates. Therefore, the adhesion of porous, electrosprayed CaP coatings was evaluated in an osseous environment by means of implantation and immediate explantation of ESD-coated dental implant screws.

A goat cadaver model was used to evaluate the adhesion of electrosprayed ACP, CA, and CHA coatings on both conically and cylindrically shaped dental implants. After euthanasia of mature Saanen goats, femoral condyles were excised and stored in distilled water until the implants were installed. Holes were drilled in the trabecular bone of the exposed femoral condyles under continuous cooling. The implants were inserted and immediately explanted by means of unscrewing, whereafter the implants were carefully brushed and cleaned in distilled water to remove adherent tissue debris. After drying the implants overnight at 40°C, SEM and EDS were carried out on all explants.

This method appears to be a simple but valuable strategy for qualitative characterization of the adhesion of CaP coatings in an appropriate manner. However, it should be realized that CaP coatings were deformed twice during implantation as well as explantation in this test, which of course does not correspond to the real clinical situation where the implant is left in place after installation. Still, it can be concluded that the mechanical strength of amorphous ACP and crystalline CA coatings was not sufficient to withstand the shear and compressive forces applied to the typical superficial pore wall structure. ACP- and CA-coated implants were covered with dense layers of CaP, which most likely originated from the compressed remnants of the reticular coatings. In contrast to ACP and CA coatings, reticular structures of CHA coatings were clearly recognizable after explantation. These findings confirm the results of scratch testing, where CHA coatings were shown to be more resistant to plastic deformation by shear stresses. Generally, it can be concluded that heat treatment at 700°C significantly increased both the adhesion and mechanical strength of electrosprayed CaP coatings to a degree where reticular surface structures were no longer easily deformed and could be (partially) maintained upon implantation and subsequent implant retrieval. Adhesion of CHA coatings can be improved as the result of oxidation of the Ti substrate (observed using XRD) after heat treatment at 700°C, which is suggested to act as an oxidic transition layer between nonoxide Ti substrates and oxidic CaP ceramic coatings. Improved mechanical strength of CHA coatings can be related to various processes that occur upon heat treatment of ESD coatings. FTIR analysis revealed that heat treatment at 700°C resulted into decomposition of carbonate groups into OH^- groups [35] for CHA coatings, which corroborates the results of El Feki et al. [47]. Carbonate anions are known to hamper crystal growth compared to carbonate-free HA by disturbing the structural stability of the apatitic lattice, which can be an explanation for the higher crystallinity and improved mechanical properties of CHA coatings compared to CA coatings. Another explanation is related to the nucleation of apatite crystals in an amorphous matrix after heat treatment at elevated temperatures, as these crystal nuclei can act as inhibitors of propagation of microcracks through the amorphous matrix. Furthermore, a decrease in submicron porosity and, correspondingly, an increase in specific surface area due to heat treatment at 700°C is expected to lead to microstructural compaction of the coating and thus to increased resistance against plastic deformation.

10.4.4 Conclusion

Mechanical properties of reticular, electrosprayed CaP coatings were characterized using a range of analytical techniques. It was observed for all these techniques that reticular ESD coatings need to be crystallized to ensure sufficient interfacial adhesion to the substrate and mechanical strength of the superficial pore wall structure for applications where shear and compressive stresses are imposed on the implant surface. Amorphous ESD coatings dissolved rapidly during fatigue testing under wet conditions and were easily deformed by shear stresses during scratch testing or unscrewing of ESD-coated dental implants from femoral condyles of goat cadavers. On the contrary, crystalline coatings heat treated at 700°C were resistant to fatigue as well as plastic ploughing deformation by means of various scratch styli, whereas the fragile surface structure of ESD coatings was maintained to a large extent after unscrewing dental implants coated with crystalline CHA coatings. The latter method of unscrewing previously implanted dental screws from osseous tissue of goat cadavers was successfully introduced as a simple method to assess the adhesion and mechanical strength of biomedical CaP coatings under conditions that mimic clinical situations as closely as possible. Based on the results, it was concluded that interfacial adhesion of crystalline CHA ESD coatings to the Ti substrate was sufficient, but that mechanical strength of the superficial architecture of ESD coatings needs to be optimized for applications where high shear stresses are imposed on the fragile coating surface of reticular ESD morphologies.

10.5 Similarities and Differences Between Plasma-Sprayed and Electrosprayed CaP Coatings

Plasma spraying and ESD are fundamentally different processes regarding experimental setups and resultant coatings. Plasma spraying uses a hot plasma in which the temperature may rise to values around 20,000°C, which results in (partial) melting of the crystalline CaP ceramic powder. In contrast, electrospraying is an aerosol-based process whereby finely dispersed, charged droplets are deposited on a heated substrate. Generally, process temperatures do not exceed 400°C during ESD, but additional heat treatments are required to crystallize the as-deposited coatings into the apatite phase.

As a consequence, coating properties in terms of chemical composition and homogeneity, average surface roughness, thickness, morphology, and crystallinity, among others are completely different for both coating techniques. Plasma-sprayed coatings must be at least 50 μm thick to cover the implant completely. The adhesion of these thick plasma-sprayed coatings tends to be quite weak, which necessitates pretreatment of the substrates by such methods as grit blasting to roughen the substrate and to increase the mechanical interlocking of the coating–substrate system. Such a surface-roughening pretreatment is not required for ESD coatings. As a result, the roughness and thickness of plasma-sprayed coatings are much greater than electrosprayed ones, as ESD coatings are formed by chemical reactions between dissolved precursor salts and decomposition products of the organic solvent. Coating growth rates using ESD are typically in the order of a few microns per hour, which enables better control of the coating thickness. In contrast to the plasma-spray process, coating thickness can be minimized to the submicron level depending on the precursor concentrations and deposition time. Another major difference between plasma-sprayed and electrosprayed coatings concerns the surface morphology, which is dense for plasma-sprayed coatings in contrast to the morphology of ESD coatings, which can be varied from dense to highly porous. Finally, electrosprayed coatings are chemically homogeneous, whereas plasma-sprayed coatings exhibit a heterogeneous crystallinity consisting of amorphous and crystalline areas resulting from partial melting of the original crystalline particles. However, plasma-sprayed coatings do not need an additional heat treatment to improve adhesion and induce crystallinity, whereas ESD coatings need to be heat-treated to obtain a crystalline, adherent coating.

10.6 Physicochemical Stability *In Vitro* and *In Vivo*

Biomedical CaP coatings can be deposited with defined chemical [14] and morphological [15] characteristics using the ESD technique. Specifically, a unique reticular coating morphology was obtained, characterized by a three-dimensional, interconnected pore network with variable pore size. This coating morphology offers the advantage of creating an implant surface with an increased, controllable surface area. As a result, phenomena such as the CaP coating dissolution rate and incorporation of osteoinductive proteins might be controlled by tailoring the surface morphology.

The ability to form apatite precipitation layers in SBF or in animal models has been regarded as evidence of bioactivity for bioceramics [48]. Therefore, dissolution and/or precipitation reactions of porous, ESD-prepared CaP coatings have been studied in a classic *in vitro* test by immersing ESD-coated Ti substrates with various crystal phases (amorphous calcium phosphate, carbonate apatite, CHA, and β-tricalcium phosphate) in SBF [35]. Because *in vitro* assays cannot completely mimic the *in vivo* situation, identical CaP coatings were also evaluated *in vivo* after subcutaneous implantation in the backs of goats to obtain insight about the dissolution and compositional behavior of porous ESD-prepared CaP coatings [35]. The following porous ESD coatings with equal surface morphology but different chemical characteristics were prepared for the *in vitro* and *in vivo* studies (commercially pure Ti disks: thickness 1.5 mm, diameter 12 mm, CaP coating thickness 2.0–2.5 μm):

- Amorphous calcium phosphate (ACP)
- Carbonate apatite (CA)
- Carbonated hydroxyapatite (CHA)
- β-Tricalcium phosphate (β-TCP)

The ACP, CA, and CHA coatings were prepared using precursor solutions with a Ca/P ratio of 1.8 [$Ca(NO_3)_2 \cdot 4H_2O$ and H_3PO_4 were precursors for Ca and P, respectively), whereas solutions with a lower Ca/P ratio of 1.4 were employed to prepare the β-TCP coatings. After coating deposition, all coated Ti substrates were heat-treated for 2 hours in air at 400°C (ACP), 500°C (CA), and 700°C (CHA, β-TCP). Uncoated Ti substrates were also used as a reference material for both *in vitro* and *in vivo* studies.

10.6.1 In Vitro *Soaking in Simulated Body Fluid*

In vitro experiments were carried out in conventional SBF with an ionic composition almost equal to that of human plasma [49]. Ionic concentrations of this SBF were 142.0 mM Na^+, 5.0 mM K^+, 1.5 mM Mg^{2+}, 2.5 mM Ca^{2+}, 147.8 mM Cl^-, 4.2 mM HCO_3^{2-}, 1.0 mM HPO_4^{2-}, and 0.5 mM SO_4^{2-}. Tris-HCl served as buffer to maintain a constant pH of 7.4. The coated and uncoated substrates (three specimens per time period per type of CaP coating) were immersed in 4 ml of SBF for 1, 2, 4, 8, and 12 weeks. SBF temperature was kept at 37°C using a waterbath and replaced with freshly prepared SBF every week. After the various immersion times, the specimens were removed from SBF, washed thoroughly with distilled water (3×) and dried at 50°C. Subsequently, all specimens were characterized using SEM, XRD, FTIR, and EDS.

The surface morphology of a porous CA coating prior to soaking is depicted in Fig. 10.7a. Upon immersing in SBF, a highly bioactive behavior was observed for crystalline apatitic coatings (CA, CHA) that induced formation of a precipitation layer consisting of densely packed CaP flakes on top of apatitic coatings during the first 2 weeks of immersion in SBF (see Fig. 10.7b for a CA coating after 1 week of soaking in SBF). FTIR and XRD analyses revealed that all precipitation layers initially consisted of OCP with its typical flake-like morphology, and Ca/P ratios of OCP-covered apatitic coatings had decreased from ~2.2 to ~1.6 as a result of the low Ca/P ratio of the OCP (1.33). Several authors have noted that OCP formation is a common feature in either simulated or real physiological environments [48, 50–53]. However, unique low angle ($<10°$ 2θ) diffraction peaks of OCP are often ignored or are difficult to detect with XRD owing to: (1) the low angle of incidence of thin-film XRD when analyzing coatings, (2) preferential orientation of OCP crystals on surfaces [54], and/or (3) small sizes in directions of the (*h*00) planes [55].

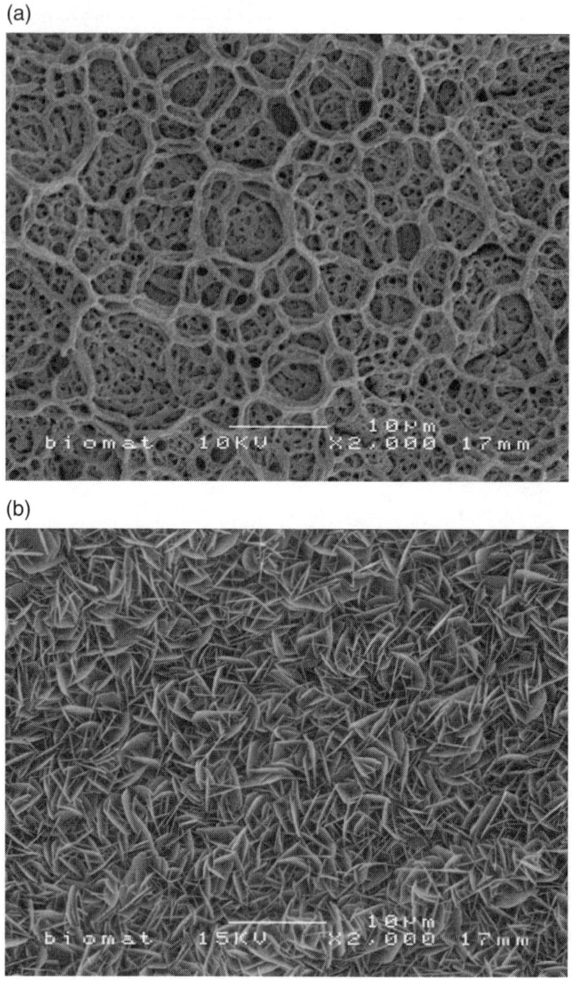

Fig. 10.7 SEM image of CA coatings prior to (**a**) and after (**b**) soaking in simulated body fluid (SBF) for 1 week. From [35]. with permission from Elsevier

A theoretical analysis of CaP precipitation in SBF by Lu and Leng [49] demonstrated that the nucleation rate of OCP is substantially higher than that of HA in SBF at physiological pH 7.4, whereas HA is thermodynamically the most stable phase in SBF. Iijima et al. [55] and Nelson et al. [56] proved that the presence of carbonate anions in surrounding fluids greatly affects the chemical nature and morphology of CaP precipitates. Nelson et al. [56] suggested that nucleation of OCP seeds was favored energetically in the presence of carbonate at concentrations <10 mM. Moreover, subsequent conversion rates of OCP toward apatite were reduced by carbonate ions disturbing the crystallization of apatitic CaP phases [16, 55], which might explain the initial stabilization of OCP precipitates on carbonated ESD coatings (ACP, CA, CHA) under conditions where apatite is the expected precipitation bulk phase. Our findings support the statement made by Xin et al. [48] that it should be reconsidered whether apatite formation is a suitable criterion by which to judge bioactivity of biomaterials, as misidentification of OCP for apatite might have confused theoretical considerations on *in vitro* bioactivity and distracted attention from other CaP phases such as OCP.

With time, OCP precipitation layers became more apatitic in nature, as reflected by (1) the gradual loss of OCP low angle reflection peaks (XRD), (2) the corresponding loss of degeneracy in the ν_4 phosphate absorption domain (FTIR), and (3) an increased Ca/P ratio, from 1.6 to 1.7 Ca/P to 1.8 to 1.9 Ca/P. OCP and apatite reveal close structural similarities, as the OCP structure is composed of apatite layers separated by hydrated layers [16, 50]. The OCP → apatite transition is mostly a hydrolytic solid-state reaction [51].

$$5\,Ca_8H_2(PO_4)_6 \cdot 5H_2O \rightarrow 8\,Ca_5(PO_4)_3OH + 6\,H_3PO_4 + 17\,H_2O$$

This gradual phase transformation from the OCP phase to the more basic apatitic CaP phase is a well known phenomenon since the work of Brown et al. [57] and has been observed by several authors *in vitro* and *in vivo* after long periods of immersion [50–58]. Actually, OCP has been frequently proposed as a mandatory precursor phase for the formation of nonstoichiometric, biological apatites [16, 51, 58]. This process was described as a long-term mineralization process yielding phase mixtures richer in apatite with higher Ca/P ratios than the transient OCP phase after maturation of biological calcification [52].

Amorphous CaP displayed delayed precipitation of poorly adherent CaP layers compared to crystalline apatite coatings, whereas heterogeneous calcification was observed on β-TCP-coated substrates (Fig. 10.8) for immersion periods of up to 8 weeks. This indicated that β-TCP and ACP coatings exhibit poor ability to induce calcification in SBF compared to crystalline apatitic coatings. FTIR and XRD analyses showed that ACP coatings were amorphous, exposing a chemically unstable surface with high solubility to the surrounding body fluid, which initially might have reduced the calcifying tendency of ACP coatings after 1 week of immersion in SBF. Eventually, the high solubility of ACP led to deterioration of the porous coating morphology, crack formation, and most likely CaP dissolution at the interface between the coating and the substrate, which explains the observed poor adherence between calcified ACP coatings and the underlying Ti substrates. The poor ability of sintered β-TCP to induce CaP formation *in vitro* corroborates a comparative study of Xin et al., who also observed that β-TCP did not readily induce OCP calcification *in vitro* and *in vivo* [48]. As before, this can be caused by the chemically unstable surface of β-TCP coatings, which might prevent formation of OCP nuclei on soluble CaP phases *in vitro*. Another factor is the absence of carbonate ions in β-TCP coatings, which can stimulate OCP formation under specific conditions depending on the Ca/P ratio and carbonate concentration of the surrounding fluids [55].

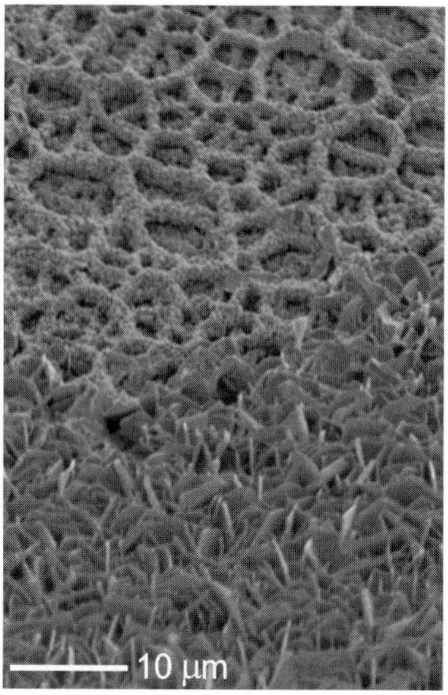

Fig. 10.8 Tilted (45°) scanning electron micrograph of β-TCP after 2 weeks in SBF. From [35] with permission from Elsevier

10.6.2 In Vivo *Subcutaneous Implantation*

Five adult goats with a mean body weight of about 50 to 60 kg were used in this study [35]. Various CaP-coated Ti disks (coated with ACP, CA, CHA, or β-TCP phase) were implanted subcutaneously in the backs of goats during four surgical sessions for implantation periods of 2, 4, 8, and 12 weeks. At the end of each implantation period, a longitudinal incision was made on both sides of the vertebral column, whereafter the implants were exposed and retrieved including the surrounding tissue. After removal, the disks were used for physicochemical characterization of the coatings as well as prepared for histological analysis. For physicochemical analysis, the explants were fixed in 4% phosphate-buffered formaldehyde solution (pH 7.4), removed from their surrounding tissue capsule, dehydrated in serial ethanol solutions, and examined by means of SEM, XRD, FTIR, and EDS. For histological evaluation, implants with the surrounding tissues were retrieved and fixed in 4% formaldehyde solution, dehydrated in serial ethanol series, and embedded in methylmethacrylate (MMA). After polymerization, 10 μm thick sections were prepared using a modified sawing microtome technique. These sections were stained with methylene blue and basic fuchsin and studied with a light microscope.

Gradual degradation was observed for all ESD coatings using XRD and SEM techniques, as indicated by a continuous decrease in intensity of CaP reflection peaks and gradual deterioration of the porous coating structure. After 4 weeks of subcutaneous implantation, no CaP reflection peaks were observed for ACP and CA coatings, but remnants of the original porous coating structure were still recognizable using SEM for both ACP and CA, emphasizing that SEM is more sensitive for detecting amorphous and/or poorly crystalline CaP ceramics in degradation studies. Thin-film XRD gives general information on the crystal nature of the entire implant surface, whereas SEM provides local details on the morphology of retrieved CaP-coated implants. Although ACP coatings were characterized as amorphous, disordered solids using XRD and FTIR, the partial maintenance of the porous coating morphology up to 4 to 8 weeks of subcutaneous implantation suggests that heat treatment at 400°C results in chemical stabilization of this ceramic coating in terms of nucleation of CaP crystallites with sizes below the detection limit of thin-film XRD. Nevertheless, the occasional detachment of surrounding layers of fibrous tissue debris from ACP coatings suggests that the surface of ACP coatings was still chemically unstable enough to hamper establishment of close contact between the tissue capsule and the implant surface. After 12 weeks, ACP and CA coatings could hardly be discerned by SEM (Fig. 10.9a) or XRD (Fig. 10.10a) as a result of severe coating degradation and coverage by surrounding fibrous tissue debris.

The CHA coatings were heat-treated at a higher temperature (700°C) and consequently revealed a lower dissolution rate than ACP and CA, maintaining the original porous coating (Fig. 10.9b) and typical apatitic reflection peaks (Fig. 10.10b) up to 12 weeks of implantation. As before, this effect was attributed to the decreased content of crystal growth inhibiting CO_3^{2-} ions and the corresponding formation of lattice-stabilizing OH^- groups after heat treatment at 700°C for CHA coatings. XRD analysis revealed that β-TCP coatings were degraded completely after 8 weeks at an intermediate dissolution rate between the rates for CA and CHA (Fig. 10.10c), although globular remnants of the reticular surface morphology were still observed by means of SEM after 12 weeks of implantation (Fig. 10.9c). As before, SEM appears to be more sensitive than XRD for detecting degrading CaP coatings. β-TCP coatings were heat-treated at a higher temperature (700°C) than CA coatings (500°C), which might have resulted in formation of relatively large β-TCP crystals.

Generally, no signs of CaP mineralization were observed; instead, coating dissolution was found for all ESD coatings according to a gradual degradation mechanism without delamination of large coating fragments. Wolke et al. [59] demonstrated that amorphous sputter coatings gradually disappeared upon subcutaneous implantation in rabbits. Crystalline, 0.1 μm thick HA sputter coatings disappeared after 8 weeks, whereas thicker (1 and 4 μm) HA coatings were maintained until 12 weeks. In contrast to these perfectly dense CaP coatings, dissolution of porous ESD coatings was accelerated by their very high specific surface, which increased the surface reactivity of thermodynamically stable phases such as CA and CHA. Thus, control over the specific surface area of ESD coatings (in terms of morphology/porosity) can be regarded as an added tool to control degradation rates of CaP coatings compared to variation of coating chemistry only, which might be of interest for applications that require sustained drug delivery profiles of incorporated biological agents such as growth factors.

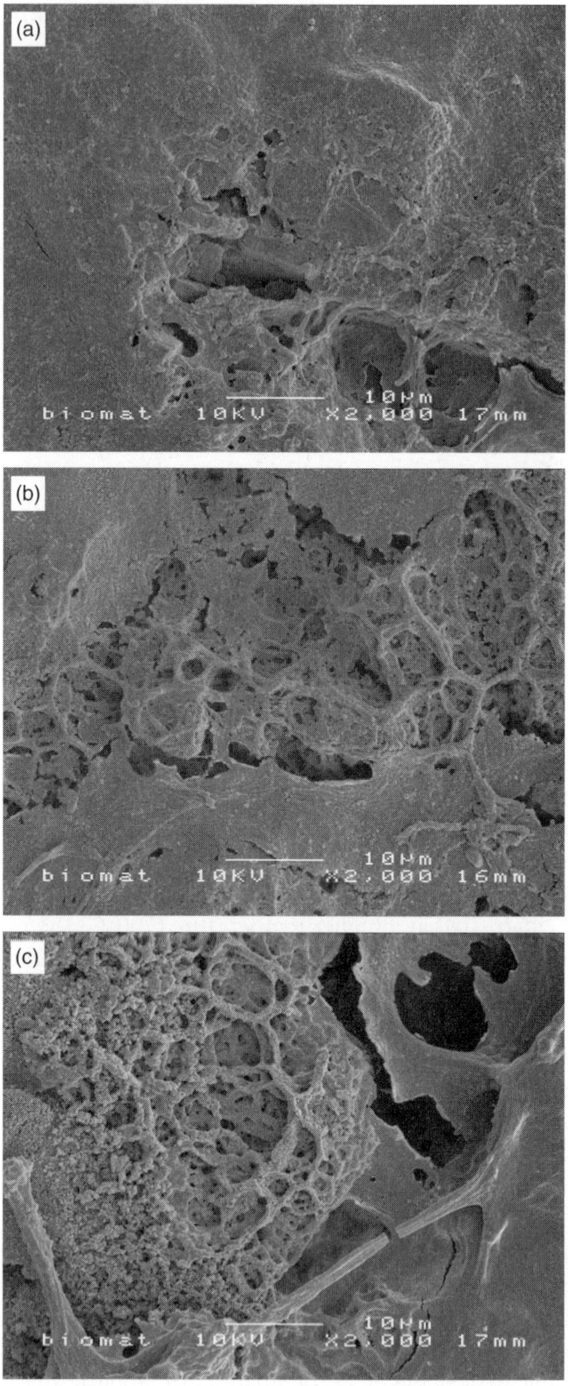

Fig. 10.9 SEM images of CA (**a**), CHA (**b**), and β-tricalcium phosphate (β-TCP) (**c**) coatings after 12 weeks of subcutaneous implantation. From [35], with permission from Elsevier

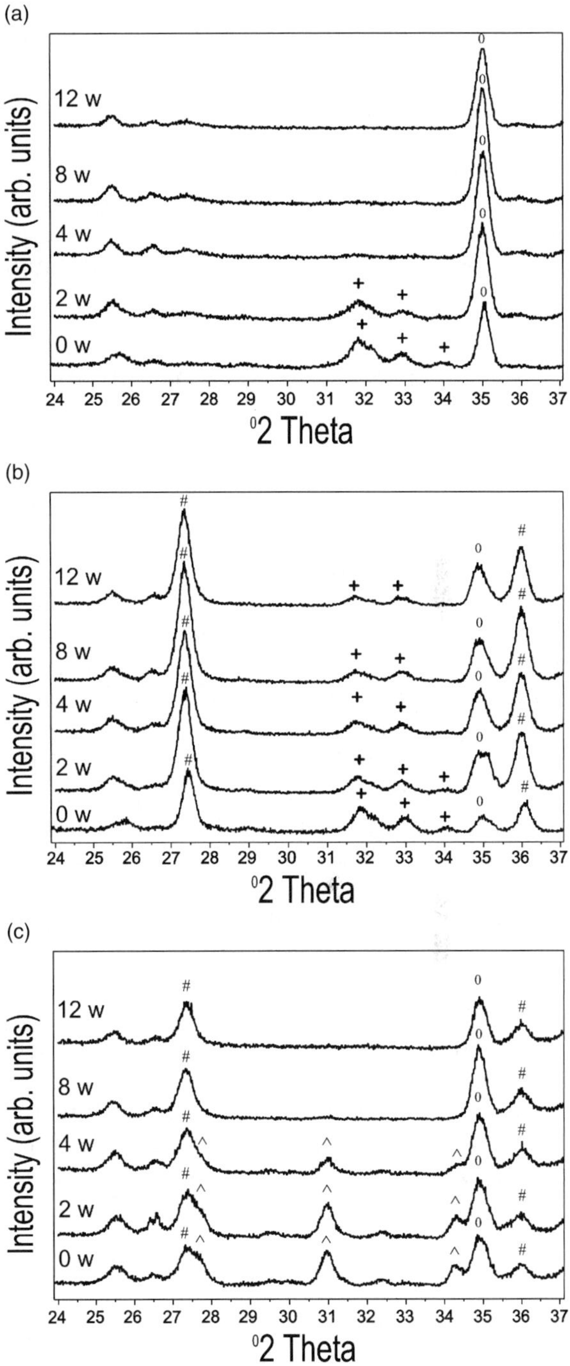

Fig. 10.10 XRD patterns of CA (**a**), CHA (**b**), and β-TCP (**c**) coatings after 0, 2, 4, 8, and 12 weeks of subcutaneous implantation. +, apatite; ∧, β-TCP; 0, titanium; #, TiO_2. From [35], with permission from Elsevier

Finally, histological evaluation demonstrated that all implanted ESD coatings evoked a biocompatible soft tissue reaction upon subcutaneous implantation for periods of 2 to 12 weeks. In response to surgical trauma and implant positioning, a normal wound healing process was observed, characterized by the formation of a thin fibrous capsule around the implants without the occurrence of a serious inflammatory reaction. Because degradation of ESD-prepared CaP coatings proceeded according to a gradual dissolution process, CaP release products did not provoke any foreign-body responses or other undesired tissue reactions, which might have been triggered by detached CaP-coating fragments [60, 61].

10.6.3 Comparison Between In Vitro *and* In Vivo *Studies*

The current subcutaneous *in vivo* study was characterized by degradation of ESD-prepared CaP coatings, the outcome of which was directly opposed to the *in vitro* soaking experiment, where abundant OCP/CA calcification of identical ESD coatings was observed. The same tendencies were described recently by Xin et al. [48], who also found less CaP formation *in vivo* than *in vitro* under almost similar *in vitro* and *in vivo* conditions. This discrepancy is inherent to the impossibility to copy the immensely complex *in vivo* environment in an *in vitro* model such as soaking in SBF. First, it should be realized that *in vivo* wound healing processes are always associated with a local decrease in pH [62], which inhibits CaP precipitation, whereas freshly prepared SBF solutions are buffered at neutral pH while performing *in vitro* soaking studies. Furthermore, the static *in vitro* conditions as employed in the current study (refreshing the SBF on a weekly basis) are completely different from the constant physiological circulation of body fluids. Ramila and Vallet-Regi [63] observed that the apatite precipitation rate and morphology were different for static and dynamic immersion of sol-gel bioglass disks in SBF, and Duan et al. [64] reported that nucleation of apatite in a dynamic soaking experiment could be detected only in the internal pore surface of porous CaP ceramics, where flow rates of SBF were lower than at the outer surface. Another major experimental difference between *in vitro* and *in vivo* studies is the presence of various biological compounds, such as proteins, in the *in vivo* environment. Proteins are known to interact with CaP ceramics as promotors or inhibitors of mineral crystal formation [65]. Several authors have already shown that serum proteins such as albumin can have an inhibitory effect on CaP crystallization *in vitro*, which could increase the solubility of protein-coated CaP ceramics over protein-free CaP under *in vitro* conditions [66, 67].

10.6.4 Conclusion

Various ESD-prepared, porous CaP coatings were (1) soaked in SBF for time periods up to 12 weeks (*in vitro*), and (2) implanted subcutaneously in goats for identical time periods (*in vivo*). *In vitro*, a highly bioactive behavior was observed for all ESD coatings, characterized by the deposition of a CaP precipitation layer on ESD coatings. *In vivo*, in contrast, all ESD coatings degraded gradually at a dissolution rate depending on the specific chemical phase, thereby enabling synthesis of CaP coatings with a tailored degradation rate. The difference between the *in vitro* and *in vivo* results can be related to the intrinsically different experimental conditions for *in vitro* and *in vivo* studies (composition and static vs. dynamic exchange of simulated/extracellular body fluids, presence of proteins, and so on).

10.7 Efficacy of Porous, Electrosprayed CaP Coatings *In Vivo*

In vitro studies have confirmed that osteoblast-like cells cultured on ESD-derived coatings have similar or improved osteogenic behavior compared to cells cultured on a radiofrequency (RF) magnetron-sputtered CaP coatings [68]. ESD-derived coatings were also found to be actively degraded by osteoclast-like cells, which suggests that they participate in the bone remodeling process [69]. Despite the promising results of the *in vitro* studies, it is known that the data obtained from cell culture experiments can never be directly extrapolated to the *in vivo* situation. However, an *in vivo* study using a so-called implant-gap model in goats proved that ESD-derived CaP coatings have osteoconductive properties [45]. On the other hand, the results showed that plasma-spray-coated implants still had a significantly more pronounced effect than the ESD-derived CaP coating. This difference in biological response is supposed to be due to a difference in the morphological and chemical structure between the plasma-sprayed and ESD-derived CaP coatings, which can influence their stability in a body environment. In view of this, optimization of the ESD-prepared CaP coatings is required. One relevant structural coating parameter that is supposed to have an enhancing effect on bone response is the coating crystallinity (i.e., the percentage of amorphous and crystalline intensities). Different crystallinities exhibit different dissolution and reprecipitation properties, which can influence bone formation at the bone implant interface. Therefore, the bone response to ESD CaP-coated screw-shaped implants with various crystallinities was studied in trabecular bone of the femoral condyle of goats [70].

10.7.1 Implant Materials, Surgical Procedure, Implant Retrieval

Tapered, conical, screw-shaped dental implants (commercially pure titanium, implant length 10 mm, implant diameter ranging from 4.0 mm at the coronal part to 3.4 mm at the apical side) were coated with the following electrosprayed CaP coatings (coating thickness 2.0–2.5 μm).

- Amorphous calcium phosphate (ACP)
- Carbonate apatite (CA)
- Carbonated hydroxyapatite (CHA)

Six samples were prepared as described in the previous section to induce different degrees of coating crystallinity. Another six uncoated Ti implants were used as a control group.

Five healthy, mature (2–4 years of age) Saanen goats were used [70]. The implants were inserted into the trabecular bone of the femoral condyle. After 12 weeks, the goats were sacrificed using an overdose of Nembutal®, and the implants were retrieved for evaluation. The femoral condyles were excised, and excessive tissue was removed. Using a diamond saw, the retrieved condyles were divided into smaller specimens suitable for histological processing. Each specimen contained one implant site with surrounding bone. Subsequently, the specimens were fixed in 4% formaldehyde, dehydrated in ethanol, and embedded in MMA. After polymerization in MMA, thin (7 μm) non-decalcified sections were prepared with an inner circular sawing microtome. The sections were made parallel to the longitudinal axis of the implant, were stained with methylene blue and basic fuchsin, and were examined by light microscopy.

10.7.2 Histological Evaluation

Light microscopic examination of the implants revealed uneventful healing of all implants. All of the implants had been inserted in cortical and trabecular bone. Histology demonstrated that some of the implants had been inserted close to the growth plate cartilage, but nowhere did the implants contact the growth plate. The drilling procedure appeared to have been accurate, as no oversized drill holes (in terms of depth and width) were observed. An overview section of a CHA-coated implant in situ is presented in Fig. 10.11.

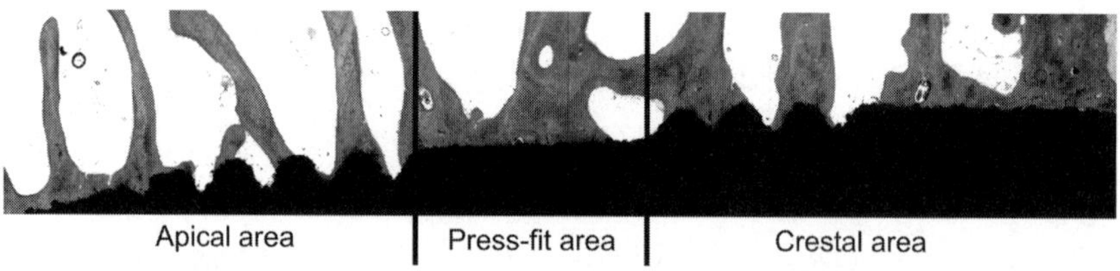

Fig. 10.11 Light micrograph of one side of an implant with CHA coating. Bone contact is visible along the surface of the entire implant. From [70], with permission from Blackwell (*See* Color Insert)

- *Crestal part of the implant*: At the crestal area, the implants were surrounded by both cortical and trabecular bone. The thickness of the cortical bone varied among specimens. No soft tissue downgrowth was observed along the surface of any of the implants. The bone was in close contact with the surrounding cortical and trabecular bone. There appeared to be no differences in bone contact between the CaP-coated and Ti implants.
- *Middle part of the implant*: The middle part of the implant was surrounded completely by trabecular bone. The newly formed bone had a typical trabecular structure and could barely be discerned from the original bone. The newly formed bone had only slightly more intense pink staining. The density and appearance of the apposed bone was similar to the original bone. Furthermore, the bone had an intimate contact with the implant surface and followed all the irregularities without the presence of fibrous tissue or inflammatory cells. Occasionally, remodeling lacunae could be observed at the bone–implant interface. A slight difference in bone contact appeared to exist between CaP-coated and bare Ti implants, with more direct bone contact for CaP-coated implants.
- *Apical part of the implant*: The apical region of the implant was also surrounded by trabecular bone. Typically, a layer of trabecular bone covered parts of the implant surface. At the lower part of the apical region, sometimes a gap between the implant and the surrounding bone was observed that lacked any sign of bone adaptation. Usually, this gap was filled with bone marrow-like tissue. No obvious differences in bone contact between the various implant groups could be seen.

10.7.3 Histomorphometric Analysis

The results of the bone contact measurements are presented in Table 10.1. Values are the mean ± standard deviation. CaP-coated corresponds to the mean of all combined CaP-coated implants. Statistical analysis was performed using two tests. An unpaired Student's *t*-test was used to compare the results of the CaP-coated implants as one group with the Ti implants, and a one-way analysis of variance (ANOVA) was used to compare the various coatings as separate groups from the Ti implants. $P < 0.05$ was considered statistically significant.

Generally, the amount of bone contact appeared to be higher for the electrosprayed, CaP-coated implants. Statistical analysis of the data revealed:

- A significant difference ($P < 0.05$) in bone contact between all grouped CaP-coated implants and the noncoated Ti implants
- No significant difference in bone contact between the separate ACP and CA coatings and the Ti implants ($P > 0.05$)
- A significant difference between CHA and Ti implants ($P < 0.05$)

Table 10.1 Percentage of bone contact after 12 weeks

Material	Bone contact
CaP-coated	64 ± 14*
ACP	66 ± 12
CA	55 ± 14
CHA	71 ± 13*
Titanium	48 ± 16

CaP, calcium phosphate; ACP, amorphous CaP; CA, carbonate apatite; CHA, carbonated hydroxyapatite
*$P < 0.05$ compared to the titanium control group

10.7.4 Discussion

The results showed that overall the CaP-coated implants had a higher percentage of bone contact than did the Ti implants. The crystalline CHA-coated implants had a significantly higher percentage bone contact compared to Ti implants. The results of the present study confirm again the osteocompatibility of electrosprayed CaP coatings. Nevertheless, only a significant beneficial effect of the CHA coating on bone–implant contact was observed. Two factors can explain the different behavior of the various CaP coatings. The first is the chemical composition of the CaP coatings, which was carbonate-containing apatite. It has been hypothesized that the bioactivity of carbonate apatite is increased compared to that of HA, as it more closely resembles the natural phase present in bone and teeth. However, the dissolution rate of carbonate apatite is increased compared to that of HA. As a consequence, the thin (2 μm) carbonate apatite coatings dissolve before they can elicit a beneficial response. An additional heat treatment at 700°C introduces hydroxyl groups to the coating, which are known to stabilize the apatite structure compared to the carbonate structure. Unfortunately, no direct proof is available for this dissolution hypothesis because our ESD CaP coatings are too thin to observe with light microscopy. However, indirect support for this theory is provided by the dissolution behavior of ESD CaP coatings during subcutaneous implantation in goats (see earlier in the chapter). Amorphous, electrosprayed CaP coatings indeed dissolve faster than crystalline coatings.

A second explanation for the improved bone contact for crystalline CHA coatings are the mechanical properties of the coating as presented earlier in the chapter [71]. Heat treatment at 700°C improves the mechanical strength of the porous surface structure of the CaP coating as well as adhesion of the coating to the underlying Ti substrate. In view of this, the 400° and 500°C heat-treated electrosprayed CaP coatings can become partially detached during implant installation, which can affect the final bone response to these implants. Finally, we must note that the results of the present study are in agreement with previous *in vivo* studies related to the influence of CaP coating crystallinity on bone behavior [70, 72, 73]. In contrast, other *in vivo* studies using CaP coatings do not confirm the effect of coating crystallinity. These studies show no influence of coating crystallinity on bone contact [74–76]. This apparent discrepancy in the literature can be explained by the type of CaP coating that was used in the experiments. Each technique to deposit CaP coatings creates unique coatings regarding their chemical composition, surface roughness, coating thickness, and morphology. Furthermore, coatings derived from various techniques require different postdeposition treatments. For instance, plasma-sprayed coatings do not require heat treatment, whereas ESD-derived coatings need heat treatment to remove the organic remnants of the solvent solution from the coating. Therefore, great care should be taken when comparing the bone performance of CaP coatings that are deposited with different techniques.

10.7.5 Conclusion

Porous, electrosprayed CaP coatings were proven to be osteocompatible. Moreover, the percentage of bone contact of the crystalline CHA-coated implant was increased compared to that of Ti implants. Regarding the amorphous (ACP) and less crystalline (CA) CaP coatings, no differences were found compared to Ti implants. Evidently, we can conclude that the degree of crystallinity influences the biological performance of electrosprayed CaP coatings.

10.8 Prospects of Future Industrial Applications

Electrostatic spray deposition, a simple, inexpensive method for inorganic and organic coatings, makes it possible to obtain thin CaP layers with an extremely wide range of chemical and morphological characteristics. Various CaP phases and phase mixtures can be deposited, and a broad diversity of coating morphologies can be produced by varying the deposition parameters related to the ESD apparatus and/or the precursor solutions. Electrosprayed CaP coatings have been shown to be biocompatible with soft tissue, and the osteoconductive nature of electrosprayed CaP coatings has been proven *in vivo*. Particular interest was given to a unique, reticular coating morphology consisting of a porous network of variable pore size. This specific coating morphology offers the possibility of varying the specific surface area of electrosprayed CaP coatings to a large extent. Consequently, the degradation rate of CaP coatings as well as the incorporation and subsequent release of biological agents (e.g., growth factors) can be influenced by chemical and physical coating properties using the ESD technique. Several studies have already shown that protein films can be deposited by means of electrospraying at low temperatures. For instance, Uematsu et al. [77] prepared electrosprayed protein thin films on aluminum-coated poly(ethylene terephthalate) (PET) substrates from aqueous solutions of α-lactalbumin. These protein coatings had a fine porous structure typical for ESD with pore diameters ranging from 40 to 600 nm, and the biological activities of the crosslinked protein films were preserved upon deposition. The large control over surface properties and the possibility of incorporating biologically active growth factors using the ESD technique offers a great advantage over conventional coating techniques, which lack this chemical and morphological variability.

Still, several problems must be solved to achieve this final goal of depositing biologically active, drug-releasing CaP coatings onto implant surfaces. First, upscaling is necessary to coat large implant surfaces, as coating areas are restricted to a few square centimeters using the current setup. Although electrospraying is a versatile technique with many possible applications, the low flow rates at which the cone-jet mode generally operates have limited the use of electrosprays. Currently, no practical applications of purely electrohydrodynamic electrosprays are in widespread use with the exception of mass spectrometry. Electrospray ionization has emerged as a powerful tool for mass spectrometry of large and complex molecules, as reflected by the fact that the 2002 Chemistry Nobel Prize was awarded to John B. Fenn for his pioneering work in this field [78].

Several researchers have been trying to increase the liquid thoughput for electrospray atomization by increasing the number of spraying cones. Rulison and Flagran devised linear arrays of six Taylor cones on capillary electrode tubes [79]. Throughout the experiments described in this chapter, a square array of four nozzles developed to increase the number of substrates that could be coated during a certain time period were used. Almekinders and Jones designed a multiple-jet electrospray atomizer of 15 cm width based on a continuous liquid feed line without single spraying nozzles [80]. Recently, investigators at Yale University (USA) reported interesting developments regarding multiplexed electrospraying systems. Deng et al. [81] developed a compact system of electrospray distributors by microfabrication of an array of nozzles (250 sources/cm^2) in silicon wafers using deep reactive ion etching techniques. Nozzles were protruding from 150 to 450 μm and were patterned with outer diameters ranging from 180 to 240 μm. By using an extractor electrode at about 0.5 mm distance from the spray sources, uniform droplets were electrosprayed simultaneously from all parallelized electrosprays, each one operating as an isolated spray on the quasi-monodisperse cone-jet mode. Duby et al. [82] reported a novel approach to multiplexing single electrosprays based on the multijet mode of electrospraying. Sharp features (e.g., grooves, ridges) were machined at the nozzle outlet to intensify the local electrical field and to anchor the single cone-jets at these features. Stable modes of operation were reported over several hundreds of volts and a broad range of flow rates. The grooved atomizer was found to be a simple, easily controlled means of multiplexing an electrospray by one or two orders of magnitude, yielding a density on the order of 50 cone-jets/cm^2. Electrospraying deposition rates and covering areas can be increased even more if these upscaled multiplexed nozzle systems are used in combination with a substrate holder connected to a computer-controlled XY table.

Relatively high temperatures are currently employed during coating deposition (> 300°C) as well as subsequent heat treatments (> 500°C) that impede co-deposition of organic molecules. High temperatures are required to decompose the precursor solvents and salts and to form the final amorphous CaP compound, whereas additional heat treatments are necessary to produce coatings with sufficient crystallinity and mechanical stability *in vivo*. A possible solution for this drawback relates to the high processing temperatures is electrospraying of stable suspensions and sols, which contain crystalline CaP nanoparticles. Huang et al. [83, 84] produced submicrometer-sized HA relics on various substrate materials by electrospraying such nanosized, stable suspensions. Starting from these suspensions and sols, a crystalline CaP ceramic is formed prior to spray generation. As a result, high temperatures during coating deposition and additional heat treatments can be avoided. Furthermore, the mechanical strength of CaP coatings can be increased by co-deposition of an organic protein component such as collagen [85] when a strong physicochemical interaction is established between the inorganic and organic composite phases. Moreover, deposition rates can be enhanced significantly compared to electrospraying of dissolved precursor salts, as the solubility of precursor salts is no longer a limiting factor when using stable suspensions and sols.

Another benefit of this suspension- and sol-based approach may be improved reproducibility compared to synthesis starting from dissolved precursor salts, which react toward solid CaP compounds after spray generation. It was shown that Ca/P ratios of the dissolved precursor salts do not correspond to Ca/P ratios of deposited coatings (see earlier in the chapter). This phenomenon depends on the mixing time of the Ca and P precursors [22], which makes the geometry of the spraying nozzle a critical process parameter. As a consequence, process control and reproducibility are complicated for the deposition of complex inorganic materials, such as carbonate apatite, by electrospraying of dissolved Ca and P precursor salts. On the contrary, compositional and crystallographic alterations of the solid CaP ceramic are not expected after spray generation during electrospraying of stable suspensions and sols.

Finally, it is possible to coat implants with complex geometries without using cast holders ("negatives") if coating deposition occurs at low temperatures. These cast holders are used to ensure heat conduction to curved implant surfaces for processing at high temperatures [71] (Table 10.2).

Table 10.2 Publications on Electrosprayed Calcium Phosphate Coatings

Author	Journal	Characterization techniques	Mechanical testing	*In vitro* testing	*In vivo* testing
Leeuwenburgh et al.	J Biomed Mater Res 66 (2003) 330	SEM, FTIR, XRD			
Leeuwenburgh et al.	Biomaterials 25 (2004) 641	FTIR, XRD, EDS			
Siebers et al.	Biomaterials 25 (2004) 2019	SEM, FTIR, XRD, EDS	Profilometry (roughness)	Cell culture (osteoblast)	
Huang et al.	J Mater Sci 39 (2004) 1029	SEM, TEM, XRD		Cell culture (osteoblast)	
Huang et al.	J Mater Sci Mater Med 15 (2004) 441	SEM, TEM, XRD		Cell culture (macrophage)	
Leeuwenburgh et al.	J Biomed Mater Res 74 (2005) 275	FTIR, XRD, EDS			
Siebers et al.	J Biomed Mater Res 74 (2005) 570	SEM, FTIR, XRD, EDS		Cell culture (osteoclast)	
Leeuwenburgh et al.	Thin Solid Films 472 (2005) 105	SEM, FTIR, XRD	Profilometry (roughness)		
Manders et al.	Clin Oral Implants Res 17 (2006) 548	SEM, FTIR, XRD, EDS			Femoral condyle (goats)
Huang et al.	J Mater Sci Mater Med 16 (2005) 1137	SEM, AFM, TEM, XRD, viscosimetry, conductivity		Cell culture (osteoblast)	
Leeuwenburgh et al.	J Eur Ceram Soc 26 (2006) 487	SEM, FTIR, XRD, EDS			
Leeuwenburgh et al.	Thin Solid Films 503 (2006) 69	SEM PDA (phase doppler anemometry)			
Leeuwenburgh et al.	Biomaterials 27 (2006) 3368	SEM, FTIR, XRD, EDS		Simulated body fluid	Subcutaneous (goats)

Table 10.2 (continued)

Author	Journal	Characterization techniques	Mechanical testing	*In vitro* testing	*In vivo* testing
Siebers et al.	Tissue Eng 12 (2006) 2449	SEM, FTIR, XRD, EDS		Cell culture (osteoblast)	
Siebers et al.	J Biomed Mater Res 78 (2006) 258	SEM, FTIR, XRD, EDS		Cell culture (osteoblast)	
Leeuwenburgh et al.	J Biomed Mater Res 78 (2006) 558	SEM, FTIR, XRD, EDS	Profilometry Tensile tests Fatigue tests Scratch tests Explantation test		
Siebers et al.	Clin Oral Implants Res 18 (2007) 354	SEM, FTIR, XRD, EDS			Femoral condyle (goats)

References

1. A. Van Zomeren, E.M. Kelder, J.C.M. Marijnissen, J. Schoonman. J. Aerosol Sci. 25 (1994) 1229.
2. A.H. Lefebvre, in "Atomization and sprays" (Hemisphere Publishing Corporation, New York: 1989).
3. W. Siefert. Thin Solid Films 120 (1984) 267.
4. A.G. Bailey, in "Electrostatic spraying of liquids' (John Wiley & Sons, New York, 1988).
5. R.P.A. Hartman, J.P. Borra, D.J. Brunner, J.C.M. Marijnissen, J. Scarlett. J. Electrostat. 47 (1999) 143.
6. H. Romat, A. Badri. J. Electrostat. 51/52 (2001) 481.
7. L. Rayleigh. Proc. R. Soc. 29 (1879) 71.
8. M. Cloupeau, B. Prunet-Foch. J. Aerosol Sci. 25 (1994) 1021.
9. Grace J.M., J.C.M. Marijnissen. J. Aerosol Sci. 25 (1994) 1005.
10. A. Jaworek, A. Krupa. J. Aerosol Sci. 30 (1999) 873.
11. P. Ducheyne, Q. Qiu. Biomaterials 20 (1999) 2287.
12. R.Z. Legeros. Clin. Mater. 14 (1993) 65.
13. J.D. De Bruijn, J.E. Davies, C.P.A.T Klein, K. De Groot, C.A. Van Blitterswijk, in Bone-bonding biomaterials, edited by P. Ducheyne, T. Kokubo T, C.A. van Blitterswijk (Reed Healthcare Communications, Leiderdorp, 1993) p. 57.
14. S.C.G. Leeuwenburgh, J.G.C. Wolke, J. Schoonman, J.A. Jansen. Biomaterials 25 (2004) 641.
15. S.C.G. Leeuwenburgh, J.G.C. Wolke, J. Schoonman, J.A. Jansen. Thin Solid Films 472 (2005) 105.
16. R.Z. Legeros, in "Calcium phosphates in oral biology and medicine" (Karger, Basel, 1991).
17. R.Z. Legeros, in "Crystallographic studies of the carbonate substitution in the apatite structure" (PhD Thesis, University of London, London, 1967).
18. C.J. Pouchert, in "The Aldrich library of infrared spectra – Edition 3" (Aldrich Chemical company, Milwaukee, 1981).
19. P. Layrolle, A. Ito, T. Tateishi. J. Am. Ceram. Soc. 81 (1998) 1421.
20. R.J. Kingsley, R. Van Gilder, R.Z. Legeros, N. Watanabe. J. Phycol. 39 (2003) 937.
21. J.T. Kloprogge, T.W. Boström, M.L. Weier. Am. Miner 89 (2004) 245.
22. S.C.G. Leeuwenburgh, J.G.C. Wolke, J. Schoonman, J.A. Jansen. J. Biomed. Mater. Res. 74 (2005) 275.
23. M.C. Siebers, P.J. Ter Brugge, X.F. Walboomers, J.A. Jansen. Biomaterials 26 (2005) 137.
24. C.H. Chen, E.M. Kelder, P.J.J.M. Van Der Put, J. Schoonman. J. Mater. Chem. 6 (1996) 765.
25. I. Taniguchi, R.C. Van Landschoot, J. Schoonman. Solid State Ionics 156 (2003) 1.
26. D. Perednis, O. Wilhelm, S.E. Pratsinis, L.J. Gauckler. Thin Solid Films 474 (2005) 84.
27. G.L. Messing, S.C. Zhang, G.V. Jayanthi. J. Am. Ceram. Soc. 76 (1993) 2707.
28. V.S. Ajaev. J. Fluid Mech. 528 (2005) 279.
29. J. Fernandez De La Mora, I. Loscertales. J. Fluid Mech. 260 (1997) 155.
30. R.P.A. Hartman, D.J. Brunner, D.M.A. Camelot, J.C.M. Marijnissen, B. Scarlett. J. Aerosol Sci. 30 (1999) 823.
31. J.G.C. Wolke, J.M.A. De Blieck-Hogervorst, W.J.A. Dhert, Klein C.P.A.T. Klein, K. De Groot. J. Thermal Spray Technol. (1) 75.
32. Z.L. Dong., K.A. Khor, C.H. Quek, T.J. White, P. Cheang. Biomaterials 24 (2002) 97.
33. R. Rohanizadeh, R.Z. Legeros, M. Harsono, A. Bendavid. J. Biomed. Mater. Res. 72 (2005) 428.
34. J.D. Haman, K.K. Chittur, D.E. Crawmer, L.C. Lucas. J. Biomed. Mater. Res. 48 (1999) 856.

35. S.C.G. Leeuwenburgh, J.G.C. Wolke, M.C. Siebers, J. Schoonman, J.A. Jansen. Biomaterials 27 (2006) 3368.
36. J.A.M. Clemens, J.G.C. Wolke, C.P.A.T. Klein, K. De Groot. J. Biomed. Mater. Res. 48 (1999) 741.
37. J.G.C. Wolke, J.P. Van Der Waerden, K. De Groot, J.A. Jansen. Biomaterials 18 (1997) 483.
38. T.W. Wu. J. Mater. Res. 6 (1991) 407.
39. B. Feddes, J.G.C. Wolke, W.P. Weinhold, A.M. Vredenberg, J.A. Jansen. J. Adhesion Sci. Technol. 18 (2004) 655.
40. S.J. Bull. Surf. Coat. Technol. 50 (1991) 25.
41. J. Wang, P. Layrolle, M. Stigter, K. De Groot. Biomaterials 25 (2004) 583.
42. K. Takahashi, T. Hayakawa, M. Yoshinari, H. Hara, C. Mochizuki, M. Sato, K. Nemoto. Thin Solid Films 484 (2005) 1.
43. P.A. Steinmann, Y. Tardy, H.E. Hintermann. Thin Solid Films 154 (1987) 333.
44. P.J. Burnett, D.S. Rickerby. Thin Solid Films 154 (1987) 403.
45. P.J.D. Manders, J.G.C. Wolke, J.A. Jansen. Clin. Oral Implants Res. 17 (2006) 548.
46. C.H. Chen, in "Thin film components for lithium-ion batteries" (PhD Thesis, Delft University of Technology, Delft, 1998).
47. H. EL Feki, C.Rey, M. Vignoles. Calcif. Tissue Int. 49 (1991)269.
48. R. Xin, Y. Leng, J. Chen, Q. Zhang. Biomaterials 26 (2005) 6477.
49. X. Lu, Y. Leng. Biomaterials 26 (2005) 1097.
50. Y. Leng, J. Chen, S. Qu. Biomaterials 24 (2003) 2125.
51. N. Eidelman, L.C. Chow, W.E. Brown. Calcif. Tissue Int. 41 (1987) 18.
52. D. Mikroulis, D. Mavrilas, J. Kapolos, P.G. Koutsoukos, C. Lolas. J. Mater. Sci. Mater. Med. 13 (2002) 885.
53. G.R. Sauer, R.E. Wuthier. J. Biol. Chem. 263 (1988) 13718.
54. X. Lu, Y. Leng. Biomaterials 25 (2004) 1779.
55. M. Iijima, H. Kamemizu, N. Wakamatsu, T. Goto, Y. Doi, Y. Morikawa. J. Cryst. Growth 135 (1994) 229.
56. D.G.A. Nelson, J.C. Barry, C.P. Shields, R. Glena, J.D.B. Featherstone. J. Colloid. Interface Sci. 130 (1989) 467.
57. W.E. Brown, J.P. Smith, J.R. Lehr, A.W. Frazier. Nature 196 (1962) 1050.
58. S. Ban, T. Jine, J.Hasegawa. Dent. Mater. J. 11 (1992) 130.
59. J.G.C. Wolke, J.P. Van Der Waerden, H. Schaeken, J.A. Jansen. Biomaterials 24 (2003) 2623.
60. J.D. Haman, K.K. Chittur, D.E. Crawmer, L.C. Luca. J. Biomed. Mater. Res. (Appl. Biomater.) 48 (1999) 856.
61. K.A. Gross, N. Ray, M. Rokkum. J. Biomed. Mater. Res. 63 (2002) 106.
62. M.E.K. Wong, J.O. Hollinger, G.J. Pinero. Oral Surg. Oral Med. Oral Patol. Oral Radiol. Endod. 82 (1996) 475.
63. A. Ramila, M. Vallet-Regi. Biomaterials 22 (2001) 2301.
64. Y.R. Duan, Z.R. Zhang, C.Y. Wang, J.Y. Chen, X.D. Zhang. J. Mater. Sci. Mater. Med. 15 (2004) 1205.
65. C. Combes, C.Rey. Biomaterials 23 (2002) 2817.
66. S. Cazalbou, C. Combes, D. Eichert, C. Rey, M.J. Glimcher. J. Bone Miner. Metab. 22 (2004) 310.
67. H.M. Kim, T. Himeno, T. Kokubo, T. Nakamura. Biomaterials 26 (2005) 4366.
68. M.C. Siebers, X.F. Walboomers, S.C.G. Leeuwenburgh, J.G.C. Wolke, J.A. Jansen. Biomaterials 25 (2004) 2019.
69. M.C. Siebers, K. Matsuzaka, X.F. Walboomers, S.C.G. Leeuwenburgh, J.G.C. Wolke, J.A. Jansen. J. Biomed. Mater. Res. 74 (2005) 570.
70. M.C. Siebers, X.F. Walboomers, J.G.C. Wolke, S.C.G. Leeuwenburgh, J.A. Jansen. Clin. Oral Implants Res. 18 (2007) 354.

71. S.C.G. Leeuwenburgh, J.G.C. Wolke, L. Lommen, T. Pooters, J. Schoonman, J.A. Jansen. J. Biomed. Mater. Res. 78 (2006) 558.
72. S. Mohammadi, M. Esposito, J. Hall, L. Emanuelsson, A. Krozer, P. Thomsen. Int. J. Oral Maxillofac. Impl. 19 (2004) 498.
73. S. Overgaard, U. Bromose, M. Lind, C. Bunger, K. Soballe. J Bone Joint Surg. (Br.) 81 (1999) 725.
74. J.E. Hulshoff, K. Van Dijk, J.P. Van Der Waerden, J.G.C. Wolke, W.Kalk, J.A. Jansen. J. Biomed. Mater. Res. 31 (1996) 329.
75. Y.L. Chang, D. Lew, J.B. Park, J.C. Keller. J. Oral Maxillofac. Surg. 57 (1995) 1096; discussion 1108.
76. J.A. Clemens, C.P. Klein, R.J. Sakkers, W.J. Dhert, K. De Groot, P.M. Rozing. J. Biomed .Mater. Res. 36 (1997) 55.
77. I. Uematsu, H. Matsumoto, K. Morota, M. Minagawa, A. Tanioka, Y. Yamagata, K. Inoue. J. Colloid. Interface Sci. 269 (2004) 336.
78. J.B. Fenn, M. Mann, C.K. Meng, S.F. Wong, C.M. Whitehouse. Science 246 (1989) 64.
79. A.J. Rulison, R.C. Flagran. Rev Sci Instrum 64 (1993) 683.
80. J.C. Almekinders, C. Jones. J. Aerosol Sci. 30 (1999) 969.
81. W. Deng, J.F. Klemic, X. Lik M.A. Reed, A. Gomez. J. Aerosol Sci. 37 (2006) 696.
82. M.H. Duby, W. Deng, K. Kim, T. Gomez, A. Gomez. J Aerosol Sci.37 (2006) 306.
83. J. Huang, S.N. Jayasinghe, S.M. Best, M.J. Edirisinghe, R.A. Brooks, W. Bonfield. J. Mater. Sci. 39 (2004) 1029.
84. J. Huang, S.M. Best, W. Bonfield, R.A. Brooks, N. Rushton, S.N. Jayasinghe, M.J. Edirisinghe. J. Mater. Sci. Mater. Med. 15 (2004) 441.
85. Y. Fan, K. Duan, R. Wang. Biomaterials 26 (2005) 1623.

Chapter 11
Biomimetic Coatings and Their Biological Functionalization

Yuelian Liu and Ernst B. Hunziker

Abstract The biomimetic coating technique can be used to deposit layers of calcium phosphate (CaP) on medical devices to improve their osteoconductivity and osseointegration.The inorganic layer generated is akin to mineralized bone matrix and can be degraded as such. The biomimetic coating technique involves the nucleation and growth of bone-like crystals on a pretreated substrate by immersing it in a supersaturated solution of CaP under physiological conditions of temperature (37°C) and pH (7.4). The method, originally developed by Kokubo and his co-workers in 1990, has since undergone improvement and refinement by several groups of investigators. Biomimetic coatings are valuable in that they can serve as a vehicle for the slow, sustained release of osteogenic agents at the site of implantation. This attribute is rendered possible by the near-physiological conditions under which these coatings are prepared, which permits the incorporation of bioactive agents into the inorganic crystal latticework rather than their superficial adsorption on preformed layers. In addition, the biomimetic coating technique can be applied to implants of an organic as well as of a metallic nature and to those with irregular surface geometries, which is not possible using conventional methodologies.

11.1 Introduction

In orthopedic and dental implantology, novel tools and techniques are being sought to improve the regeneration of bone tissue. Numerous attempts have been made to enhance the osteoconductivity of titanium prostheses, including modifications in their surface properties and coating with a layer of calcium phosphate (CaP).

Y. Liu (✉)
Section of Oral Implantology, Department of Oral Function, Academic Centre of Dentistry Amsterdam (ACTA), Louwesweg 1, 1067 EA, Amsterdam, The Netherlands; ITI Research Institute for Dental and Skeletal Biology, University of Bern, Switzerland
e-mail: y.liu@acta.nl

B. León, J.A. Jansen (eds.), *Thin Calcium Phosphate Coatings for Medical Implants*, 301
DOI 10.1007/978-0-387-77718-4_11, © Springer Science+Business Media, LLC 2009

Hydroxyapatite (HA) and related CaPs are known to be biocompatible and osteoconductive [1, 2]. HA ceramics have been widely employed in orthopedics for nearly two decades. They are relatively inexpensive, non-toxic, minimally resorbed and of acceptable compressive strength; they attach well to hard tissues and conduct bone apposition. The major drawback of HA ceramics is their low tensile strength (brittleness) [3–6].

HA is the most important representative of the bioactive CaP ceramics. There is abundant evidence in the literature that sintered HA is well incorporated into living bone and that it does not undergo any significant biodegradation once it has become bonded to it (a feature that may be disadvantageous as well as advantageous) [5–8]. Although the static mechanical strength of sintered HA is comparable to that of cortical bone, this material is prone to fatigue failure under conditions of high tensile loading, which renders it unsuitable for applications in load-bearing situations.

Until recently, layers of CaP were deposited on the surfaces of metal implants under physical conditions that were highly unphysiological. The methods employed have been various and include plasma spraying, high-velocity oxygen-fuel spraying, electrophoretic deposition, sol-gel deposition, hot isostatic pressing, frit enameling, ion-assisted deposition, pulsed laser deposition, electrochemical deposition and sputter coating [1, 6, 9–18]. Titanium prostheses that have been coated with plasma-sprayed layers of HA have been used with promising results in joint reconstruction. The plasma-spraying technique is, however, conducted at extremely high temperatures ($> 1000°C$). The mineral layers generated are composed of large, partially molten HA particles, which are not only prone to delamination but are also poorly degraded in a biological milieu.

The technique whereby such layers are produced has recently undergone a revolutionary change [19–21], which has had profound consequences for their potential to serve as drug-carrier systems. Hitherto, CaP layers were deposited on the surfaces of metal implants under highly unphysiological physical conditions, which precluded the incorporation of bioactive agents. These agents could only be adsorbed, superficially, on preformed layers. Such superficially adsorbed molecules are released too rapidly in a biological milieu to be effective in their osteoinductive capacity. Now, it is possible to deposit CaP layers under near-physiological conditions of temperature and pH by the so-called biomimetic process, during which bioactive agents can be co-precipitated [22–24]. Because these molecules are integrated into the inorganic crystal latticework, they are released gradually *in vivo* as the layer undergoes degradation. This feature enhances the capacity of these coatings to act as a carrier system for osteogenic agents, such as members of the transforming growth factor-β superfamily (TGFβ), for example, bone morphogenetic proteins (BMPs) and the growth and differentiation factors (GDFs). Ideally, the CaP coatings should be well attached to the carrier surfaces, osteoconductive, osteoinductive, resorbable, inexpensive and surgically easy to handle. They should promote cell adhesion, proliferation and differentiation, and should also protect and predictably release the entrapped bioactive agent, thereby facilitating tissue ingrowth and establishing a mechanically stable environment for bone regeneration.

11.2 Biomimetic Coatings

Biomimetics, which literally means the mimicry of biology, is a branch of science in which biologists and engineers jointly endeavor to produce "bioinspired" materials that can be used for tissue engineering. This broad new field has ancient roots. The replacement of bodily parts dates back at least 2500 years, to the time when the Etruscans substituted missing teeth with artificial ones carved from the bones of oxen. The first recorded use of dental amalgam to repair decayed teeth was in China in the year 659 AD. As human life expectancy has increased, the need for better coping with diseased, damaged or destroyed bodily tissues or parts has heightened.

11.2.1 Biomimetic Coating Techniques

Several years ago, attempts were made to coat medical devices with layers of CaP under more physiological or "biomimetic" conditions of temperature and pH [2, 19, 20, 22, 23, 25], primarily to improve their biocompatibility and biodegradability. The mineral layers generated by biomimetic methods are comparable to biological mineral, whereas those produced by traditional methods are composed of large, partially molten HA particles. The latter are not only prone to delamination but are also poorly degraded within a biological milieu.

The biomimetic coating technique involves the nucleation and growth of bone-like crystals on a pretreated substrate by immersing it in a supersaturated solution of CaP under physiological conditions of temperature (37°C) and pH (7.4). The method, originally developed by Kokubo *et al.* in 1990 [19], has since undergone improvement and refinement by several groups of investigators [23, 26–30].

The coating solution contains HCO_3^-, HPO_4^{2-}, Ca^{2+}, Mg^{2+}, Na^+, K^+ and Cl^-, which are present in most bodily fluids. The implant is first immersed within five-times-concentrated simulated body fluid (SBF) under high-nucleation conditions, viz., in the presence of Mg^{2+} (7.5 M) (Table 11.1) to inhibit crystal growth, for 24 hours at 37°C. A thin (< 3 μm thick), dense, amorphous layer of CaP is thereby uniformly deposited on the implant surface, and this serves as a seeding substratum for the subsequent growth of a substantial (30–50 μm thick) crystal latticework. The latter is prepared by immersing the coated implant in a supersaturated solution of CaP (pH 7.4) (Table 11.1), for 48 hours at 37°C. Under these conditions, the coating is composed of crystals of octaCaP (OCP) (Fig. 11.1).

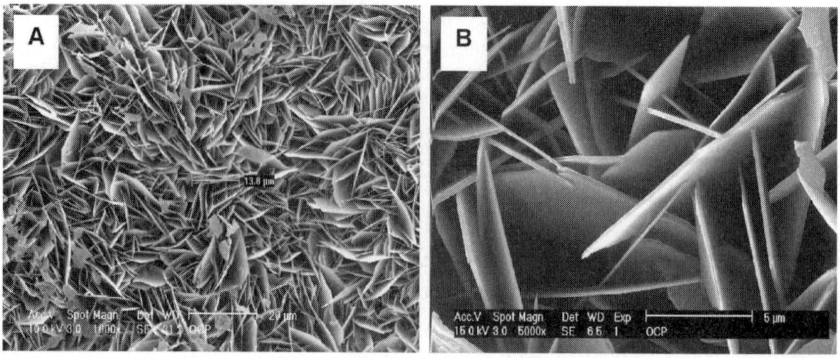

Fig. 11.1 Scanning electron micrographs of an OCP coating at low (**A**) and high (**B**) magnification

Table 11.1 Composition of human blood plasma, simulated body fluid, five-times-concentrated SBF, and the supersaturated solution of CaP

Fluid	Na^+	Mg^{2+}	Ca^{2+}	Cl^-	HPO_4^{2-}	HCO_3^-
HBP	142.0	1.5	2.5	103.0	1.0	27.0
SBF	146.7	1.5	2.5	147.8	1.0	4.2
SBF×5	733.5	7.5	12.5	740.0	5.0	21.0
CPS	140.4	0	3.1	142.9	1.86	0

HBP, human blood plasma; SBF, simulated body fluid; SBF×5, five-times-concentrated SBF; CaP, calcium phosphate; CPS, supersaturated solution of CaP
The concentrations are given in millimolar units

Table 11.2 Composition of various fluids with different concentrations of Mg^{2+} and HCO_3^-

Fluid	Na^+	Mg^{2+}	Ca^{2+}	Cl^-	HPO_4^{2-}	HCO_3^-
HBP	142.0	1.5	2.5	103.0	1.0	27.0
SBF	146.7	1.5	2.5	147.8	1.0	4.2
SBF×5	733.5	7.5	12.5	740.0	5.0	21.0
Modified SBF×5	702.0	2.5	12.5.1	714.5	5.0	10.0
SBF×5 (no Mg^{2+})	733.5	0.0	12.5	740.0	5.0	21.0
SBF×5 (Mg^{2+} ×3)	733.5	4.5	12.5	740.0	5.0	21.0
SBF×5 (Mg^{2+} ×8; no HCO_3^-)	733.5	12.0	12.5	740.0	5.0	0.0
SBF × 5 (no Mg^{2+}; HCO_3^- ×8)	733.5	0.0	12.5	740.0	5.0	33.6

Coatings of different structures can be generated under different ionic conditions (Table 11.2) and at temperatures of 45°C or 50°C [21, 26, 27, 31, 32]. The structure of the coating can also be influenced by the time of coating.

The biomimetic coating process is simple to perform, is cost-effective, and can be applied even to heat-sensitive, non-conductive and porous materials of large dimensions and with complex surface geometries. An additional advantage of the biomimetic method is that biologically active molecules, such as osteogenic agents, can be co-precipitated with the inorganic components. As a consequence, the proteins are truly incorporated into the crystal latticeworks and not merely deposited on their surfaces. In forming an integral part of the CaP coatings, the protein molecules are liberated not in a single burst (as when superficially adsorbed) but gradually, which bodes well for an enduring osteogenic effect at the implantation site. The disadvantage of such coatings is that they are of low cohesiveness and are degradable, both *in vitro* and *in vivo*; and they adhere poorly to the underlying substrate. However, in a clinical situation, their biodegradability could be advantageous, particularly if they are serving as a vehicle for drug delivery.

11.2.2 Characterization of Coatings

- *Coating thickness:* The thicknesses of coatings can be determined *in situ* using a magnetic induction probe (Minitest 2100; Electrophysik, Cologne, Germany), the measuring range of which lies between 0 and 100 μm.
- *Fourier-transform infrared spectroscopy:* The coatings are peeled away from the carriers and then mixed with potassium bromide (0.6–0.8 mg of sample material per 280 mg of potassium bromide), prior to the analysis by Fourier-transform infrared (FTIR) spectrometry. The types of chemical bonds existing in the coatings can be established by means of this technique.
- *Scanning electron microscopy and energy-dispersive x-ray spectroscopy:* Prior to examination by scanning electron microscopy (SEM), the coated carriers are sputtered with carbon particles to a thickness of 12 to 16 nm. SEM yields information concering the crystal structure of the coatings, whereas energy-dispersive X-ray spectroscopy (EDX) furnishes data relating to their chemical structure.

11.2.3 Typical Results Obtained Using the Standard Biomimetic Coating Process

Coatings are typically 10 to 15 μm in thickness. Coating thickness can be modified by changing the volume of the coating solution and the duration of the coating process. SEM reveals OCP coatings to be composed of thin, plate-like crystals (Fig. 11.1), whereas carbonated apatite ones consist of amorphous or nanocrystalline material (Fig. 11.2).

FTIR spectroscopy discloses that carbonated apatite coatings have two prominent absorption bands at 1410 and 1460 cm^{-1}. Two C-O bands stemming from CO_3^{2-} groups appear at 1470 and 1425 cm^{-1}. P-O bands stemming from PO_4^{2-} groups appear at 1115, 1042, 970, 610 and 570 cm^{-1}, and P-OH bands stemming from HPO_4^{-} groups appear at 920 and 870 cm^{-1}. OCP coatings are additionally characterized by bands at 906 cm^{-1} and 852 cm^{-1} (Fig. 11.3) [29].

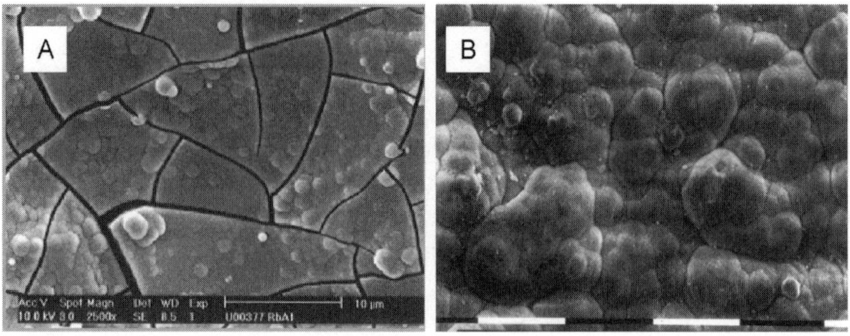

Fig. 11.2 Scanning electron micrographs of an amorphous (**A**) and a nanocrystalline (**B**) carbonated apatite coating

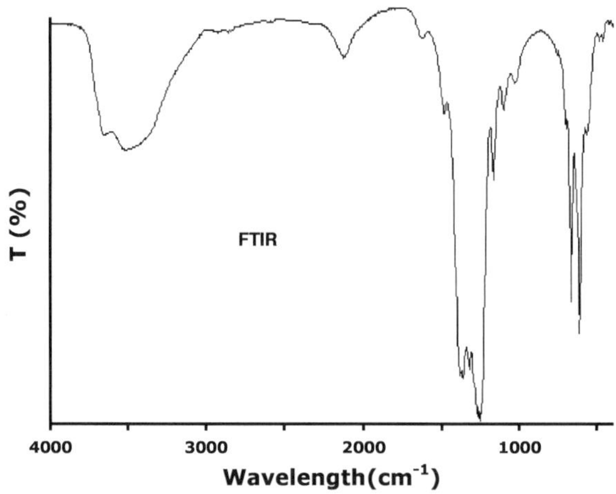

Fig. 11.3 Fourier-transform infrared (*FTIR*) spectrograph of an OCP coating

11.2.4 Incorporation of Osteogenic Agents into Biomimetic Coatings: Biological Functionalization

Although biomimetic CaP coatings improve the osteoconductivity of metal implants, they do not render them osteoinductive, a feature that is required to expedite the osteogenic process and accelerate implant integration. This property can be conferred by introducing an osteogenic agent into the system [33–37]. Using conventional coating methods, osteogenic agents can be deposited only superficially on preformed coatings: by adsorption [33, 38–40], by binding to biofunctional proteins [41], or by chemical treatment [42]. The disadvantage of this mode of attachment is that the biologically active molecules are released rapidly upon exposure to a physiological environment. Consequently, their osteogenic effects are of short range and short-lived. Using the biomimetic technique, osteogenic agents can be incorporated into the crystal latticework of the coatings. Consequently, they are released more slowly over a longer time-span.

11.3 Biomimetic CaP Coatings as a Delivery Vehicle for Osteogenic Drugs

The advent of the biomimetic coating technique has broadened the potential of CaP layers to serve as a carrier system for osteogenic drugs, permitting them to be rendered osteoinductive. Granted this facility, investigators must select an appropriate osteogenic agent.

Members of the TGFβ superfamily, such as certain TGFβs and GDFs, and especially BMPs, probably represent the most promising candidates for this purpose. Interest in this latter group of agents dates back to 1964. Urist [43] demonstrated that demineralized, dried and pulverized bone could stimulate the formation of osseous tissue at an ectopic site (muscle) in rabbits. The osteogenic fraction of the bone matrix was later isolated and subjected to amino-acid sequencing. This analysis revealed BMPs to be structurally similar to TGFβs, and they are now classed as a subgroup of this superfamily [44–47]. More than 15 of the 30-odd members have been isolated and synthesized by recombinant DNA technology [48–50].

Interest in BMPs obviously preceded the advent of the biomimetic coating technology, and various materials have thus already served as their carriers, including collagen, synthetic and natural ceramics, demineralized bone matrix (DBM), and polyglycolic acid [47, 51–56]. Human recombinant BMP-2 used in conjunction with each of these carrier systems is released in two kinetically distinct phases: an initial rapid phase of a few hours' duration and a second slower phase spanning several weeks. Collagen retains the largest fraction of BMP-2 during the initial phase and synthetic HA particles the smallest (10%). The other carriers retain 30% to 50% of their load during this phase. With the exception of synthetic HA, the mineral-based carriers retain the largest fraction of BMP-2 during the second phase, which reflects their high affinity for this agent. However, none of the materials serves as an optimal drug-delivery system.

The potential of biomimetic CaP coatings to serve as a carrier system for BMP-2 is now being investigated by our group [57–59]. The drug has been successfully co-precipitated with the inorganic components and, thus incorporated, retains its biological activity *in vitro* [58, 59]. Experiments using an ectopic (subcutaneous) model for bone formation in rats have revealed BMP-2 to be osteogenically potent. Furthermore, bone-forming activities are sustained for a considerable period of time, which indicates that BMP-2 is indeed released gradually (as anticipated) and not in a single burst [57].

Instead of incorporating BMP-2 itself into a carrier system, the drug could be substituted for a plasmid containing the gene for BMP-2. The rationale behind such an undertaking would be that whereas a protein is ultimately degraded, a gene would become incorporated into a host cell and remain active for a longer period [60–62]. The gene for BMP-2 has been delivered to orthotopic ossification sites in rats and dogs via viral and non-viral carriers [48, 63]. It has not yet been incorporated into biomimetic implant coatings.

11.3.1 In-Vitro *Testing of the Osteogenic Potential of Biomimetic Coatings Bearing BMP-2*

Titanium-alloy disks were coated biomimetically with a layer of CaP into which various amounts of BMP-2 were incorporated (1–3 μg/disk). The osteogenic potency of BMP-2 thus incorporated was assessed by monitoring the alkaline-phosphatase activity of rat bone-marrow (RBM) stromal cells cultured directly on the coated disks. BMP-2 incorporated into CaP coatings was more potent in stimulating the alkaline-phosphatase activity of RBM stromal cells cultured thereupon than was the freely-suspended drug in stimulating the same cell population cultured on a plastic surface. Hence, the osteogenic potency of BMP-2 incorporated biomimetically into CaP layers is not only retained but enhanced in this situation, probably by virtue of a localized concentration effect.

11.3.2 In-Vivo *Testing of the Osteogenic Potential of Biomimetic Coatings Bearing BMP-2*

11.3.2.1 Ectopic Ossification Model in Rats

We investigated the potential of BMP-2 incorporated biomimetically into CaP coatings to induce and sustain bone formation at an ectopic (subcutaneous) site in rats over a course of 5 weeks. For this purpose, one experimental and three control groups were set up: titanium-alloy implants bearing a co-precipitated layer of CaP and BMP-2 (experimental group); naked titanium-alloy disks (negative control for the effects of a CaP layer and of BMP-2); titanium-alloy disks bearing a layer of CaP (negative control for the effects of BMP-2); and titanium-alloy disks bearing a layer of CaP and superficially adsorbed BMP-2 (positive control for superficially adsorbed BMP-2). Six implants per group were implanted subcutaneously in the dorsal region of rats, two per animal. Samples were retrieved at 7-day intervals over a period of 5 weeks for histological and histomorphometric analyses.

Ectopic bone formation occurred only in the experimental animals (Fig. 11.4). Bone tissue first became apparent 2 weeks after implantation, and thereafter was deposited continually until the end of the 5-week monitoring period. Ossification occurred by a process of intramembranous (direct) growth, there being virtually no evidence of an endochondral mechanism having been followed. The total volume of bone formed increased significantly ($P < 0.005$) from 5.8 mm^3 per implant after the second week to 10.2 mm^3 per implant after the third, when the net daily rate of bone formation was highest (0.8 mm^3 per implant per day). Bone tissue was deposited not only on the implant surfaces but also at some distance therefrom, maximally at 340 μm by the end of the third week. This distance had decreased to 200 μm by the end of the fifth week,

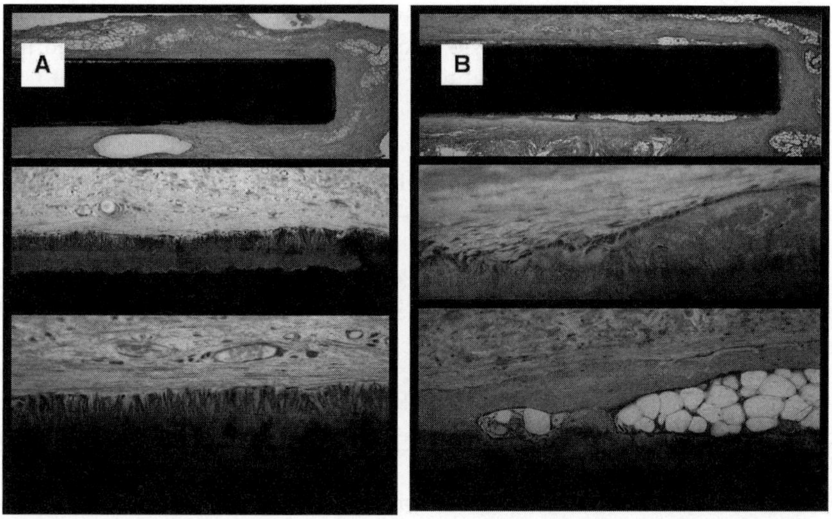

Fig. 11.4 **A** Light microscopy images (low-, intermediate-, and high-magnification views) of a titanium alloy disk bearing an OCP coating 5 weeks after implantation at a subcutaneous site in a rat. No bone tissue has been deposited (80 μm thick section stained with McNeal's tetrachrome, basic fuchsine, and toluidine blue O). **B** Light micrographs (low-, intermediate- and high-magnification views) of a titanium alloy disk bearing octaCaP coating into which bone morphogenetic protein2 (BMP-2) had been incorporated, at 5 weeks after subcutaneous implantation in a rat. Bone tissue has been deposited both directly on the coated disk and at some distance therefrom, within the connective tissue capsule (80 μm thick section stained with McNeal's tetrachrome, basic fuchsine, and toluidine blue O) (*See* Color Insert)

indicating that bone remodeling processes were underway, which would be a normal occurrence under physiological conditions. The biomimetic coating was degraded gradually during the course of the 5-week monitoring period, by the end of which time one-third of its volume remained. The implication is that one-third of the initially incorporated amount of BMP-2 (1.7 μg per implant) likewise remained and that bone formation could have continued for several more weeks after the end of the experimental period. The findings of this study demonstrated that BMP-2 incorporated biomimetically into CaP coatings is capable not only of inducing at a low pharmacological level the formation of bone at an ectopic site but also of sustaining osteogenic activity for a considerable period of time.

11.3.2.2 Orthotopic Ossification Model in Miniature Pigs

To clarify the potential beneficial and adverse effects of BMP-2 on the osteoconductivity of titanium-alloy implants, we considered two basic types of surface: a sand-blasted, acid-etched one and a sand-blasted, acid-etched one coated with a layer of CaP. These two surfaces served as the baseline controls. In the first category, BMP-2 was adsorbed directly onto the metal surface; in the second, it was either adsorbed onto, incorporated into, or incorporated into and adsorbed onto the CaP coating. The implants were inserted into the partially edentulous maxillae of adult Goettingen miniature pigs. The neoformation of bone along the implant surface and up to a distance of 175 μm therefrom (the immediate peri-implant space) was monitored quantitatively 1, 2 and 3 weeks after surgery (i.e., during the early phase of healing when any interference with the osteoconductivity of the implants would be apparent).

Our findings revealed the osteoconductivity of the implants to be greatly influenced by BMP-2 and its mode of delivery. The net volume of bone deposited within the immediate vicinity of the coated implants (up to 175 μm therefrom) could be increased by the presence of BMP-2 during the first two postoperative weeks but was decreased by its presence during the third. Bone coverage of the coated implants was lowered by the presence of BMP-2 at each weekly juncture. The net volume of bone deposited both directly on and within the immediate vicinity of uncoated implants was lowered by the presence of BMP-2 at each time point. In general, implant osteoconductivity was most severely compromised when BMP-2 was present as an adsorbed depot (subject to a burst-release profile) and less so when it was delivered via a slow-release system (incorporated into a CaP coating).

Data relating to the degradation of the implant coatings are summarized in Table 11.3. Coatings bearing incorporated and adsorbed BMP-2 underwent the most extensive degradation during the 3-week monitoring period, followed by those bearing only an incorporated depot of the drug. Coatings bearing no BMP-2 underwent the least degradation during the 3-week monitoring period, followed by those bearing only an adsorbed depot of the drug.

During the first week of implantation, coatings bearing incorporated and adsorbed BMP-2 were degraded by 74% and those bearing only an incorporated depot of the drug by 60%. Coatings bearing only adsorbed BMP-2 were degraded by 17% and those bearing no BMP-2 by 5%.

By the end of the second week, coatings bearing incorporated and adsorbed BMP-2 had been degraded by 88% and those bearing only an incorporated

Table 11.3 Changes in the thickness of OCP coatings bearing incorporated, adsorbed or no depot of BMP-2 at various times after implantation at a maxillary site in miniature pigs

	Mode of BMP-2 loading		Coating thickness[a] (μm)		
Coating	Inc.	Ads.	Week 1	Week 2	Week 3
Coating 1	+	–	22.26 ± 4.26	2.58 ± 1.36	1.08 ± 0.45
Coating 2	–	+	45.53 ± 4.36	16.82 ± 5.45	13.35 ± 4.17
Coating 3	+	+	14.63 ± 2.46	6.52 ± 2.82	0.46 ± 0.20
Coating 4	–	–	52.00 ± 1.83	27.72 ± 7.69	15.31 ± 3.14

Data are represented as mean values ± standard error

Inc., incorporated; Ads, adsorbed

[a]Initial coating thickness = 54.7 ± 8.73 μm

depot of the drug by 95%. Coatings bearing only adsorbed BMP-2 had been degraded by 70% and those bearing no BMP-2 by 50%.

By the end of the third week, coatings bearing either incorporated and adsorbed BMP-2 or only an incorporated depot of the drug had been almost completely degraded. Those bearing only adsorbed BMP-2 or no BMP-2 had been degraded by about 75%.

11.4 Biologically Functionalized Biomimetic Coatings

That biomimetic CaP layers are biocompatible and osteoconductive is well known. Indeed, it was for these attributes that this type of coating was chosen to act as a carrier for BMP-2. Although BMP-2 is itself osteoinductive, its osteogenic potency is markedly enhanced after incorporation into biomimetic CaP coatings [58]. This finding is accounted for by the drug's slow rate of release from these coatings over a protracted period of time. BMP-2 is liberated gradually because it forms an integral part of the inorganic crystal latticework. BMP-2 deposited superficially on the surfaces of preformed CaP coatings is released in a single rapid burst, and the drug, being highly water-soluble, diffuses away from the implantation site too quickly to be able to exert its osteogenic effect [57].

The forces governing protein adsorption onto the surface of a preformed CaP coating are believed to be chiefly electrostatic in nature [64], but the mechanisms underlying the incorporation of protein molecules during their co-precipitation with CaP are more complex and poorly understood. Protein molecules possibly participate in the formation of the three-dimensional crystal latticework or at least influence its growth. They may act as tied molecules, in which case they would be effectively bonded, or serve as seeds for crystallization and possibly influence the number of nucleation sites generated [65, 66]. Protein molecules may also be aggregated and penetrated by mineral ions during the formation of a coating. Although bovine serum albumin influences the structure of the CaP latticework into which it is incorporated, BMP-2 does not have this effect. Hence, the mechanism of incorporation may be different in each case. However, incorporated BMP-2 does modify the physical properties of biomimetic coatings. *In vivo*, proteins are known to strengthen mineralized tissue and to stabilize its mineral contents. In our studies, the rate of release of Ca^{2+} from biomimetic coatings was indeed slowed by the presence of incorporated BMP-2, which may improve the coating's attachment to the underlying titanium-alloy implant. Indeed, BMP-2-containing coatings have been shown to be mechanically more cohesive than those composed purely of CaP. BMP-2 incorporated into the body of the inorganic latticework possibly reinforces the coating by surrounding the brittle CaP crystals, which is analogous to the situation in dental enamel. This property of mechanical cohesiveness is important during the surgical implantation procedure, which generates high shear forces that could rupture the coatings. That the coated implants furnished a mechanically stable environment *in vivo* was evidenced by the finding that ectopic bone formation in rats occurred via intramembranous growth. In previous studies involving this model, ossification followed a predominantly endochondral course, which requires a less stable mechanical environment. Our studies with this model [67] also yielded evidence of the high biocompatibility of BMP-2-containing coatings, in that bone-marrow tissue was sometimes observed to contact the coatings directly, without intervening bone. Bone-marrow tissue contains immunocompetent cells, which are highly sensitive to foreign material. Dental implants bearing a BMP-2-containing CaP coating osseointegrated more rapidly at an orthotopic site in adult miniature pigs than did uncoated ones [68].

11.5 Conclusions

Biomimetic coatings are valuable in that they can serve as a vehicle for the slow, sustained release of osteogenic agents at a site of implantation. This attribute is rendered possible by the near-physiological conditions under which these coatings are prepared, which permits the incorporation of bioactive agents into the inorganic crystal latticework rather than merely their superficial adsorption onto preformed layers. In addition, the biomimetic coating technique can be applied to implants of an organic as well as of an inorganic nature and to those with irregular surface geometries, which is not possible using conventional methodologies.

References

1. K. De Groot, J Oral Implantol 12 (1986) 485.
2. K. De Groot, J Biomed Mater Res 23 (1989) 1367.
3. T. Kitsugi, T. Yamamuro, T. Nakamura, S. Kotani, T. Kokubo and H. Takeuchi, Biomaterials 14 (1993) 216.
4. C. P. Klein, A. A. Driessen and K. De Groot, Biomaterials 5 (1984) 157.
5. C. P. Klein, J. G. Wolke, J. M. De Blieck-Hogervorst and K. De Groot, J Biomed Mater Res 28 (1994a) 961.
6. C. P. Klein, P. Patka, J. G. Wolke, J. M. De Blieck-Hogervorst and K. De Groot, Biomaterials 15 (1994c) 146.
7. H. Zhang, S. Li, Y. Yan and Y. Wang, Biomed Mater Eng 10 (2000) 213.
8. H. Schliephake, D. Scharnweber, M. Dard, S. Robetaler, A. Sewing and C. Huttmann, J Biomed Mater Res 64A (2003) 225.
9. K. De Groot, R. Geesink, C. P. Klein and P. Serekian, J Biomed Mater Res 21 (1987) 1375.
10. J. G. Wolke, K. Van Dijk, H. G. Schaeken, K. De Groot and J. A. Jansen, J Biomed Mater Res 28 (1994) 1477.
11. J. G. Wolke, J. P. Van Der Waerden, K. De Groot and J. A. Jansen, Biomaterials 18 (1997) 483.

12. J. G. Wolke, K. DE Groot and J. A. Jansen, J Biomed Mater Res 39 (1998a) 524.
13. J. G. Wolke, K. De Groot and J. A. Jansen, J Biomed Mater Res 43 (1998b) 270.
14. J. A. Jansen, J. G. Wolke, S. Swann, J. P. van der Waerden and K. De Groot, Clin Oral Implants Res 4 (1993) 28.
15. J. W. Vehof, J. Van Den Dolder, J. E. De Ruijter, P. H. Spauwen and J. A. Jansen, J Biomed Mater Res 64A (2003) 417.
16. L. Agata De Sena, M. Calixto De Andrade, A. Malta Rossi and G. DE Almeida Soares, J Biomed Mater Res 60 (2002) 1.
17. J. Wang, J. De Boer and K. De Groot, J Dent Res 83 (2004) 296.
18. J. Wang, P. Layrolle, M. Stigter and K. De Groot, Biomaterials 25 (2004) 583.
19. T. Kokubo, H. Kushitani, S. Sakka, T. Kitsugi and T. Yamamuro, J Biomed Mater Res 24 (1990) 721.
20. T. Kokubo, Biomaterials 12 (1991) 155.
21. P. Li, (US Patent 6139583) (2000).
22. H. B. Wen, J. R. De Wijn, C. A. van Blitterswijk and K. De Groot, J Biomed Mater Res 46 (1999) 245.
23. Y. Liu, P. Layrolle, J. De Bruijn, C. Van Blitterswijk and K. De Groot, J Biomed Mater Res 57 (2001) 327.
24. Y. Liu, E. B. Hunziker, P. Layrolle, C. van Blitterswijk, P. D. Calvert and K. De Groot, J Biomed Mater Res A 67 (2003d) 1155.
25. K. De Groot, J. G. Wolke and J. A. Jansen, Proc Inst Mech Eng [H] 212 (1998) 137.
26. F. Barrere, C. A. van Blitterswijk, K. De Groot and P. Layrolle, Biomaterials 23 (2002a) 1921.
27. F. Barrere, B. C. Van, G. K. De and P. Layrolle, Biomaterials 23 (2002b) 2211.
28. F. Barrere, P. Layrolle, C. A. van Blitterswijk and K. De Groot, J Mater Sci Mater Med 12 (2001) 529.
29. F. Barrere, P. Layrolle, C. A. van Blitterswijk and K. De Groot, Bone 25 (1999) 107S.
30. B. Gondolph-Zink, Orthopade 27 (1998) 96.
31. P. J. F. Layrolle, K. De Groot, J. D. De Bruijn, C. A. Van Blitterswijk and H. Huipin, (US Patent 6207218) (2001).
32. P. Li and P. Ducheyne, J Biomed Mater Res 41 (1998) 341.
33. I. Ono, H. Gunji, F. Kaneko, T. Saito and Y. Kuboki, J Craniofac Surg 6 (1995) 238.
34. J. P. Fiorellini, D. Buser, E. Riley and T. H. Howell, Int J Periodontics Restorative Dent 21 (2001) 41.
35. T. Kawai, A. Mieki, Y. Ohno, M. Umemura, H. Kataoka, S. Kurita, M. Koie, T. Jinde, J. Hasegawa and M. R. Urist, Clin Orthop (1993) 296.
36. A. H. Reddi and N. S. Cunningham, Biomaterials 11 (1990) 33.
37. C. M. Agrawal, J. Best, J. D. Heckman and B. D. Boyan, Biomaterials 16 (1995) 1255.
38. I. Ono, H. Gunji, K. Suda, F. Kaneko, M. Murata, T. Saito and Y. Kuboki, Plast Reconstr Surg 95 (1995) 1265.
39. S. A. Esenwein, S. Esenwein, G. Herr, G. Muhr, W. Kusswetter and C. H. Hartwig, Chirurg 72 (2001) 1360.
40. X. Wang, Y. Jin, B. Liu, S. Zhou, L. Yang, X. Yang and F. H. White, Int J Oral Maxillofac Surg 23 (1994) 115.
41. K. Endo, Dent Mater J 14 (1995) 185.
42. H. M. Kim, F. Miyaji, T. Kokubo and T. Nakamura, J Biomed Mater Res 32 (1996) 409.
43. M. R. Urist, Science 150 (1965) 893.
44. G. Aldinger, G. Herr, W. Kusswetter, H. J. Reis, F. W. Thielemann and U. Holz, Int Orthop 15 (1991) 169.
45. K. Elima, Ann Med 25 (1993) 395.
46. M. B. Lee, J Clin Periodontol 24 (1997) 355.
47. K. Takahashi, Nippon Yakurigaku Zasshi 116 (2000) 232.
48. R. T. Franceschi, Crit Rev Oral Biol Med 10 (1999) 40.

49. A. Yamaguchi, Nippon Rinsho 60 Suppl 3 (2002) 40.
50. A. H. Reddi, Clin Orthop (1998) S66.
51. D. D. Lee, A. Tofighi, M. Aiolova, P. Chakravarthy, A. Catalano, A. Majahad and D. Knaack, Clin Orthop (1999) S396.
52. G. Schmidmaier, B. Wildemann, F. Cromme, F. Kandziora, N. P. Haas and M. Raschke, Bone 30 (2002) 816.
53. L. A. Salata, V. Franke-Stenport AND L. Rasmusson, Clin Implant Dent Relat Res 4 (2002) 27.
54. J. O. Hollinger AND K. Leong, Biomaterials 17 (1996) 187.
55. G. N. KING, Curr Pharm Biotechnol 2 (2001) 131.
56. C. A. Kirker-Head, Adv Drug Deliv Rev 43 (2000) 65.
57. Y. Liu, E. B. Hunziker, C. Van De Vaal and K. De Groot, Key Engineering Materials, Trans Tech Publications 254-256 (2004) 619.
58. Y. Liu, E. B. Hunziker, P. Layrolle, J. D. De Bruijn and K. De Groot, Tissue Eng 10 (2004) 101.
59. Y. Liu, E. B. Hunziker, K. De Groot and P. Layrolle, in Bioceramics 15, edited by B. Ben-Nissan, D. Sher and W. Walsh (Trans Tech Publications, Sydney, 2002) p. 667.
60. D. A. Oakes and J. R. Lieberman, Clin Orthop (2000) S101.
61. H. Ohgushi and A. I. Caplan, J Biomed Mater Res 48 (1999) 913.
62. A. A. Scaduto and J. R. Lieberman, Orthop Clin North Am 30 (1999) 625.
63. T. D. Alden, P. Varady, D. F. Kallmes, J. A. Jane, JR. and G. A. Helm, Spine 27 (2002) S87.
64. W. Becker and B. E. Becker, J Am Dent Assoc 124 (1993) 37.
65. M. Shirkhanzadeh and G. Q. Liu, Materials Lett 21 (1994) 115.
66. A. G. Coombes and J. D. Heckman, Biomaterials 13 (1992) 217.
67. Y. Liu, K. De Groot and E. B. Hunziker, Bone 36 (2005) 745.
68. Y. Liu, L. Enggist, A. F. Kuffer, D. Buser and E. B. Hunziker, Biomaterials 28 (2007) 2677.

Chapter 12
Prospects for Future Applications

The successful integration of medical and dental implants into the bone can be envisioned as a race against time among the processes of wound healing, fibrosis and microbial invasion. The stake in this contest is to accomplish a harmonious interface between the implanted material and surrounding bone tissue as characterized by the development of natural tissue structures.

Currently, we know that CaP ceramic is a material that possesses intrinsic properties to favor the realisation of the above-mentioned harmonious interface. Unfortunately, the mechanical properties of CaP ceramic are not appropriate to be used in loaded applications, which support their use as coating material on an underlying mechanically strong material. Basically, the main advantage of bioactive CaP-coatings appears to be the rarity of reported adverse results. This fact provides the surgeon with forgiveness for shortcomings in implant design as well as surgical technique using CaP-coated implant systems.

This book has presented an overview of several thin film deposition techniques that can be used to deposit thin CaP coatings onto implant surfaces. Physicochemical, mechanical, and biological properties of the various newly obtained thin CaP-coatings were discussed. The final goal of this book was not to make a preferred statement about any of the described techniques. In general, each technique has its own merits for a specific application, e.g. liquid-based coating techniques are more appropriate for the coating of complex 3-D structures, while line-of-sight techniques, like laser and sputter coating, are very suitable for orthopedic and oral implants.

Further, it has to be emphasized that despite the proven efficacy of CaP-coatings for bone-bonding purposes, universal acceptance of CaP-coated systems has not been achieved. Several factors have been suggested in literature to be responsible for this phenomenon, such as commercially based pricing strategies which determine that non-coated devices are currently cheaper. In addition, the large variability in quality of plasma-sprayed hydroxyapatite coatings from different companies and even between different batches has caused concerns about the long-term reliability of CaP-coated systems.

In view of the above mentioned, it is imperative that for the clinical breakthrough of thin CaP-coated devices quality reports are available for each batch in order to avoid the use of coatings of poor quality. In addition for market acceptance, prospective randomized clinical trials have to be performed that proof the safety and clinical efficacy of the applied thin CaP-coatings. An additional issue in this lack of acceptance is that our knowledge about how bone formation is stimulated by calcium phosphate ceramics is still rudimentary. Therefore, more attention should be paid to the various events involved in the bone formation process around implants provided with a thin calcium phosphate coating. Experiments have to involve both cell biological and physicochemical studies. The cell biological studies will provide information about the role of adhesive proteins and extracellular matrix production on the calcium phosphate surfaces. The physicochemical approach will provide information about the interfacial phenomena, i.e. the relation of Ca^{2+} dissolution and extracellular matrix deposition. For the interfacial characterization use has to be made of conventional techniques, but also advanced surface analysis techniques have to be used, as described by Feddes et al. in Chapter 3 . Furthermore, it is essential that the *in vitro* findings are related to experimental animal and human clinical studies.

Another important concern is the crystallinity of the deposited thin coatings. Crystallinity is required in order to prevent early dissolution of the coating. Currently, the most frequently used technique to induce crystallinity is by making use of post-annealing procedures. A disadvantage of this procedure is that discoloration can occur of titanium implants, which is due to titanium oxide formation at the implant surface. Although, this change in color has no effect at all on the final biological response to the implant surface, it makes the implant less "attractive".

A further challenge to be beaten is the scaling up of these techniques, which have been up to now only intensively tested in the rather well-controlled laboratory environment.

A final positive remark to the development and use of thin calcium phosphate coatings is their possible contribution to the studies of the lower limit of thickness in their bone regeneration capabilities down to the nanometer range. The high degree of control of thickness and lateral resolution of nanocoatings may open up new applications and improved performance of innovative medical devices.

Under the assumption that all above-mentioned items can be solved, there appears to be a promising future for the use of thin calcium phosphate coatings to facilitate bone healing around medical implants.

Vigo, España, Betty León
Nijmegen, Gelderland John A. Jansen

Index

Printed in the United States of America